Pain

Also by Javier Moscoso

J. Moscoso, *Diderot y D'Alembert. Ciencia y técnica en la enciclopedia*, 2005, Madrid, Nivola.

Barona, Moscoso, Pimentel, eds, *Para una historia de la objetividad. La Ilustración y las ciencias*, Valencia, Biblioteca Valenciana, 2002

J. Moscoso, *Materialismo y religión. Ciencias de la vida en la Europa ilustrada*, Barcelona, Serbal, 2000.

J. Moscoso, A. Lafuente, eds, *Monstruos y seres imaginarios en la Biblioteca Nacional*, Madrid, Doce Calles, 2000.

Lafuente y J. Moscoso, eds, *El compás y el Príncipe. Ciencia y Corte en la España moderna*. Valencia, Consejería de Cultura de la Generalitat valenciana, 2000.

Diderot, *El sueño de d'Alembert*, Spanish Edition and translation by J. Moscoso, Madrid, Compañía Literaria, 1996.

Pain

A Cultural History

Javier Moscoso
Research Professor of History and Philosophy of Science, Spanish National Research Council

Translated from the Spanish by Sarah Thomas and Paul House

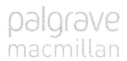
palgrave
macmillan

First published 2012 by
PALGRAVE MACMILLAN

Palgrave Macmillan in the UK is an imprint of Macmillan Publishers Limited,
registered in England, company number 785998, of Houndmills, Basingstoke,
Hampshire RG21 6XS.

Palgrave Macmillan in the US is a division of St Martin's Press LLC,
175 Fifth Avenue, New York, NY 10010.

Palgrave Macmillan is the global academic imprint of the above companies
and has companies and representatives throughout the world.

Palgrave® and Macmillan® are registered trademarks in the United States,
the United Kingdom, Europe and other countries.

ISBN 978–1–4039–9118–8

This book is printed on paper suitable for recycling and made from fully
managed and sustained forest sources. Logging, pulping and manufacturing
processes are expected to conform to the environmental regulations of the
country of origin.

A catalogue record for this book is available from the British Library.

A catalog record for this book is available from the Library of Congress.

10   9   8   7   6   5   4   3   2   1
21 20 19 18 17 16 15 14 13 12

For Arturo, *la alegría de mi vida*

Contents

Illustrations

Acknowledgments

During the writing of this book, I have become indebted in very different ways to many people and institutions. The Spanish Ministry of Science and Technology, the Wellcome Trust Center for the History of Medicine, and the Spanish National Research Council have supported this work through visiting positions and research projects.[1] At the same time, the inauguration in February 2004 of the exhibition *Pain: Passion, Compassion, Sensibility* at the Science Museum in London, UK, was what brought about this book's existence. None of it would have been possible without the offer I received then from Palgrave Macmillan to put on paper what we had attempted to exhibit in the Science Museum of London with objects from the Henry Wellcome collection as well as from many other European and American institutions.

This book also would not have been possible without the assistance and generosity of numerous friends and colleagues. I hope they will be able to forgive that here I can only mention them in the most random of orders. My most heartfelt thanks to Fernando Broncano, Javier Ordóñez, Montse Iglesias, Carlos Thiebaut, Jesús Vega, David Teira, Reyes Mate, Claudia Stein, Roger Cooter, Juan Pimentel, Manolo Lucena Giraldo, Javier Echeverría, Irina Podgorny, Ada Galán, Helena de Felipe, Celia Martínez, Belén Rosa de Egea, Juan Manuel Zaragoza, Concha Roldán, Josep Corbí, Antonio Sánchez, Fanny Hernández, Carmen Ramírez, Leticia Fernández-Fontecha, William Schupbach, Ken Arnold, Fernando Vidal, Nike Fakiner, Alberto Fragio, Eva Botella, Lola Sarabia, Lucía Díaz-Marroquín, Felipe Pereda, Mercedes García-Arenal, Eduardo Manzano, Victoria Diehl, María Gómez Garrido, Marina de la Cruz, Pura Fernández, Rafael Huertas, María Cifuentes, Inés Vergara, Paola Martínez, José Luis Villacañas, Cristina Santamarina, Rosa Peris, Miguel Marinas, José María González García, Beatriz Pichel, Mercedes Peris, Sally Bragg, Cristina Garaizábal, Agustín Serrano de Haro, María Iñigo, and Mar Cejas. To all these friends and colleagues, I would also like to add the anonymous referees from Palgrave and, of course, Sarah Thomas and Paul House, who rendered my Spanish into English with patience and dedication.

The one who should go first is always left until last. For many years she has patiently endured the diversion of my energies to this project. For this, and for so many other things, the last note of gratitude must be for Reyes, *esposa de mi piel, compañera de la vida.*

Introduction

Pain, which almost always lacks justification, does have a history. If we took the teachings of Lucretius seriously, we would have to concede that the historians who have washed their hands of the passions could only write the history of concealment and lies, given that, according to this Latin thinker, truth only flourishes in moments of uncertainty and danger.[1] When the German philosopher Friedrich Nietzsche wrote *The Gay Science* in 1888, he also understood that the intellectuals of his time had left aside the sentiments that give color to existence.[2] Albeit timidly, the new humanities have begun to include emotions among their new objects of study. Some scholars have recently written books and articles on hatred, fear, compassion, rage, boredom, resentment, or love.[3] For the proponents of these approaches, excluding desire, aversion, happiness, mourning, hope, fear, modesty, shame, rage, hatred, or love in the study of culture would be akin to replacing the history of humanity with a rational reconstruction where, against all evidence, social actions appear devoid of emotions or instincts.[4] Proponents of the so-called "affective turn" generally quote a text by Lucien Febvre written in 1941 as the starting point of this new trend. In this text, the French historian denounced the fact that elements of social behavior as basic as fear, hatred, cruelty, or love had been excluded from the recounting of political decisions or economic activity. Since all emotions, however, even those traditionally considered more irrational, guided both individual decisions and collective actions, history could not be separated from life or distanced from the present.[5] On the contrary, the demand for large-scale research into humankind's fundamental feelings was clearly politically inspired. It urged a new form of confronting the past that, taking on the blood and guts of the human condition, would put yesterday's lessons to today's use. Distanced from all those philosophical systems that had made the human being an entelechy whose veins do not flow with blood, but rather with the diluted residue of reason, the new human sciences, as they were then known, projected

1

a philosophy of social perception of, and collective reflection on, the forgotten passions of the past.[6]

Even though the history of human suffering has an obvious emotional dimension, the temporal modulation of human pain cannot be located either in the history of the passions or in the history of the sciences. For one thing, it does not refer to the acquisition of knowledge, but to the production of meaning. Halfway between the world of emotions and the realm of sensations, the history of pain refers back to the history of experience; that is, to the history of what is at once familiar and strange, one's own and another's, individual and collective. This word choice is not arbitrary, for under the umbrella of this term, experience, the body does not separate from the soul, the material from the spiritual, the self from the other. Sensorial elements do not exclude emotional reactions, nor do the visible forms of cruelty or harm exhaust the sphere of historical research.[7] Although we live in a world that has obliged us, and still forces us, to think in exclusive categories, the history of pain cannot be written using them.

The history of this experience has begun to be explored in relation to the internal development of medical or physiological theories of suffering, or in connection to the pharmaceutical remedies used to alleviate it.[8] Researchers have also focused on the history of torture, education, or some branches of medicine, like surgery or obstetrics. In other cases, they have paid attention to the changing attitudes or cultural responses to personal pain and the suffering of others. The inquisitive gaze has increasingly fallen on the practices and representations of violence, including in this category military campaigns, religious wars, or modern terrorism.[9] Just as historians of science have attempted to account for the progressive objectification of subjective perceptions, cultural historians, inspired by the new opposition to clinical medicine, have sought in the history of human suffering the triumph of a new humanitarian model for managing pain and death. In both cases, little has been done to disentangle the social dimension of this experience or to examine its historical forms of collective visibility. Unlike the most internal and the most cultural approaches, this book attempts to unravel the persuasive and rhetorical procedures that have historically conditioned the experience of harm. This is a text about the successive (but not progressive) forms of materializing or objectifying pain, about the rhetorical modes that have allowed, across the centuries, the cultural understanding of human suffering.[10] In this regard, it is not a book on history proper, neither is it a book on cultural history, despite its title, but rather a book on the historical epistemology of (a certain type) of experience, on the rhetoric and persuasive means historically employed to generate conviction about the reality of pain.

Following the philosopher Wilhelm Dilthey, the anthropologist Clifford Geertz has distinguished between the mere flow of life, the delimited unit of this flow, and this unit's expression through language, science, or art. Here it is sufficient to differentiate between the mere experience and its intersubjective articulation. The latter, unlike the former, has a beginning, a development, and an end; it constitutes a unit that may, in turn, resolve itself into a variety of cultural expressions.[11] The photos we may take on a journey, for example, do not exhaust what we saw and lived during our adventure. The (real or imaginary) album in which we paste our memories is yet another way of structuring and giving meaning to a partial or biased selection of all we have experienced. We could also have kept a diary, perhaps accompanied by little fetishes, like a museum pass, the bill from a restaurant, or a train ticket. In any case, the relationship between the journey and its photographs – which can be arranged by theme, or place, people, or style – is not merely *causal* in the sense that the first (the journey, the experience) determines the form of the second (its representation, its expression). Undoubtedly, if we travel to Paris the photos will be of this city and no other, but our previous knowledge, expectations, and evaluations will also modulate the moment and mood in which we decide to portray ourselves. Put in a trivial way: one lives, thinks, and feels in accordance with commonplaces and learned values. The hundreds of tourists who flock to the Mona Lisa with their cameras are, perhaps, not (only) interested in the painting, but also in its emotional appropriation. Many of them could even have arrived at the museum with the sole intention of taking a photo that, in their places of origin, will acquire a new individual meaning and a different collective value. Cultural historians have rightly pointed out that images are not transparent, and consequently cannot be interpreted as mere representations of the states of things. This is equivalent to saying that expression (pictorial expression, for example) neither literally accounts for experiences nor exhausts their content. On the contrary, these expressions should be interpreted as indices of evaluative, emotional, and intellectual elements. Therefore, as far as the history of experience is concerned, the problem does not consist of knowing how to access the private contents of consciousness, but rather of how the experience of human suffering has historically been articulated; that is, how a journey along the path of pain may have crystallized into a material album of harm.

Although many historians hold that the history of *subjective* experience is closely linked to the history of private life and that, consequently, the best sources for unraveling its secrets would be those documents that we could consider most *intimate,* we should also keep in mind that what makes diaries, autobiographies, and confessions possible is the desire to transcend one's own perspective, to find consolation in mutual company, or to give meaning to personal experiences.[12] A large part of the discussion on psychological disorders or nervous conditions reflects a similar tension between the (subjective) certainty of what the patient feels and the (objective) truth of what science diagnoses. A history of pain too closely linked to private life would tend to disintegrate into a variety of gestures, representations, expressions, remedies, and symptoms. At the same time, no history of pain that aspired to be a long-term history could base itself on the same primary sources across a period of centuries. This is the reason why our task as historians cannot consist of a mere accumulation of cases, but rather of a reconstruction of the forms in which experiences materialized into structured units that, at the same time, may have remained fixed in science or art. And we must say "may," because the presence of pain does not in and of itself guarantee its social perception. From this perspective, the historian not only interprets cultural forms as material expressions of lived experience, but also brings unnoticed experiences into the sphere of public awareness.

One of the most seminal works in drawing attention to such unnoticed experiences was Elaine Scarry's *The Body in Pain*. Although Scarry's book was published in 1985, it is worth clarifying some of the commonplaces upon which her argument is constructed. After a quarter century, the task cannot be to debate a work that, based on its trajectory and merits, has attained the status of a modern classic, but rather to underline some of the suppositions on which the argument is founded. Although Scarry's work connected pain's supposed inexpressibility, its political consequences, and what she called "the nature of human creation," the book also found a source of inspiration in the elusive relationship between the mute experience of pain and the human representation of suffering. Much like this book, Scarry's was written halfway between experience and expression. However, that is where all similarities end. Her characterization of the experience of physical pain, which continues to echo as a mantra practically across the entire academic spectrum, owed a great deal to a commonsensical philosophy inherited from modernity, to its hackneyed dichotomies and its intellectual topologies. In a general sense, her understanding of pain was based on two problems belonging to the philosophy of mind in the second half of the twentieth century: first-person authority and the problem of other minds. In the first case, Scarry assumed the indubitable nature of painful experience for any person who suffers it. In the second, she symmetrically defended the difficulty of producing knowledge about the pain of others. In the first case, pain appeared as the greatest conviction, while in the second, it reflected the greatest of uncertainties: "pain comes unsharably into our midst as at once that which cannot be denied and that which cannot be confirmed."[13] Pain's resistance to language was only one consequence of its "unsharability;" the inevitable conclusion of the private nature of the contents of consciousness – or as Scarry terms them, our "interior states." In her view, given that physical pain lacks "referential content," since it does not refer to any object outside itself, it "resisted objectification in language."[14] Curiously, at the only moment when Scarry appears convinced that pain was "originally an interior and unsharable experience," a paradoxical mention of Wittgenstein's philosophy appears.[15] And we must say "paradoxical," because for this Austrian philosopher the mere possibility of a private language, and by extension a private experience, interior and unsharable, would be completely devoid of sense. Wittgenstein's argument, to which I will return in the fifth chapter of this book, rested on the circumstance, later pointed out by other philosophers, that pain, like other states of consciousness, is not only known but also learned through the mediated experience of others. For Wittgenstein, unlike for Scarry, "you learn the concept 'pain' when you use language."[16] Scarry's great intuition, that pain has to do with meaning, weakened when we accept that meaning should always be referential (which is obviously not the case) and when we miss its collective nature.

That pain is an experience is not open to discussion. Although the International Association for the Study of Pain (IASP) defines it in that way – as "a sensory and emotional experience" – the evidence in favor of this characterization not only depends on this particular scientific definition from the mid-1970s, but on the innumerable testimonies and processes that made it possible.[17] As we will see in the last chapter, behind this phrase the entire history of pain associated with incurable and terminal illnesses lives on, along with the numerous testimonies of patients, especially soldiers, afflicted by untreatable injuries. The IASP's definition has allowed a cultural re-evaluation of pain, as well as of its supposed biological universality. In this new model, pain results from the interaction of physiological, psychological, and cultural elements. At the same time, the patient's subjective narrative becomes an unquestionable fact of clinical practice. So far there is nothing objectionable. After all, the presence of cultural or evaluative elements in the study of pain has made possible the substitution of the old myth of the progressive objectivization of subjective experience with a holistic approach that recognizes the subjectivity of experience as an objective fact of science and culture. However, the question of clarifying where the "culturality" of pain resides remains unsolved. From the already generalized agreement that experience itself is modified in accordance with cultural guidelines and patterns arises the need to direct research toward the study of these very guidelines and patterns. From the conviction that pain can not only be taught, but also learned, follows the necessity to track the cultural forms that the experience of harm takes on. After all, if pain is (also) a cultural experience, what are its historical variations? How can they be studied? In a word, where are the socially mediated tools that allow the expression and modulation of this experience? The cultural history of pain navigates between two great dangers. The first has to do with the dissolution of the object of study in its historical appearances; for if the experience of pain is culturally determined, why keep thinking that we are dealing with a unique experience? Mustn't we recognize the existence of as many experiences as cultures, or, as a last resort, subjects? The second danger consists of writing a finalist history, inscribed, for example, within the context of the civilizing process or other teleological dynamics. Given that pain's salience as a privileged object of research and medical practice only took place in the twentieth century, there has been a prevailing tendency to turn the conceptualization and management of chronic pain into the inevitable conclusion of the entire history of human suffering.

From a structural point of view, pain is a drama. Although this affirmation possesses the advantage of its evidence – and although many academics have observed theatrical elements in the history of human suffering – the jargon of representation or performativity has appeared, except on particular occasions, as an accessory to the historical narrative, as a rhetorical addition with which to color the direct or indirect testimony of doctors and patients, but also of masochists or torturers. To affirm that pain exists under the form of a social drama means, however, that its historical variations share some common elements; it implies recognizing that, independently of its cultural expressions, there is a constant traveling down the path of suffering and facing harmful experience.[18] Pain's drama appears in a sequential form; it displays a dynamic structure that includes a moment of rupture that demands reparation. This shares the basic form of a rite of passage: the person in pain lives in a liminal space, in an indeterminate region; as long as the suffering does not cease, the sufferer wanders between separation and reconciliation. The majority of those who suffer, even if in solitude, consider their pain this way: in a transitory form, which sooner or later should stop or be remedied. Here experience takes on its most dramatic and literal sense, which implies displacement and peril. For both those who suffer and those who look on, pain – if it must be considered as such – is a drama that situates us in a borderland. Liminality – a concept we have borrowed from the anthropology of experience – constitutes a recurring motif in the history of human suffering. The person who suffers lives among shadows, like the nuns of the seventeenth century whom we will study in the second chapter; or between the human and the superhuman, like the virgin martyrs of the sixteenth century that we shall see in the first; or even between consciousness and unconsciousness, like the anesthetized men and women we will study in the fifth. Sometimes the border is physical, for he who suffers – as Don Quixote well knows – also travels. Other times, however, the distance is merely symbolic: it doesn't affect the victim, but rather the witnesses, who should not situate themselves too far from or too close to the real stage of violence.

As concerns its dramatic nature, pain mobilizes all the elements of theatrical representation. The experience of harm has its actors, plot, stage, costumes, props, scenography, and, of course, its audience. Far from lacking a voice, or posing a challenge to language, the theater configures the literary form of harmful experience.[19] Its cultural expression is not merely demonstrative; for just as the person who displays photos from their travels does not want to prevail but rather convince, those who express their pain make it, in accordance with learned rhetorical forms, at the same time patent and public. Their cries, their words, their actions, seek to transform certainty into truth through a concurrence of persuasive elements. Although the philosopher Cioran asserted that it was impossible to dialog with physical pain, each and every page that follows here contradicts this supposed impossibility.[20] The theater of cruelty, the anatomical theater, the baroque theater of emulation, the Enlightenment spectacle of violence, the operating theater linked in the early modern period to the rhetoric of dental surgery or obstetrics, the comedy of the masochist or the mentally ill person in the last decades of the nineteenth century, all point always in the same direction. In the drama of pain, the one who hurts plays a role that generates conviction under the strict observance of persuasive rules.

In a book that spans 500 years, history cannot remain uniform in its sources or its methodological approaches. The genealogy of culture, which analyzes pain's historical modulations, is merely the counterpoint to the (historical) epistemology of experience. In the first case, cultural materializations are understood as expressions of our affects, or, as it were (following Nietzsche) as "symptoms of the body." In the second case, the challenge consists in untangling the (historical) forms that configure and modulate the experience of harm. Only in a very inappropriate sense can these structuring forms be called *categories*. To begin with, they are not formal representations; they do not serve to construct anything, but rather to bestow a collective meaning upon the experience of harm. Understood as persuasive schemes, they constitute what have been denominated, since the times of Aristotle, as topics, *topoi*.[21] This word, which today is almost synonymous with "stereotypes," should be understood in its literal sense: as a commonplace that is everyone's and belongs to us all. Confronting the problem of rhetorical reasoning, and after taking a roll call of the arguments particular to each of its varieties, Aristotle dedicated a good part of his treatise to the study of common arguments; and although he never managed to offer a definition, he referred to these *topoi* as general sources of reasoning.

Representation, imitation, sympathy, trust, testimony, correspondence, coherence, narrativity, or reiteration – concepts which provide the titles of various sections of this book – are some of the forms that enable the configuration of pain into an intersubjective reality that can be analyzed. These topics, *topoi*, that I propose here as part of a general understanding of harmful experience are not *emotional styles*, but rather schemas, even commonplaces; so common that the reader will find them trivial. None of them completely exhausts the persuasive schemas that allow interrelating a person's pain, the pain of others, physical pain, and moral suffering, but they do provide a starting point. If pain is, as the physiologist Bichat suggested, "the cry of life," what interests us in this expression is not only the cry, as an abbreviated formula of suffering's resistance to language, but what this very expression suggests about the crystallization of life's flow.[22] The person in pain learns to feel within an intermediate space, a common space, which delimits and conditions his or her sensation and evaluation of harm. In this common space, experience is articulated in such a way that one can, among other things, recognize pain *as pain* and suffering *as suffering*; but it also makes possible, on the contrary, taking pleasure in harmful experiences. The history of religious asceticism and of sexual masochism, but also of chronic pain, of the late medieval representation of violence or of the placebo effect would all be incomprehensible without this duality between the unified form of experience and the cultural modulation that allows the breaking of the (supposedly objective) correspondence between physiological pain and its subjective expression.

For those who are in pain, the probability that their experience will be culturally meaningful increases depending on whether it can be imitated or represented. Everyone knows this. It also helps if their suffering and anguish produce sympathy or commiseration among those present. If the sensations do not correspond to any visible or known cause, some problems will arise. And if they do correspond, the best scenario is that the groans and laments are uttered within certain limits and in strict proportions. If all else fails, their narrative account should at least have internal coherence and be consistent with previous cases. That the pain is conscious or unconscious is not as important as whether its presence is socially recognized. But if nothing works; if their pain cannot be observed; if it doesn't produce sympathy; if it doesn't correspond to any organic lesion or disorder; if it lacks narrative coherence; if it doesn't exist socially, then we must take refuge in the accumulation of the greatest possible number of similar cases. Each of these persuasive forms, including this last one, through which philosophy recognizes that repetition is the best way to express difference, constitutes a rhetorical strategy, an argumentative topic by which to transform the certainty of an experience into a social and inter-subjective truth.

1
Representations

Pain and history

The high altar of the church of Santa Mayorga de Campos, in Valladolid, Spain, features an altarpiece dedicated to the patron saint of Orense, Saint Marina. Twelve panels divided into two sections depict the most noteworthy events of her life and circumstances of her death, while a third series shows various moments from the Passion of Christ.[1] The altarpiece, dated around 1500, covers Marina's life from the confirmation of her faith to her death in Antioch, beheaded on the orders of the prefect Olybrius. According to the hagiographical writings of the *Golden Legend*, the life of this noble maiden took an unexpected turn when she caught the prefect's eye and he sent his servants to bring her to him with the intention of seducing her: "if she is freeborn, I shall make her my wife; if she is a slave girl, I shall take her as my concubine," he told his footmen.[2] Faced with her refusal to give in to his advances, Olybrius had her sent to prison and chained up in shackles. The prefect prepared to interrogate her: "it is a contradiction that a maiden so fair and so noble as you should have a crucified man as her God," he said. When she again rejected him, he commanded her to be lashed with rods, and that her flesh be torn with iron combs "until the blood flowed out of her body, like water flows out of a spring" (see Figure 1).

There is a certain logic in beginning this book with the representation of physical suffering because, beyond verbal articulation, we know about the pain of others through the observation of their bodily gestures, attitudes, and expressions: in other words, through a set of expressive signs that can, in turn, be transferred to the world of images. Before words come to our aid, the evaluation of another's emotions depends on cries, grimaces, and tears. At least from the *Physiognomy* of the seventeenth-century French artist Charles Le Brun, to Darwin's *The Expression of the Emotions in Man and Animals* of 1872, facial gestures and corporeal signs have constituted a gateway to emotional states, whether these grimaces were interpreted in accordance with the theory of evolution or the aesthetics of taste.[3] Contrary to the universalizing approaches of Darwin and Le Brun, who, for different reasons, considered that the same emotions always triggered the same gestures, twentieth-century anthropology studied how expressive signs vary in their forms, intensity, and acceptability in different social contexts. One of the pioneering books in this direction pointed out how different ethnic groups in contemporary North American culture responded differently to pain.[4] Although the methodology of this study has been repeatedly called into question, the idea that bodily responses are learned as regulated codes within our cultural heritage is no longer debated; the same stimulus does not always correspond to the same gesture, nor do the same gestures or attitudes derive in all cases from the same emotional state.[5] The history of tears is a good example of the various uses that can be associated with an act that is at once cultural and physiological.[6] Where, how much, and in what circumstances it is permissible to cry, whether to express happiness or as a sign of pain or mourning, depends on social contexts that transform sobs into comprehensible actions. The same reasoning also applies to the case of pain. The images and icons that have reached us over the years may serve as indicators of the norms and rules that allowed bodily behavior and expressions to be culturally revealing. However, in the Marina altarpiece, as in most representations of extreme violence related to the lives of the saints from the end of the Middle Ages, the faces of the victims remain unaltered, and neither the facial expression nor any other element allows us to infer, beyond the visualization of the punishment, the magnitude of their physical suffering. Facial expressions are perhaps the first and most basic way of knowing a person's state of mind; but these visual features, or the lack thereof, must be relocated within the cultural framework that created them, and which makes them simultaneously possible and meaningful. If we only took into consideration these expressive features, the visual representation of virgin martyrs could not be part of the history of pain. After all, nothing in their peaceful faces or their calm gestures allows us to infer any presence of harm.

The altarpiece of Saint Marina is one of the numerous notable images related to physical suffering produced toward the end of the Middle Ages. From the plains of Castile to the Carpathian Mountains and from the Mediterranean to the North Sea, many artists dedicated some of their greatest works to the representation of extreme cruelty or violence, either related to Christian martyrs, the life and death of the Savior, or the torments and punishment of Purgatory and Hell.[7] The spectacle of suffering within judicial doctrine, political authority, religious struggles, or the dance of death was expressed repeatedly through a finite set of iconographic elements related to the mutilation, violation, or dissection of the body. Various historians have posited that these representations arose as a reflection of the violence experienced in legal punishment, religious wars, popular revolts, and public executions. For the art historian Lionello Puppi, for example, since the majority of artists had direct knowledge of the processes of execution and torture, the violence represented should be understood as a mere expression of religious atrocities or punitive arts developed in a time of apocalyptic anguish, Satanism, endemic famine, and frequent outbreaks of plague.[8] Men and women at the end of the Middle Ages found these images above all in churches, but also in many other places connected in one way or another with the world of the spectacle.[9] Dürer's *Four Horsemen of the Apocalypse* could not be a better expression of this collective gloom provoked by continual references to the triumph of death. For Mitchell B. Merback, on the other hand, the realism of these images cannot be considered a mere reflection of criminal justice. On the contrary, painting was rather an ideal *model* in which the past was merged with the present, and the then with the now. Far from being just a reflection, representation constituted an iconic model with a great deal of pedagogic content.[10]

The artistic expression of medieval suffering very likely stood somewhere between these two positions. On the one hand, representations of pain were part of lived experience; hence their meaningful nature. In an almost trivial sense, artists painted what they saw. On the other hand, however, images of extreme violence did not exactly reflect the world; rather, they built it, or to use a more appropriate expression, they dramatized it. The violence represented resembles the violence experienced, not because the former imitates the latter, but because both are governed by the same rules. The pain of the martyr was expressed in a theatrical context where the scenes depended on norms, conventions, and ritualized acts.[11] As in punitive practices, suffering took place within a comedy of gestures, at times linked to the dramatic use of masks.[12] Much like in Brueghel the Elder's very well known painting, *The Road to Calvary*, nothing allows us to distinguish the sacred from the profane, the joyful from the painful, biblical experience from lived experience. From the beginning to the end, the protagonists of medieval altarpieces, like those found guilty in penal trials, passed through a liminal world where their words and gestures, like their scenery and clothing, were regulated. At the moment of execution, the celebration of blood resembles the liturgy; or, the reverse: the Eucharist is devised as a collective recreation of a public execution. Whether we speak of represented violence or the representation of violence, blood and pain govern the rules of memory.

This correspondence between the spheres of represented and real violence is not immediately obvious. The images adorning the walls of medieval churches do not reflect historical reality – how could they? On their own they are not a mirror of punitive violence or the pedagogy of arms; they do not represent states of things, but states of mind. Their referent is not exactly reality, but rather experience. They do not show us history, but emotions. Their purpose is not to reveal the drama of existence, but to open the doors onto a participatory and collective action, of a dramatic nature, that configures and constitutes experience. As twenty-first-century spectators, unable to refer these images to the traditional elements associated with the arts, such as beauty or proportion, we locate them in an unclassifiable and distant place. We refuse to look at them under the pretext of not understanding them; or, on the contrary, we use them as instruments of knowledge, consumerism, or lasciviousness. Since at least the end of the nineteenth century, violence deemed gratuitous has frequently been presented as a form of obscenity. In early modern Europe, however, the abusive reiteration of bodily torments has a very different meaning. The virgin martyrs, Christ's Passion, the massacred victims of religious wars, or, more extremely, the dissected bodies represented in anatomical plates, are part of an iconographic pattern that interprets violence within an evaluative framework that transforms the protagonists into beings that wander through illogical and almost unreal spaces. On the border between life and death, between the one and the many, the concrete and the ideal, their gestures have not been laid down as a testimony of lived experience, but rather as part of an intricate, theatrical mechanism that feeds memory, keeping alive recollections of faith, passion, and knowledge.

Virgin martyrs

The altarpiece of Saint Marina, currently in the Fine Arts Museum in Oviedo, Spain, resembles countless others featuring similar themes and motifs made in Europe toward the end of the Middle Ages. This work, attributed to the Master of Palanquinos, much like the "Martyrdom of Saint Barbara" by the Dominican monk Master Francke, represents the victory of faith through the punishment of the body.[13] In both pictorial sets, the torture of the flesh aims at the violation of chastity. In keeping with the worship of virgin martyrs from the end of the Middle Ages, torture introduces an element of lust. Since faith and virginity are mutually protective – to lose one's faith would imply losing one's virginity, just as to lose one's virginity would imply losing one's faith – martyrdom was designed to break the former in order to corrupt the latter.[14] Since the prefect Olybrius was obsessed with both, torture acquires the configuration of sexual violence. Dishonor is insinuated through the humiliation of the flesh: a recurring motif in the religious iconography of the time that has one of its most emblematic examples in the flagellation of Christ painted by the Catalonian painter Lluis Borrassà [c. 1360–1425] (See Figure 2).

As in medieval trials related to sexual purity, where innocence was revealed when torture was unable to fulfill its natural effect, the re-composition of the body, unharmed after each blow and unaltered after each trial, suggests an extreme victory of faith.[15] When the crowd begs Marina to give in and submit to the prefect, so as not to lose her beauty or her life for remaining faithful to her religion, the virgin humbly accepts her punishment. Violence is a threat to her integrity, but ugliness does not concern her. Unlike the prefect, whom she thinks of as a "shameless dog" or an "insatiable lion," Marina's beauty depends on the strength of her spirit and not on the state of her body. Her calmness contrasts sharply with the angry, distorted faces of her torturers. The just and the condemned stand on opposite ends of the whip. Peace is on one side, violence on the other. Disfiguration, as a sign of moral depravation, only affects the footmen who whip her or the prefect who desires her. The altarpiece highlights the young woman's spiritual beauty through a body that remains intact and unaltered after each torture and returns to its natural state after each blow. Her beauty, a constant reference in both literary characterizations and artistic representations, turns her body into a witness of truth and a tabernacle for salvation. Her purity embodies the dignity of a Church that uses martyrdom as a tool for evangelization. Neither her nudity nor her torn flesh manage to corrupt her spirit. Not even when a gigantic dragon devours her, in a flight of fantasy that even Jacopo da Vorágine considered "farfetched," is her dignity tarnished or her body disturbed. Quite the reverse: the young woman manages to escape unharmed from the beast, bursting its stomach open after crossing herself.

Even when the martyrdom of virgins includes a clear sexual element, gender is not the determining factor. Altarpieces were not intended for sexual arousal, but rather for representation of emotional states.[16] Their narrative structure, far beyond the carnal limits of the libido, creates a harmful space, at once real and imaginary, where wounds are dramatized and interpreted. It does not concern women exclusively. In Catalonian gothic painting, for example, Bernat Martorell [c. 1400–1452], one of Borrasà's followers, produced an altarpiece on George of Cappadocia. The story of this young Christian, beheaded on the orders of Diocletian on 23 April, AD 303 for refusing to renounce his religion and embrace paganism, constitutes one of the great icons of Mediterranean culture, both within and outside Christianity. As in the cases of Saint Marina and Saint Barbara, the ruler ordered that he be tied to a horse, that his flesh be torn, that flaming torches be applied to burn his innards and salt be rubbed into his wounds. Like them, the knight accepted his punishment without tears or complaints. His hieratical countenance showed only an expression of determination and confidence. In the absence of any sign of suffering or gestures of surrender, the judge ordered that he be fried in a colossal pan of molten lead. Martorell depicted the saint on different panels: whipped, with his hands tied, dragged by a horse, and, finally, beheaded. At no moment, however, does his face show any sign of fear, pain or doubt (See Figure 3). His impassivity serves as proof of his supernatural resistance. Swords cannot cut him nor poison harm him. Like in the evisceration of Saint Erasmus, a painting by the Flemish artist

Dieric Bouts (c. 1410–1475) that hangs in Louvain Cathedral, George accepts his torment serenely, almost with pleasure. Far from feeling the slightest pain, he seems to be as comfortable in the pan of boiling lead, *"as if he were taking a bath"* (see Figure 4).

The panels of the altarpiece of Saint George, like those of Saint Marina, depict the triumph of faith through the rending of the flesh. Whether in the context of devotion or worship, the saints' stories contain the mode in which they ought to be memorized and the way in which they should be interpreted. It does not matter if they lack verisimilitude or contradict their literary sources. Since their function is not merely representational, it is inconsequential that the facts attributed to the young Galician Marina, who would become the patron saint of Orense, really correspond to the life of Margaret of Antioch. The one may easily usurp the life of the other. There was, indeed, a Marina in Galicia, but the events that marked her life had little to do with those shown by the Palanquinos Master. The Galician saint, forced to pretend to be a man for most of her life, was accused of making a farmer's daughter pregnant. She was expelled from the monastery and bore the shame of her supposed sin with integrity, subsisted off charity and handouts until, in the moment of her death, the monks discovered that he whom they had taken for a licentious monk was in fact a holy woman.[17] The same uncertainties applied to the deeds attributed to George of Cappadocia. The way in which he killed the dragon, whose foul-smelling breath caused the death of many inhabitants of Silca, a non-existent place, did not form part of the legend until well into the ninth century. In both cases, the lack of historical coherence affects neither the purpose nor the aim of the tale. The altarpiece does not transcribe facts, but rather articulates experiences that are expressed through a pictorial narrative. The succession of scenes inverts the logical order that suggests that the meaning of a story is posterior to the story itself, a moral conclusion or lesson extracted from historical teaching, as in a parable. On the contrary, the altarpiece centers on the constitution of a collective experience by means of stories than can be quite similar, or even interchangeable.

The stories of Margaret of Antioch and George of Cappadocia do resemble one another. Both saints abandon their privileges of birth and convert to Christianity. Both lose their lives confronting the local authorities. Although they are not the only martyrs to defeat a dragon, this heroic deed became the main motif of their iconography. In both cases, the sign of the cross served as the mark of the struggle. From a martyrological point of view, both suffered similar torments, which they accepted with the same determination. They were both beheaded, after their miracles of physical resistance inspired mass conversions. Finally, both their stories feature a supernatural intervention bringing punishment and death to the unjust. As in many other similar cases, the succession of scenes obeys the parameters of what the anthropology of experience has called a "social drama:" a gradual process of rupture and collective reconciliation.[18] The scenes reflect a story of separation and reunion; they record a ritual – more specifically, a rite of passage. As in the particular ceremonies of birth, marriage, or death, the altarpiece panels depict a journey of initiation that begins with a physical and moral partition from familial bonds and community ties. Once the frontier of rootlessness has been crossed, the saints move toward a place that is somewhere between the sacred and the profane; they inhabit a space between the worldly and the supernatural; mutilated, dismembered, and fragmented, they float between two worlds. This intermediary space, represented as an enormous entrance, threshold, or limit – a place where history and community do not yet exist – is characterized by disorder and disproportion. The true lives alongside the false, the real with the ethereal, natural with supernatural, and the dead with the living.[19] Not even sexual attributes remain stable or unaltered. In the case of Marina, the young Galician woman who lived her days as a man, the drama also allows for the concealment, disguise, or transposition of gender. The world in which the story takes place is filled with intermediary species, imaginary places, and impossible spaces. The Master of Palanquinos, for example, does not hesitate to attribute to the devil the features of different beasts, emphasizing his ugliness with a large horn protruding from his forehead, and fire-spewing jaws emerging from his knees, his genitals, and his long dendriform tail. The heads of the martyrs always appear surrounded by a halo of sanctity. They are young, but look old. Torture does not destroy them and pain does not affect them. Quite the reverse, the mutilation of their bodies always concludes with the reunification of their limbs and the miraculous curing of their wounds. In the impossible space through which they wander, pain expresses its most cruel and most bloody form. One torment is added to the next in a passionate succession of wounds, blows, tears, fractures, and macerations. The only possible relationship between the offense and the sentence is that the tortured be absolutely innocent and the punishments absolutely disproportionate.

In the context of this ceremonial sequence, the magnitude of the torment determines the intensity of the miracle: the more inhumane the former, the more superhuman the latter. The acknowledgment of this supernatural intervention rests on the repeated failure of the expressive signs that, in all honesty, should correspond to the injuries. The torture does not produce the logical effect or the desired aim. Neither the burning torches, the boiling baths, the mutilation of the body, nor the evisceration of the organs weakens the faith, corrupts the soul, or destroys the body. Against all odds, it is not faith that helps to bear the torments, but rather the transition of these tortured bodies along the path of penances that reinforces their faith. Sacrifice makes possible the physical and the symbolic re-joining of the limbs severed from the saint's body and from the body of the Church. In both cases, what had been previously dismembered must be now reunited and re-membered.[20] Given that all justice springs from harm, the degree of pain makes its reparation increasingly urgent. Throughout the process, as in other similar rituals, blood plays a central role.[21] "There is no festivity without sacrifice," wrote the philosopher Nietzsche when examining the origins of tragedy. Some of the most common ways of administering pain in the lives of the saints, such as flagellation, had always been linked to purification rituals and practices. Others, the most dramatic, make explicit the disproportion between crime and punishment. More generally, they demonstrate the need to subject the body to the greatest possible pain. For those who suffer it, martyrdom constitutes a heavenly blessing, a sign of being chosen. The most vehement of them even dreamed of going in search of the martyrs, "to share in their crusade and in their martyrdom."[22]

All these elements serve to underline the well-documented connection between pictorial representation and medieval theater.[23] The altarpiece does not merely imitate the narrative fragments of *The Golden Legend*: rather, it emphasizes the ritual dramatization of violence. In the same way that the varied liturgies prior to the Council of Trent contained musical and interpretative elements – to the extent that it is difficult to know whether the theater was imitating the liturgy or vice versa – the altarpiece makes possible the reconstruction of the drama and the materialization of experience. These connections between hagiography and the theatrical sphere are numerous. Many spectacles staged in the Toledo cathedral in the fifteenth century, for example, included text, music, and theater. The most elaborate among them used machinery and technological resources to simulate, for example, a saint's apparition or an angel's flight. Those actors playing the parts of demons were dressed in animal hides while the others were costumed according to their characters. Throughout Europe, mainly in the representation of the Passion or the saints' martyrdoms, these effects were so realistic that substitutes for human blood often splattered church floors. Animal entrails replaced the organs of the martyrs, and actors simulated, sometimes putting their lives at risk, beatings, and torments. Along with *Corpus Christi*, the most popular liturgical drama, these spectacles had subjects as varied as Adam and Eve, the Adoration of the Magi, or the Last Judgment.[24] In this theatrical representation of spiritual life, hagiographic topics enjoyed a pride of place. In Spain, these plays became known as "*Comedias de santos*" and, together with the so-called "*Autos sacramentales*," lived on until the seventeenth century.[25]

The proliferation of these plays, as well as the resulting entrance of visual and popular culture into European cathedrals and churches, explains the successive decrees regarding the regulation of their use and the canonization of their structure. After the Reformation, many Lutherans fought against both the proliferation of religious images and liturgical dramas. The Calvinists soon followed this trend: "the Holy Bible was not given us to serve us as a pastime,"

stated the synod of Nimes in 1574.[26] In Spain, in the context of the condem-
nations of the Council of Trent, the Provincial Council of Toledo drew up a
decree in 1565 for regulating spectacles, and the Jesuit Juan de Mariana [1536–
1623], magister at the powerful Colegio Romano, denounced the theater in
his *De spectaculis*, a recreation of the classical text by Tertulian: "There is no
public spectacle without violence," the Christian author stated.[27] Despite these
critiques, pictorial art and theatrical representation often featured the same
protagonists. The French painter Jean Hortart, for example, attended these representations in Lyon, often taking part in the costuming; many other painters
participated in the *mis-en-scène* of liturgical drama.[28]

The use of the word "theater," which appears in some of the most relevant
works on the spectacle of violence in Early Modern Europe – such as Giovanni
Luychen's *Il Teatro delle crudeltà* or Richard Verstengan's *Le Théâthre des cruantés*,
discussed below – is not purely coincidental. The theater and the altarpiece
take part in the pedagogical function of medieval art and its gestural culture.[29]
On the one hand, they helped a largely illiterate public to understand the mysteries of the Passion or the lives of the saints. In this sense, they serve as mirrors
of geographical, historical, and moral knowledge. But they also make the representation of a drama possible; they allow for the remembrance of an experience
through a ritual exercise that was, in turn, based on the premise that "only what
does not cease *to give pain* remains in one's memory."[30] The spectacle of violence
configures the brutalized form in which human beings remember themselves as
animals. Facial expressions, hand movements, bodily positions, the attitude of
those portrayed as well as their clothing, all shape a regulated set of expressive
signs that facilitate the unfolding of the narrative. The pedagogic and evangeli-
cal aspects, ludic plots, and emotional elements gave pain a collective meaning
in the context of liturgical representation. It was not the first time in the West
that experience was built on the crudest ritualization of harm, but it was the
first time that these rituals were accompanied by images and sculptures of large
dimensions or by engravings and woodcuts reproduced through mechanical
procedures.

"Whenever man considered it necessary to make a memory for himself, it was
never done without blood."[31] So wrote the philosopher Friedrich Nietzsche in
his *Genealogy of Morals* in the second half of the nineteenth century. In his view,
the main moral concepts such as blame, conscience, and duty, were bathed in
blood. For Nietzsche, religions and legal systems were, in their deepest nature,
mnemonic systems supported by a cruel and disproportionate violence that
had in the past constituted mankind's great festive happiness. One hundred
years later, some of these ideas were brought up to date, first by the French
historian Michel Foucault, and later by a number of scholars of literature and,
more specifically, ancient and medieval theater. For Jody Enders, for example,
the history of theater coincides, in its structural elements, with the history

of torture; both emerged within what Isidoro de Sevilla called the *spectacle of cruelty*. For Anthony Kubiak, theater, as a civilizing activity, was also based on the perception of terror. Despite their different historical moments and approaches, all these authors point out the inextricable connection between aesthetic experience, moral standards, the revelation of truth, and the production and contemplation of pain. They also all, in their way, underscore the elusive relationship between linguistic expressiveness and the expressions of the body. Each of them endeavors to locate the impenitent procession of suffering within the cultural bastions of law and aesthetic experience. The representation of violence coincides with the violence of the representation because, sadly perhaps, pain was never an excrescence of culture, but one of the foundational elements of its most deep-rooted values.[32]

The theater of cruelty

The visualization of physical suffering, while not exclusive to early modern Europe, found then a centrality perhaps only comparable to the proliferation of images of extreme pain characteristic of the second half of the twentieth century or the beginning of the twenty-first. Then, as now, the theatricality of representation lessened or glorified violence. The meaning of such visual representation depends on its material format and its means of distribution; for only through technological mediation does pain become history, a narrative built with emotional fragments as diverse as devotion, commiseration, piety, fear, indignation, shock, terror, or lasciviousness. In this respect, nothing has changed over the last 500 years. On the one hand, the history of pain, and even more so its visualization and iconic representation, is not necessarily concerned with real events, but rather with experiences that are merely imagined. On the other hand, the pain of history, this constitutive form of experience, makes use of visual representations to turn emotions into narratives.

We could distinguish five broad spheres in which physical suffering acquired a certain visual pre-eminence in early modern Europe: the realm of punishment, the theological context, military activity, anatomical representation, and the practice of medicine. The theological context would include the representation of suffering in Hell and Purgatory, hagiography, asceticism, the martyrdom of the saints, as well as the scenes of the Passion. Military activity would comprise disputes between states, social movements, wars of religion, popular uprisings, and conflicts arising from conquest and colonization. The legal realm would include the use of pain in public executions, trials, and judicial interrogations. In all these cases, the representation of suffering is first inscribed in an imaginary context composed of visual and narrative elements; secondly, it forms part of an abstraction that simultaneously refers to the quotidian and the extraordinary, the private and the public, the distant and the close, the historical and the fabled. Finally, the representation of pain remains faithful to two guiding principles. First, pain is shown as reiterative, monotonous, and interminable; second, suffering is expressed in the modality of the greatest possible pain.

Then, as now, violence made use of technological equipment. The visual culture of pain at the end of the twentieth century could not have existed without the proliferation of standardized and mechanical means of reproducing images. At the end of the Middle Ages, the invention of the printing press and the subsequent emergence of iconography acquired a central role in religious struggles, political revolts, and, as we shall see below, in anatomical texts. The best engravers of the Early Modern period, such as Peter Brueghel, Jacques Callot, Lucas Cranach, and Dürer himself, participated in this technological implementation of the spectacle of violence. Private experience seemed to be inextricably linked to its forms of public distribution. Or rather on the contrary: the social distribution of these images permitted and configured the formation of experiences.[33] Following the Council of Trent, the use of images was established and partially regulated, to the point that Protestant attacks against the veneration of saints, their representation, or their relics actually helped bring about their flourishing.[34] In this relationship between pain and memory, there coincided three distinct iconographies: those dealing with images and objects of religious devotion, with engravings of religious wars, and with anatomical illustrations. All three were built upon a punitive disproportion that used pain as both an emotional and cognitive tool. In all three, the body, whether it was the criminal's body, the martyr's body, or the dissected corpse, was called upon to become an example. They were put to very different uses, as varied as the ways in which they were consumed, but these three groups maintained important similarities. To begin with, neither the moral ideal, nor the punitive example, nor the anatomical model was a representation of the quotidian, but rather of the supernatural or the intangible. All three cases privilege violence as a means of gaining access to a space that is simultaneously close at hand and inaccessible. Finally, the invisibility of these ideal models was presented under the rubric of full and collective certainty. It is in the representation of pain that the emotional and the epistemic meet. In all three cases, truth was made manifest through the destruction of the flesh.

Despite differences of use, this regulated way of representing harm has remained inscribed in our collective imagination. Freed from mnemonic constraints, imitative values, or religious uses, the representation of pain is still expressed today according to the rules of a rite of passage. Now, as before, suffering bodies inhabit indeterminate spaces and dystopian geographies. Some of the most emblematic images of the visual culture of the late twentieth century share this characteristic. It might be the photograph, taken from behind, of a Haitian youth wandering naked through the ruins of Port-au-Prince; or perhaps the self-portraits of the artist David Nebreda. Violence is expressed in the ritualized form of geographic uncertainty and temporal universality. Our icons refer to well-established patters in the rhetorical construction of the model. Their different cultural values do not undermine their iconographic similarities. On the contrary, we have learned to represent our pain within an inherited framework, consisting of values and practices that we no longer recognize as our own. We have changed the sheets, but we have our dream of violence in the beds of others.

Wars of religion

One of the works of particular importance here is the *Theatrum Crudelitatum haereticorum nostri temporis* (Theater of the Cruelties of the Heretics of Our Time), initially published in Latin in 1587 and later translated into French, and widely distributed in England, Scotland, France, and the Low Countries. Its author, Richard Rowlands [1550–1640], an English Catholic in exile, had changed his name to Verstegan after leaving prison. The 29 engravings included in this work had a certain similarity to those made by Théodore de Bry for the illustrated edition of Bartolomé de las Casas's *La destrucción de las Indias*, and the engravings of Pérrissin and Tortorel on wars and massacres in France.[35] For the Anglo-Dutch Verstegan, a friend of the Jesuits, a spy, trafficker, and publicist of the Reformation, who achieved his fame through a travel book, the images and engravings that accompanied his text did not fulfill a documentary function; they were not intended to serve as a historical record, but as a model of an emotional response.[36] His work served the purpose of denunciation through an evaluative description of events, both in the book's design and its execution. The aim of the book was stated from the outset. He had not written his work to entertain or to please. Quite the opposite, his intention was "to make tears fall from the eyes, lamentations fill the mouth, sighs the heart and weeping the chest."[37] Verstegan sought in his readers an emotional reaction rather than a cognitive effect. He did not wish to make an account of events, but to make use of them. His purpose was not to inform, but to shock; to encourage a collective communion centered on the representation of injustice. The Cardinal Gabriela Paleotti, author of a treatise on art based partly on the work of Charles Borromeo, explained his work in the same terms:

> To hear the narration of the martyrdom of a Saint, the fervor and the perseverance of a virgin, the passion of Christ Himself, this is something that moves us deep inside; but to have in front of our eyes, in living color, the tortured saint, the martyred virgin and elsewhere Christ nailed to the Cross, increases our devotion so much more. And that those who do not recognize these facts are made of words or marble.[38]

The collective feelings of all those who were not made of words or marble could be unleashed in different ways. Verstegan's book abounds in interpretative and rhetorical resources designed to encourage the conviction of injustice and the outrage of innocence. First of all, faith in history, in the veracity of the events narrated, becomes confused with the history of faith, that is, with the temporal evolution of Christianity. Those of his contemporaries who thought that the times of martyrdom were a thing of the past – like those of the knight-errantry – were mistaken. Rather, representation of the massacre becomes one more instance in the continuing battle between the followers of good and the supporters of evil. After the arrival of the Messiah, there was no distinction between the old and the new martyrs.[39] Measured against the magnitude of their torments, their suffering, abnegation, and innocence are universal and eternal. The maximum pain to which both new and old were subjected transcends their specific historical circumstances to such an extent that today's martyrs can be seen to arise as an inevitable consequence of those of yesterday. The images of the *Theatrum* connect past and present, transforming the story represented there into an example of the permanent struggle against the evils of the world. Much like Tortorel and Pérrissin's prior works, Verstegan's text also found inspiration in Appian of Alexandria's *History of Rome*, a text which described the massacres committed under the Triumvirate of Octavius Caesar, Antony, and Lepidus, and whose translation was very popular in the sixteenth century. Thus the new martyrs could, in death, relive an experience; that is, they could die in accordance with the patterns and models inherited from the Christian persecutions in the times of Nero and Diocletian.[40]

Verstegan also employs a rhetorical device that consists of dividing the engravings into different numbered scenes that, in turn, refer to an explanatory text. As with treatises on anatomy, first we see and then we read. Some authors have suggested that the use of these numberings might be related to the specific structure of Ignatius of Loyola's *Spiritual Exercises* and, more generally, to the way in which the Jesuit students of the Roman College numbered their materials of study.[41] This same correlation between images and texts can also be found in some of the frescoes that adorned Jesuit colleges during the second half of the sixteenth century. One of the most notable cases is a set of hagiographical scenes painted by Niccolo Circignani, *Pomaracio*, in the church of Saint Stefano Rotondo, in Rome, with which Verstegan was probably familiar. There are, however, many examples of similar numerations in the context of the representation of the Christian martyrs' torments. In Antonio Gallonio's book, *De sanctorum martyrum cruciatibus*, for example, a treatise published in Rome in 1591, the correspondence between image and text also relies on visual calls, very much like endnotes.[42] In the first part of the book, Gallonio has placed the images that accompany the nine chapters, which take up 376 pages. Each image refers the reader to a brief explanation of the scene, included in a note, and to a more detailed account that accompanies the prints. The work as a whole offers a new repository, an encyclopedia of punishment and torment where, unlike our ritualized forms of publically confronting disgrace, the visual representation of drama precedes its verbal description. The result produces a dual experience in which the emotion awakened by the visual observation of suffering is first transformed into a definition and only later into a story. Even when the life of each saint is only briefly reported, the circumstances of his or her death become an intangible and limited example of a collective murder. Taken individually, each martyr adds a new form of dying, as abominable as all the others, to the global testimony that the book aims to express.

Finally, both the texts and images are markedly repetitive; not only in their overwhelming reiteration of scenes but through a prose which frequently tends toward the endless concatenation of adjectives:

> This is how you will see the heretics in this Theater, bloodied, dirty and dusty, returning from the hunting of Catholics, blood pouring from their mouths and ears, as, having defeated, disemboweled and flayed them, they bury themselves in their blood, they dive in up to their ears turning them to pulp, feeding on their flesh and, when they are satiated, they call the beasts to make the most of the massacre.[43]

The reiteration of the greatest possible pain, in words as well as images, turns the narrative into an abusive display, a never-ending enumeration of a sequence that comes across as overwhelming and inconclusive. The number of bodies mutilated for the sake of faith, despite seeming excessive, is never enough. One of the most striking cases in this respect was the publication, in 1634, of the *Sacrum sanctuarium crucis et patientiae*. In this work, the Jesuit Father Biverus described all testified forms of crucifixion with the aid of engravings.[44] Throughout its almost 700 pages, his account includes more than 100 different ways of fixing a body to a pole. Martyrs appear tied, nailed, shredded on vertical, horizontal, or inverted crosses; on ships, in deserts, on trees, on palm trees; naked, clothed, mutilated, burnt, pierced with arrows, decapitated, clamped, lanced; with their body upside-down or in the ground, stoned, or impaled. Collective crucifixions are added to the individual ones, increasing the horror of the massacre and the multiplication of innocence: women, children, the elderly. In a few cases, the crucifixion of the martyr takes place atop the image of an already crucified Christ. In one of the strangest cases, the arms of Tarbula and her maids are nailed to one cross and their legs to another. Their bodies had already been sawed apart (see Figure 5).

Verstegan's *Theatre* was written in the context of Renaissance Europe's wars of religion, both Catholic and Protestant. For our purposes, it is irrelevant to emphasize the torments suffered by the Catholics at the hands of the Protestants after the Reformation or, as is the case of *History of The Martyrs Prosecuted and Killed for the Truth of the Gospel* by Jean Crespin, focus on the crimes committed by the Church of Rome against the Protestants. In neither case does the representation of the massacre follow the patterns of lived experiences.[45] On the other hand, these texts were not written to inform or provide knowledge. They were written to cry over. This is why the verisimilitude of the events is at times of less interest than the visualization of suffering. The scenes that accompany Pérrissin's work on the massacre of the Huguenots clearly possess these characteristics (see Figure 6). Dozens of undistinguishable bodies are thrown into the river or beaten to death. Many others are knifed. Some are tortured. In its crudeness, very similar to Dürer's painting *Martyrdom of the Ten Thousand*, the engraving requires no further explanation. The indiscriminate violence extols the innocence and purity of heart of those who, by themselves, count as nothing. Then, as now, the visual and textual representation of the massacre walks a fine line between the one and the many. If it were not offset this way, the scene could only display an implausible set of unconnected crimes. As with the martyrologies of Biverus or Gallonio, the artist may very well highlight some cases, but must be careful not to misrepresent the whole. The specific circumstances of this or that martyr are only of interest within the broader context of the massacre. The victims' bodies have been swept from the face of the Earth, not because of their own deserving, but as a result of universal injustice. The mass killing may take place in Antwerp, or in Poitiers, but the bodies are no more than an instance, just another example of the triumph of faith. This is the only measure. The number of dead, on the other hand, is insignificant. There are simply many, too many. Or, as in Dürer's painting, they are 10,000!

Unlike the narrative techniques of our contemporary world – which always begin with the recounting of the fallen, only later to provide us with the identities of some of the dead and, in extreme cases, question those who also could have died but did not – the late medieval theater of cruelty presents cadavers as an amassed whole. It does not count them, but situates them as accumulative episodes in the history of faith. Dürer's painting, for example, could show the legend of the martyrs sentenced on Mount Ararat on the orders of the Persian King Saporat, but the painter has also introduced contemporary elements in this recreation of the ancient world, thus establishing continuity between past and present. Among all the bodies depicted, only one can be clearly identified: his own. Quite remarkably, Dürer included his portrait in the midst of the massacre so as to lay claim to the work's authorship. *"Made by Albrecht Dürer, German,"* he writes. Commissioned by Frederick the Wise to accompany his collection of relics in Wittenberg, the image of Saporat also reflects the prevalent fear of the Turks that existed at the beginning of the sixteenth century, following the fall of Constantinople in 1453.

The way in which human beings have been subjected to execution and torture constitutes a museum of horror that has begun to be uncovered through studies in the history of art and of punitive practices. The art of castigation forms part of the macabre history of forced pain and of the economy of suffering, which have been treated in very different ways in accordance with scholarly tendencies. The studies of Michel Foucault, Pieter Spierenburg,

Richard J. Evans, and Edward Peters have traced the tortuous history of execution procedures from the Middle Ages to the penal reforms of late eighteenth century.[46] Some time ago, the historian Natalie Zemon-Davis considered the riots of violence of the sixteenth century within the context of purification rituals.[47] She held that images, books, or bodies should no longer be examined through the lens of religion, but rather situated in a broader profane context. Violence should not be considered using religion, but anthropology. She was right. Compared with contemporary theaters of cruelty, these martyrs from the wars of religion appear deprived of all characteristics except their collective innocence. Like the virgins of the medieval altarpieces, these assassinated victims inhabit an emotional and cognitive frontier. They are neither alive nor dead. They do not belong to the here or to the now. They are neither one nor many. Their existence is at the same time visual and textual. On the one hand, the fragmentation of their bodies keeps alive a story which, to put it simply, has no real substance. On the other hand, the textual narrative merges with the visual resources as a means of ennobling emotion and facilitating memory. Despite the cruelty of the chosen punishments, the body is not victimized, but rather extolled. Its mournful yet calm face does not follow any natural logic. Its most immediate imitative model could be found in other paintings and engravings, but the contrite attitude that uses pain as a process toward salvation has a very different reference. Both as a whole and taken individually, "martyrs exemplify" a correspondence between pain and salvation, a relationship that was strengthened after the twelfth century, when the birth of Purgatory coincided with the first great appearance in the West of moral suffering described in terms of physical ailments.[48] It would not be until the seventeenth century that theologians would question the supposedly eternal nature of the punishments of Hell and, until the eighteenth century, that political philosophy would endeavor to establish a principle of proportion between crime and punishment. Meanwhile, cruelty was expressed by means of an imitative and disproportionate procedure, through the repetition of punishment, with a performative purpose and highly dramatic content.[49]

The pain of Christ

The imaginary recreation of the virgins' and martyrs' torments not only configures experience qualitatively, it also provides a scale with which to measure the anguish of our pains or the intensity of our groans. Martyrdom establishes a form of mediation, but also a process of measurement; an imaginary standard that allows us to distinguish the more from the less. The physical resistance of these venerable beings determines how much our ailments may hurt and how exaggerated our lamentations can be. Compared with theirs, our hardships are meager and our complaints out of proportion. The vicissitudes and accidents of our lives are measured in light of the magnitude of their wounds and the impassibility of their faces. Far from the nineteenth century's attempts to measure emotions, the medieval representation of violence establishes a unidirectional topology, from the greater to the smaller and from the divine to us. The martyrs and saints take up tertiary positions in this scale, which descends from the (superhuman) Passion to (human) suffering; they can mediate between one and the other because they wander in between those residences. Although they provide the ruler used to measure pain, they do not set up, however, the standard of the scale. Though their pain may be excruciating, it cannot be compared with the Passion of Christ. Only this latter is beyond all measurement. It is not even disproportionate, for there can be no possible proportions in the depiction of a pain that aspires to bring about the beginning of a New History. The Jesuit Biverus, whose catalog of crucifixions was mentioned previously, states this relationship explicitly in one of the emblems accompanying his work: rather than the compass or the set square, it is the cross that provides the imaginary scale of all human pains and sufferings (see Figure 7).

One of the most emblematic images of the religious representation of pain in the modern world, the polyptych of Issenheim by the German master known as Mattias Grünewald [1470–1528], shares many of these characteristics. Art historians have explained how these eight scenes, painted around 1515, functioned together in accordance with the requirements of the liturgical year. Historians of medicine, on the other hand, have placed the emphasis on the health-care procedures that inspired the work.[50] Mounted on an articulated structure, the patients could watch the panels, which measure more than two meters, open and close in a dramatic representation of high symbolic content. Together with the *predella*, the eight panels, arranged with three different openings, covered important biblical events interspersed with images of the life of Anthony the Great. The temptations of this saint, who lived as a complete recluse on the outskirts of Coma, Egypt, until his death in the year 356, were a frequent source of inspiration for the Great Masters. Peter Brueghel the Elder, for example, produced various pieces on this subject; so did Hieronymus Bosch, who surrounded the saint with women and pigs as symbols of lechery. The hermit responded to the temptations of the flesh with voluntary fasting, constant discipline, and compulsive prayer. He never ate anything before sundown and then only once every two or four days. He conceived of his body in terms of prison and punishment, a tradition that goes back to Plato's *Phaedon*, which was spread throughout Europe by neo-platonic movements, and which became part of the development of Christianity during the Middle Ages.[51] Determined to visit Paul of Thebes, Anthony journeyed to Alexandria. On his way, the Devil appeared to him accompanied by horrible and monstrous creatures that "tore him with their teeth, horns, and claws."[52] He then saw a miraculous bright light that cured his wounds. Anthony called out to the light: "Where were you, Jesus? Dear Lord, where were you? Why were you not here earlier to help me and heal my wounds?"

The altarpiece's central scene of Christ's crucifixion begins with a grotesque enumeration of the most terrible pains that can possibly be applied to the flesh: thorns penetrating the forehead; fingers that twist under the pressure of nails and tear the joints; dislocated extremities; the torso hunched; the skin extraordinarily lacerated and reduced to fragments of a recent history of abuses, blows, and humiliations that have become pustules and wounds. The image of this crucified man is not unlike other fourteenth- and fifteenth-century depictions of pain, but it does serve as an extraordinary iconic model on the meaning of physical agony and, by extension, on the interpretation of collective suffering. In the year 1502, shortly before the Antonians of Issenheim commissioned this work, an anonymous sculptor from Breslau produced a carving in polychromed wood with a height of 116 centimeters. Unlike Grünewald's Christ, this *Christ in Distress* appears peaceful, with an engrossed face, a resigned attitude and a contrite expression (see Figure 8). In the absence of source documents allowing us to identify the scene, we may surmise that the artist was inspired by *Job on his Dunghill*, an iconographic model based in turn on the precedent of the battered boxer by the Greek sculptor, Lyssipos. Tormented by his misfortune, once his possessions, his children, and his health have been lost, the wise Job, the man who has lost everything except the conviction of his innocence, resists impassively. His wife upbraids him: *"Curse God and die,"* she screams.

Whether the figure of Job served as the inspiration for this work, or whether it refers to a different tradition, nothing allows us to locate the Polish Christ within the known life of Jesus. In this it resembles Grünewald's painting. Despite their many differences – and the fact that the polyptych may be considered a liturgical work whereas the Breslau sculpture is more of a devotional image – neither piece is concerned with historical or textual truths. On the contrary, the iconographic depiction emphasizes the physical and symbolic signs of evil inscribed on the pestilent skin of the leper or on the fetid pustules of the victim of compulsive ergotism. In the first case, the creature abandoned in the swamp of misery is not unlike other representations of lepers in similar attitudes and positions. In the second case, Grünewald has also portrayed a person suffering from what was then called "Saint Anthony's fire." In the lower corner of one of the panels, the one depicting Anthony being attacked by monsters and devils, the painter has superimposed on the swollen, ulcerated, agonizing figure the saint's own words: *"Ubi eras bon Jesus?"* The polyptych integrates within the same scene the fears of the sick and the torments of the hermit. Both look for consolation in the intermediary space of eternal alliances. Although neither of them wishes to suffer, their pain bears witness to a will greater than their own. "O my Father, if it be possible, let this cup pass from me,"[53] Jesus said on the Mount of Olives. The *cup* is precisely what Grünewald represents: the limit between pain and Salvation, between life and death, between the new and the ancient history, between the Old and the New Testament, between His Will and the will of an Other, who is also He.

The successive visualization of these intermediary spaces allows the articulation and modulation of experience, teaching how harm has to be felt and how pain should be understood.[54] Within the same symbolic space, the living commune with the dead, angels with demons and saints with monsters. The Virgin, the prophets, the heavenly choirs merge with fallen angels, blessed souls, and Roman soldiers. Bodies wander between life and death, between the human, the infra-human, and the superhuman. All of them inhabit borderlines and impossible spaces as a result of a temporal, emotional, or figurative disproportion. Not only devils, omnipresent figures in the modern teratological tradition, make up the morphological pattern for the *intermediary species*.[55] The other characters also live and die away from the community: in a desert like John the Baptist, in a cave like Paul the hermit, in a sepulcher like Anthony the Great, or on a cross, like the Son of God. Their gestures and attitudes share the stage with their symbolic representations. The lamb, the water, the bread, the crown, the halo, the crosier, the raven, the cloak, the arrow, or the blood merge into a landscape which is, at the same time, illuminated and gloomy. Last, but not least, Grünewald's painting is interspersed with religious texts. In some cases, these written testimonies appear on leaves that surface in the middle of a landscape or in half-open books whose pages can be read accidentally. In the first panel, as we shall see, the words are uttered and accompanied by indicative signs.

Like a theater of voices and expressive gestures, the painter depicts the rule that makes the universal experience of pain more comprehensible: "*He must increase, but I must diminish*," the painter writes in the mouth of John the Baptist.[56]At the same time, he has decided to incorporate its meaning into the scene, modifying its spatial perspective as much as its temporal coherence. On the one hand, he has shrunk the size of the witnesses. On the other hand, he has placed at the foot of the cross a prophet who was already dead, beheaded, at the time of Christ's Passion. The modification in the proportion of the figures and the unlikely presence of John the Baptist at Calvary are calculated choices. From a theological standpoint, the new rule that John the Baptist spoke of in Aenon put an end to the times of the prophets. The crucifixion, the entrance of God into History, laid the basis for a new alliance that no longer depended on the law, but on faith. Unlike those old prophets who spoke of the promised land without having seen it, here we have one who does not speak from hearsay, who has actually stood before the Father, who has had Him before his very eyes; as opposed to the old Alliance based on the Word, a new pact is invoked based on the (direct) experience of Christ's pain. This new pact aspires to provide a new measure of all human suffering, a considered way of regulating how to feel and how to suffer. Pain, which is not only taught but also learned, will acquire different modulations if it is experienced from outside or from inside this new beginning. The provisions of this new pact do not eliminate it, but they relativize it and, up to a point, even trivialize it. From the new Sinai, redemption allows for the sustained happiness of those who suffer: "*because they will be consoled;*" the good fortune of the poor and the hungry, "*because they will be satisfied.*"[57] Faith does not eliminate the feeling of harm, but it does relocate experiences of hurt in accordance with past suffering, with the received example, with the magnitude of the Passion, and, above all, with the promise of future redemption.

The anatomical theater

Like the images of the Christian martyrs, often portrayed along with the instrument of their martyrdom or holding their mutilated limbs in their hands as a reminder of their torment, the anatomical model also bears signs on the flesh of the violence that has just been inflicted upon his or her body. The culture of dissection that flourished in Europe during the sixteenth century was inspired by a manual and cognitive exercise. *Divide et impera* was the instruction of the time. Whereas the knowledge of the ancients depended on books and literature which allowed them to "*listen to the dead with the eyes,*" according to the famous verse by the Spanish poet Francisco de Quevedo, the new anatomists want to see not just with their eyes, but also with their hands. In the famous frontispiece of *De humanis corporis fabrica* by Andrea Vesalio [1514–1564], for example, the surgeon picks up the scalpel and dissects the insides of a woman amidst the murmurs of those crowding around the table.[58] In *La storia de Nastagio degli Onesti*, a group of canvasses painted by Botticelli around 1483, a knight extracts his lover's heart with his own hands and throws it to his dogs.[59] Once the torture is over, the young girl gets up again and a new pursuit begins. The lover's conquest, described in terms of the chase or the hunt, also points out the new cognitive practices. Distanced from the passivity of the medieval studios, the new anatomical practices no longer depend on revelation, but on *venatio*, the hunt, on the pursuit and stockpiling of nature's secrets.

The formation of the new anatomical atlas implied an unprecedented reshuffling not only for the living, but also for the dead; not only for the eyes, but also for the hands. The externalization of the interior was carried out by means of a manual exercise which, breaking the skin, led the scalpel toward the inside of the organs. The plates from the so-called *Anatomical Renaissance*, connected to the schools of medicine in Padua, Bologna, or Leiden, intended to show the mutilation that had just taken place inside another theater: the anatomical one. In most cases, the anatomist's hand moved from the sternum to the abdomen while a second transverse incision opened the flesh in the shape of a cross, so that the skin could be divided into four and its upper parts could be nailed or tied to the shoulders. Although dissection generally took place with the criminal laid out upon a *tabula*, a dissecting table, on other occasions the corpse was suspended with pulleys. This form of exploration, developed in Bologna, would later allow the Italian anatomist Berengario da Carpi, in his comments on a 1521 text by Mondino Dei Luzzi, to present a crucifixion scene in an anatomical treatise.

The dramatization of anatomical plates results in a varied set of iconographic elements: muscles separated from the bones, skin freed of flesh, dissected figures showing their own insides, reflexive skeletons, submissive and cooperative corpses. In all cases, we know that pain is there, but it cannot be seen. It constitutes a precondition of a form of representing harm that eliminates it, however, from the end result. The anatomized body shares in the dramatic idealization of physical suffering exhibited by other visual approximations of violence. The connection between pain and knowledge melds with the victory of faith, with the triumph of death or, in the extreme, with the Man of Sorrows, who shows, through the scars on His skin and the signs on His body, the most visible traces of His recent story. Although all anatomical representations have many common features, historians of art and medicine have underscored in this context the depictions of the flaying of Marsyas. This story was disseminated in the early modern period through Book VI of Ovid's *Metamorphoses*, and would come to serve as an anatomical model *par excellence*. The visual recreation of this story constitutes one of the most recurrent motifs in Renaissance and Baroque art.[60] José Ribera [1591–1692], *el españoletto*, painted a version in 1637 – a mere four years after finishing his *Martyrdom of Saint Bartholomew*. Titian produced another version of the subject, in which he portrayed himself contemplating the scene. The image was echoed in Raphael's frescoes and in the work of other artists like Guilio Romano and Melchor Meier. Scholars have counted more than 100 depictions of the scene in engravings, canvasses, and frescoes from the sixteenth and seventeenth centuries. The flaying of Marsyas, which also has a religious counterpart in the martyrdom of Saint Bartholomew in Armenia, was not only a recurrent motif in the arts but was also profusely used in anatomical treatises.[61] Perhaps the most famous plate was included in Versalius's *Fabrica*, but similar images are found in the works of Charles Estienne or in the plates Nicholas Beatrizet engraved for the Spaniard Juan de Valverde's *Anatomía* in 1566 (see Figure 9).

According to Greek legend, the satyr Marsyas began to play the flute when Athena, who had invented the instrument, threw it into a pond after noticing that playing it distorted the proportions of her face. When he became an expert, the satyr challenged Apollo, the patron of the arts, to a musical duel. It was ruled that the winner could treat the defeated party as he wished. Once Apollo was declared the winner, and the mathematical beauty of his lyre preferred over the grotesque expression of the satyr – who was also unable to sing and play at the same time – the god condemned Marsyas to be tied to a tree and flayed alive. "Music," he cried, "does not deserve so much pain." Despite his laments, Apollo tore Marsyas' skin from his body until not a single fragment was left intact. Blood flowed everywhere until his skin was gone and his internal organs and lung tissues became visible. The tears of the fauns, satyrs, and nymphs formed a river in the region that Ovid called Phrygia, in Asia Minor.

In the cultural history of pain, the figure of the *écorché*, the flayed victim, has two clear implications. First of all, this type of figure, very similar to the bronze sculptures inherited from antiquity, enabled learning the disposition of the muscles and the internal structure of the body. As in the case of the so-called Belvedere Torso, a marble statue attributed to Apollonius of Athens, used in Vesalius's *De corporis fabrica* and later in Valverde's Anatomy, the Renaissance anatomist frequently represented corpses in the manner of heroes or gods from antiquity. In the second place, this type of representation, beyond its role as an anatomical model, also constitutes a penal example. It is an instance of medical arts, but also of political powers.[62] As in the case of the criminals Lorenzo da Bonconvento and Francesco da Buderio, dissected by Vesalius on 22 January 1540 in the anatomical theaters installed in the church of Saint Francis in Bologna, the physical exploration suggests an inversely proportional relation between the construction of the anatomical model and the personal identity of the dissected criminal. On the one hand, the dissecting table exhibits the dead body to the shamelessness of the public's gaze. On the other, it serves to reinforce the convict's loss of identity, and consequently to increase a punishment that, against all logic, can only be administered to a corpse.

In both cases, the visual depiction of the body could not be obtained through a transposition of the anatomical features of the cadaver, but rather through the ideal representation of its structure. Renaissance anatomists did not draw what they saw, but what they knew; their images did not adapt to the world, but to the referential universe of their classical legacy. The formation of the anatomical Atlas was a complex exercise that belonged to what Chancellor Francis Bacon termed the "sciences of the trained eye." In view of a dissected body, condemned to serve as anatomical evidence, the plates lead our attention astray from the particular and the specific, back to the general and necessary. The corpses of anatomical treatises do not reflect corporeal accidents, but aspire to provide an ideal body that does not exist in nature. Only inasmuch as Valverde, for example, has managed to fuse in a single plate the anatomical model, the aesthetic rule, the punitive example, and the religious ideal, we may vindicate the universal necessity of the image. The loss of skin is just one of the necessary moments in the creation of a science freed from subjective constrictions, which is, nevertheless, built from the most private experience.

The images of extreme violence of our post-modern world share certain elements with those that proliferated at the end of the Middle Ages. In both periods, pain can only be depicted in accordance with established parameters and rules of obliged compliance. The virgin martyrs, the anatomical treatises, the theaters of cruelty or the scenes of the Passion do not represent pain. On the contrary, the visualization of physical suffering assumes, for those who stand in front of the altarpiece, the engraving, or the plate, an evaluative exercise. In all cases, the protagonists inhabit imaginary spaces. They all wander, as intermediary beings, through transitional worlds, between the human and the divine, the particular and the ideal, the one and the multiple and, as in the case of anatomical models, between the singular and the universal. Unlike our contemporary depictions of radical evil, the anatomical, religious, or punitive images of Early Modern Europe can only exhibit violence *in its effects*, without the cries and gestures that usually accompany the abuse of the body. Neither the martyrs of the religious wars nor the criminals of the anatomical plates have chosen to become moral examples or anatomical models, but when the time comes, the virgins do not surrender and the criminals do not complain.

Our means of representing violence also express pain by means of a theatrical drama. But, unlike the early modern imaginary, our iconic models do not produce a punitive example, an aesthetic rule, an anatomical model, or a moral standard. Our blood is no longer medieval. The intensity of our torments may be similar, but our forms of victimization, of empathetic identification, our compulsive consumption of harm, our desire to safeguard or to eroticize crime, are not present in the pictorial or literary depictions of late Middle Ages. On the contrary, the way in which violence was inscribed on the early modern body lacks, in our eyes, credibility. We recognize the force of the image while simultaneously denouncing its ingenuity. In the twenty-first century, beatings land on the skin by means of a news caption. In the late Middle Ages, on the other hand, pain was never the end of the story, but the beginning; it was not shown for entertainment or to encourage consumption, but as an educational process which allowed the establishment of communitarian ties and shared histories. Violence can be extreme in both cases, but whereas modern cinema actors seek to adapt their expressions to the horrors of our world, the martyr's countenance remains unmoved. We recognize the expression of the greatest possible harm that might be inflicted upon a body, but there is nothing to suggest a counterintuitive recreation of a form of pain that cannot be explained or understood with any logic or accepted from the standpoint of any rule. The quintessence of the cultural construction of violence in our contemporary world – the crude and stark depiction of *Radical Evil* – did not exist in the early modern world. Their mutilated bodies did not feature the gratuitousness or the obscenity of the reiteration of a pain built precisely on the absence of explanation; a pain that is presented under the pretext of information, consumption, entertainment, or lewdness. Our contemporary body is destructive, whereas the medieval body was constructive. Its beatings and lacerations transcended the reduced space of narrated events to recreate an imaginary state in which to merge the emotional and the collective understanding of pain.

2
Imitation

Pain is not transparent. It could certainly be said, of images that suggest its presence, that their motives are not concerned with physical suffering, but with melancholy, cruelty, anguish, torture, fear, or violence. The marks of pain are elusive inasmuch as the same bodily gestures do not always refer to the same emotions; likewise, the same feelings can be manifested by different expressive means. Various kinds of concealment proliferate between the experience and the expression of pain. The theater of the body is subject to restrictions and rules; its scenic development depends on artifice, adornment, and effects that provide collective credibility to private sensations. And vice versa: these rules also allow public experiences to configure personal feelings. If in the previous chapter the problem was to seek out emotion in elusive representations that expressed pain in an indirect and complex way, in this chapter, the difficulty consists of accounting for a pain that dissolves in rhetorical complications and expressive adornments. As opposed to the late medieval image of the martyr who represented a pain that could not be identified and was allegedly not felt, now pain, plunged into a new form of collective invisibility, still cannot entirely reach public perception.

The relationship between feelings and the images thereof that we saw in the previous chapter is no less problematic than the relationship between words and things that we shall see in this one. Unlike the sixteenth century, when it was still possible to *see* with words and *speak* with images, the seventeenth century opens a rift between language and the world. The French historian Michel Foucault traced the main lines of this border and chose a literary hero, Don Quixote, as the first modern character. This is what is striking about modernity: its most eminent protagonists are imaginary beings.[1] Even though Foucault dedicated a few pages to gestural language (of action), he made no reference to the intermediate space between language and the world. His book, concerned with the cognitive conditions of representation, lacked emotions. Not only does this word not appear a single time in the entire text, Foucault also seems to suggest that the new epistemic order only conceived of the passions as part of a linguistic cartography. However, the early modern world, which separated words from things, the soul from the body, men from beasts, reality from fiction, and certainty from doubt, was also concerned with meeting places; with real or imaginary, natural, or cultural spaces that would serve as a point of connection between these dichotomies. When the philosopher René Descartes wrote his *Passions of the Soul*, he traced a border between love and hate, the mind and the heart, the I and the we, in which passions were expressed like musical notes, capable of moving the body by means of the soul or, vice versa, of affecting the soul by means of the body. And he was not alone. Many other moralists and philosophers, as well as physiologists and what we would today call political philosophers, appeared in his wake. The most famous of these, Thomas Hobbes, first separated us from one another and later made us into dangerous enemies. Only one emotion, fear, prevented a fratricidal war. Upon this emotion the entire construction of politics was built. In the twentieth century, cultural historians have stressed a variety of aspects of the relationship between thoughts and passions. The study of theatrical forms, expressive means, of manuals for professional procedures to awaken emotions in the public all took place at the same time that Descartes wrote his *Discourse on the Method*. Perhaps we can doubt that the world is a stage, but in the theater it is best not to doubt. That is its magic. Dualism may be a philosophical proclamation, but the rhetorical figure of the early modern period is not the dichotomy, but rather the oxymoron: an apparent contradiction in terms that, being abominable for philosophy, appears everywhere in the more expressive atmosphere of literature and the arts.

Foucault was entirely right to choose the protagonist of a novel as the symbol of modernity. He was also right to transform the character into a *homo viator*, pursued by words and crisscrossed by signs and similarities. The story of Don Quixote – the gentleman from La Mancha who went mad reading books on chivalry and wandered around a good part of Spain's geography in his delirium, freeing the world from giants and sorcerers – possesses many of the programmatic elements of the new epistemological order: the elusive relationship between words and things, between imagination and memory, or between reality and fiction. Foucault did not manage to glimpse a single emotion in Cervantes' book. However, *Don Quixote*, whose first part was published in 1604, reflects the tensions between physical pain and moral suffering, personal pain and the pain of others, internal drama and external tragedy. Its multiple narrative layers lead right to the very heart of suffering, fear, moral defeat, physical pain, and real or imaginary means of curing it – whether we think of illness, punishment, war wounds, religious asceticism, or punitive flagellation. The fact that Foucault did not perceive any of this does not lessen his contribution. He was concerned with a different problem. Nor was he alone in this oblivion.

Of the more than 500 titles quoted by the scholar Francisco Rico in his edition of *Don Quixote*, only a few are dedicated to pain.

Don Quixote will serve us as a through-line for a cultural evaluation of harmful experience, its regimes of visibility or opacity, its simultaneously public and private character. The purpose is not to add yet another chapter to the already numerous studies on Cervantes, but to examine the means and artifices that allow the modulation of experience to such a point that even the most transparent, immediate and visible of emotions, pain, disappeared in the midst of rhetorical artifice. As opposed to the widely accepted idea that the same feeling can be evaluated differently depending on cultural context, this chapter argues in favor of the most logical, although perhaps the least intuitive, conclusion: the blows may be the same, but the sensation, which does not exist outside its dramatic elements, does differ from one context to another. It is simply not the same sensation. There is no emotional reality *out there* that can be reinterpreted in accordance with cultural location or historical moment. Rather, there exists a plurality of effects that can materialize in different experiences, which only retrospectively may be considered under the same referential framework. It does indeed seem like magic. But it is a highly rationalized magic that is expressed in two cultural paradoxes: invisible pains and public secrets. We who live in the twenty-first century know a great deal about both of these categories. Our technological world has no shortage of iconic and expressive artifices for making emotions visible; or, for that matter, for making them disappear beneath the mantle of oblivion. We are capable of outpourings of public grief at the death of a beached whale, yet we are also capable of ignoring whole populations that are subject to tropical disease, ethnic wars, or endemic famine. Unlike the previous chapter, where the martyr's response, against all public evidence, denied his or her pain, now the public, against testimonial evidence, also denies it. We have moved on from an image without emotion to an emotion with no image. In one case, what is seen does not exist; in the other, what exists cannot be seen.

What allows for this new regime of visibility is the most basic form of representation: mimesis, or, to use the historically appropriate word, imitation. Unlike the late medieval theater of cruelty, characterized by dramatic and mnemonic elements, baroque theater is imitative. Don Quixote's behavior, like that of the Spanish pious women that we will examine in the second section of the chapter, cannot be understood without this unrestricted desire to break with one's own existence to live, so to speak, the life of others. Rebuked by his neighbor, Pedro Alonso, whom the nobleman has mistaken for Rodrigo de Narváez, Don Quixote replies irately: "I know who I am." To which he adds that not only could he be Valdovinos or Abindarráez, but also "all the Twelve Peers of France and even the Nine of Fame." He is not wrong; the actions of the nobleman, like those of the devout women, are inscribed and written upon the existence of others. Don Quixote lives as others do, he behaves as others do, he feels and he suffers as others do – others who are not he. His personal identity is not built on doubt, but on a certainty that requires a permanent theatricalization, a *mis-en-scène* in accordance with the interpretative nature of his persona.

Invisible sensations

Against all appearances, the adventures of Don Quixote are part of a literary fiction that uses woe as the driving force for the story. In *The Rise of the Novel*, the scholar Ian Watt explains how the success of the new narrative forms that prevailed in England in the eighteenth century came about through an emotional communion with the novels' victims.[2] The reader's identification with the protagonists of these stories enabled the new urban bourgeoisie to shed a fair amount of real tears for the misfortunes of imaginary beings.[3] *Don Quixote*'s misadventures do not form part of the culture of sensitivity, but rather of a literary imagination that constructs a reading through the reiteration of misfortune. Suffering articulates and directs the narrative, thus making the story possible. In *Don Quixote*, which Dostoyevsky called "the greatest and saddest of all books,"[4] the protagonist's own, personal story reveals unhappiness and suffering; it positions the reader, or the audience, as a privileged spectator of ills and dangers. Discourse is identified with the drama to such a point that the person who hears it knows, if not how to remedy the ills, at least how "to feel sorrow for them."[5] Cervantes' novel, which abounds in reflections on trouble and misfortune, permits a new evaluative framework in which the two protagonists interpret the ills of others and feel their own. One of the two, Sancho, is unable to explain how it is possible to spend one's life in search of adventures and find no more than "kicks and tossings, stones and fists."[6] For Don Quixote, knights errant "are subject to a good deal of hunger and misfortune, and even other things that are felt more easily than said."[7]

That which is "felt more easily than said," those normally abhorrent feelings that Don Quixote himself silences or hides out of modesty or shame, have nothing to do with moral suffering, that emotion which, according to Marcus Aurelius' *Meditations,* can be governed by the will. Rather, these feelings have to do with physiological pain, with the suffering of the organs, the rupturing of the body.[8] For reasons that will be explained later, this form of suffering has gone unnoticed for entire generations of readers of *Don Quixote*. Compared with the numerous studies related to mockery, humor, heroism, tragedy, geography, or history, the pain of the man who faced down so many dangers, and who achieved so many heroic and courageous deeds constitutes little more than an occasion for laughter if not a literary fiction. It is as though the reasons that led Sancho to give his knight the sobriquet of "the Knight of the Sorrowful Face" were a matter of little importance, as though the conditions surrounding Don Quixote's adventures had more to do with the melancholy of the soul than with the fate of the body.[9] At best, Don Quixote's pain has been put off in favor of other forms of moral suffering. The natural history of his soul – the modern prison of the body – has left little room for the vicissitudes of his arms, his ribs, his hands, or his teeth.

There are two readings of *Don Quixote* that are partially in conflict with my own. Later I will explain why this disagreement is only of a partial nature. For the time being I should like to explain the discrepancy. For Mikhail Bakhtin in *Rabelais and his World*, *Don Quixote* constitutes an exemplification of what the Russian critic calls "grotesque realism:" a form of subverting the social and moral order inspired by the lowest bodily strata. In his reading of the novel, Bakhtin explores the relationship between the protagonists through a division of functions that allows him to situate, on the one hand, the soul and, on the other, the body's sewer, the belly. Thus, whereas Don Quixote fulfills the prerogatives of the head, Sancho is identified with the demands of the stomach; whereas one has a spiritual existence, the other is unable to raise his conscience even a foot off the ground; whereas one devotes himself to his cause, motivated by virtue, the other is driven by his own interests; whereas one was born to live dying, the other was born to die eating; and whereas one considers that until death, everything is life, the other knows that the disgrace of his defeat, the loss of his honor, or the enchantment of his beloved can be even worse than death. Don Quixote and Sancho exist in the same relation as the high in opposition to the low, parody as opposed to ceremony, carnival versus Lent, the carnal against the spiritual, the sacramental versus the excremental.[10] From Bakhtin's point of view, the parody of the book consists in the reversal of the hierarchical order whereby inns become castles, flocks become armies and prostitutes become noble ladies. The regenerative power of grotesque realism emerges in the denial of ascetic ideals by the lowest corporal strata. Sancho's lead role is therefore providential, for it is only through his foolish and trivial consciousness that the mockery of the chivalrous ideal defended by his master can come to pass; an ideal that, the great majority of the time, only ends up increasing pain and enabling disgrace.

For the ethnologist Roger Bartra, in a more recent essay on melancholy in Baroque culture, the suffering of *Don Quixote* is not found in the vicissitudes of the body, but in the sicknesses of the soul.[11] Using the *Examen de Ingenios para las ciencias* (1575) by Huarte de San Juan, and, above all, a modern reinterpretation of the old humoral theory, Bartra explains the behavior of the knight – who recognizes himself as "the most unfortunate of men"[12] – in the context of the transformation of melancholy that took place during the Renaissance. Although Bartra recognizes a Christological background to Cervantes' novel, he also states that Don Quixote transforms medieval indolence so that the reader is forced, along with Sancho, to recognize that the worst thing that can happen to a man is "to let him die, just like that, without anybody killing him or any other hands ending his life except those of melancholy."[13] The harsh humor of the novel is based on the incongruence between the will of the heart and the impossibility of the task, so that the knight's misfortunes do not come from pain but from defeat and absence.

Bakhtin's and Bartra's interpretations, which present us with a Don Quixote consumed by the sorrow that *afflicts his troubled heart*,[14] lose sight of the extent to which Cervantes represented his protagonist in confrontation with the tyranny of matter. But the power of mockery to crush indolence and complacency should not make us forget that the arduous tasks of decapitating serpents, defeating armadas and undoing spells could not be done with merely the will, but also require the will of the body; the hand that Don Quixote offers to Maritornes, not for her to kiss but so that she "mayest gaze upon the composition of its sinews, the consistency of its muscles, the width and capacity of its veins."[15] Melancholic humor and grotesque reality do not substitute physical suffering, but prejudge the way in which readers evaluate pain and confer on it an emotional meaning. It is sometimes forgotten, however, that Cervantes' book is also a text about "the pounding which has not ceased,"[16] the lasting scars which "won't fall away from my memory any more than they'll fade from my back."[17] Likewise, it is also forgotten that Quixote and Sancho's wanderings are so marked by misfortune, weariness, and wounds that the protagonists themselves see their relationships, company, and business in accordance with the many blows and punches they have received together. Within the framework of literary fiction, the suffering of the main characters is one of the least debatable elements. Not so much from the reader's point of view, for whom it is diluted in Cervantine humor, but from the point of view of Don Quixote himself, who is, at times, unable to sleep or to speak a word, still less lie down with a woman, on account of his pain: "because I lie so bruised and broken," he said to Maritornes, "that even if I with all my heart desired to satisfy thine own desires, I could not."[18]

When asked about the living conditions of a knight-errant, in a text which openly contradicts the more popular image of the mad adventurer who interprets the world according to what he has read, Don Quixote bases his judgment not on the authority of books, as he normally does, but on a reasoning built on his own lived experiences: "I wish only to suggest, given what I suffer" that the work of a knight-errant "is undoubtedly more toilsome and more difficult, more subject to hunger and thirst, more destitute, straitened and impoverished." At least for once, chivalric literature is based on experience rather than life based on literature. It is the reality of suffering that feeds the imagination, not the memory that configures experience. It is the present pain, the recognition that "experience has often shown me that my flesh is weak and not all impenetrable"[19] which allows him to affirm that "there can be no doubt that knights errant in the past endured many misfortunes in the course of their lives."[20]

Throughout the book, there is ample evidence of the degree to which the hero suffers. Once dressed in his armor, Don Quixote is knocked from his horse by "a gallant blow" when trying to lance a merchant, and he is beaten by a mule trader's servant, "so furiously that...he thrashed Don Quixote as if he were threshing wheat."[21] His body is so damaged that he is left broken and delirious. This is nothing, however, compared with the misfortunes that befall him on his second outing, beginning with the tremendous walloping he receives when charging against the windmills. After the ingeniously titled *molimiento* – which incorporates the term for both windmill and bodily ache – it is his squire's turn to suffer at the hands of the friars of San Benito, who leave him with "no hair in his beard unscathed, they kicked him breathless and senseless and left him lying on the ground."[22] Meanwhile, Don Quixote receives a cut from the Biscayan that takes off half his ear and leaves him in very bad shape. Knight and servant both suffer even more greatly at the hands of the Yangueses, who beat them "with great zeal and eagerness...leaving the two adventurers looking bad and feeling worse."[23] To these misfortunes, we would have to add the tremendous beating Don Quixote was given by the muleteer that left him "so badly battered that if the first blow had been followed by a second, he would have had no need for a physician to care for his wounds," or the blow he was given by the candle "and all its oil" when he still lay on his back, "unable to move simply because he was so badly beaten and so covered with poultices."[24] To which the muleteer "raised his arm on high and delivered such a terrible blow to the narrow jaws of the enamored knight that he bathed his whole mouth in blood; not content with this, he jumped on his ribs, and with his feet moving faster than a trot, he stomped them all from one end to the other."[25] Or the stones that were thrown at our hero by the goatherds, of which one entombed "two ribs inside his body,"[26] whereas another "came flying and hit his hand, striking the cruet so squarely that it broke into pieces, taking along three or four teeth from his mouth and smashing two of his fingers."[27] Stones also rained down from the hands of the galley slaves, together with the blows one of them gave him with a shaving bowl, breaking it across his back. Likewise, he was maltreated by Cardenio and even, toward the end of Part One, by Maritornes, who, when she left him hanging by one arm, "caused him so much pain that he believed his hand was being cut off at the wrist or that his arm was being pulled out of its socket."[28]

Although the Second Part of the book does not abound quite so much in the physical suffering of its hero, this does not prevent him from being "trampled and kicked and bruised by the feet of filthy and unclean animals."[29] Or from a cat leaping "at his face and [sinking] his claws and teeth into his nose and the pain [being] so great that Don Quixote began to shout as loudly as he could."[30] It is not strange, therefore, that, upon the knight's arrival in Barcelona, a Castilian who had read the First Part of the novel calls out to him and asks how he could have made it there without dying from the numerous beatings he had suffered. In view of so much woe, Don Quixote confesses he was born "to be a model of misfortune, the target and mark for the arrows of affliction."[31] Neither is it strange that in the face of the comments by Sansón Carrasco that the authors of the story could have included many more beatings, blows, and punches, the man from La Mancha replies that "they also could have kept quiet about them [...] if they belittle the hero."[32]

The American scholar David B. Morris, in *The Culture of Pain*, has pointed out that, following the unfortunate episode with the windmills, Don Quixote, who is riding a little bent and sideways in the saddle as a result of the fall, comments that if he is not complaining of the pain "it is because it is not the custom of a knight-errant to complain about any wound even if his innards are spilling out because of it."[33] Although Morris uses this text as a confirmation of the heroic evaluation of pain in the context of the formation of the European chivalric conscience, he forgets that Don Quixote does complain that he is in pain from his injuries, and a great deal. So much so, in fact, that in fewer than two pages following the cut to his ear from the Biscayan and until he finds remedy at the hands of some goatherds, the knight protests three times about the pain, refuting on various other occasions his own rule.[34] He also complains bitterly after the beating he receives at the inn, even exaggerating his own pain and frightening himself by his own appearance: "what he thought was blood was nothing but the sweat pouring out of him because of the distress he had experienced in the tempest that had just passed."[35] In the framework of the different forms of configuring reality, pain is one of the least debatable elements. Not so much from the point of view of the reader – who does not pay attention to the evidence presented – as from that of Don Quixote himself.

Esther Cohen traces the roots of indifference toward pain, the ability to bear painful sensations with what she terms *impassibility* in the context of the cultural development of the *apatheia* of the stoics; in other words, the ability to control one's emotions, which are inevitably produced by bodily sensations – a Christianized tradition, which only allowed women the expression of pain but which denied it to, for example, the characters of the epic poems and books on chivalry of the Low Middle Ages.[36] In the Renaissance, however, there were many authors who left traces of their pain and suffering. In the case of *Don Quixote*, far from being an incidental element in the development of the novel, pain found a place in all areas of the narrative structure. It was, to begin with, an extra-literary reality; it is not for nothing that the work of Cervantes contains many perfectly identifiable elements of what was a society steeped in the continuous anticipation of suffering and death. The life of the galley slaves, the

Holy Brotherhood, the prisoners of Algiers, military campaigns, banditry, and asceticism are all perfectly recognizable in the work. Furthermore, the pain of the needy and the afflicted, the pain of all those who have been "thwarted in their desires and deceived in their hopes"[37] makes the work of a knight-errant more necessary than ever.

Beyond the extra-literary reality of the novel, in the sphere of literary reality, of the parameters that determine what is and what is not at the very heart of Cervantes' discourse, and excepting the dreamed elements (such as the delusions in the cave of Montesinos), the conscious lies (such as the mockery of the dukes or Sancho's lie about Dulcinea), or the theatrical elements (such as the puppet show, the story within the story, or the novels within the novel), the reality of pain does not obey a simple formula within the realm of physiology. Rather, pain lives within the framework of a complex interpretative structure that permits, at the same time, its presence and its omission. Of course, pain is felt, in the first place, as the effect of a violent action against the bodily economy. Most of Don Quixote's pain comes from punches, lashings, rapier thrusts, stonings, and attacks with other implements such as oil lamps, which leave the hero on the ground. The evaluation of this kind of pain may have variations, in such a way that he may be left beaten to a pulp but not insulted,[38] and even may think that the "wounds received in battles bestow honor, they don't take it away."[39] Whatever the case, it is unquestionable that we are dealing with abhorrent feelings. We also have the opposite situation, where appearances are not the cause but rather the effect of states of consciousness: where giants appear when there are only windmills, helmets when there are only basins, or armies instead of flocks of sheep, our knight can modify sensory experience even in those aspects which, like pain, would seem less disposed to bend to the influence of the will. Moreover, his suffering, whether in its origin, its evaluation or its remedy, is always mediated by spells and enchantment. To begin with, Don Quixote suffers real wounds at the hands of imaginary beings, which he himself turns into the only source of his torments. Not only were the hands of the mule driver "attached to the arm of some monstrous giant,"[40] but the source of his greatest misfortunes was a cohort of scoundrels and rogues, of sorcerers who pursue him, have pursued him and will continue to pursue him "until they throw him and his high chivalric exploits into the profound abyss of oblivion."[41]

If the physical pain in this novel has passed unnoticed for generations of readers, it is not only because moral affliction, psychological suffering, decrepitude of the mind, delirium, or the breaking of the soul have been given preference over the miseries of the body. Nor is it because we have thought that the protagonist of these misadventures lacks a body. There are sufficient, albeit not many, descriptions of what he looks like and of his movements, which turn what others see as automatic actions into voluntary ones. Throughout the pages of the book, Don Quixote appears fully aware of his physiological condition and the state of his limbs: "I see very clearly, Sancho, that I am not handsome, but I also know that I am not deformed; it is enough for a virtuous man not to be a monster to be well-loved."[42] If we have been unable to put ourselves in the space opened up by our protagonist's wounds, if we have forgotten his suffering or if we have given it value only in the context of irony and calculated mockery, it is not because we have preferred the will of the mind to the state of the body. It is because of the presence of a psychological state that makes the real invisible and turns it into a mere appearance; it makes black appear to be white, makes the diabolical angelic and the pestiferous fragrant; a perceptual transformation that is described in *Don Quixote* as "enchantment."

The enchantment of pain in the early modern period is that it cannot be seen, but is rather assumed to exist as an inevitable, even festive, element of real life or literary action. Don Quixote's pain becomes diluted in a reading that converts the misfortune and misadventure of others into a source of humor, mockery, and joke. The supposed disenchantment of the world, which the sociologist Max Weber considered the quintessence of modernity, is no more than a chimera. The *Entzauberung* does not entail the disappearance of magical elements; rather, it situates magic within the realm of imperceptibility, far from the new critical standpoint. Above all, in the case under consideration here, the early modern world was *encantado*, thrilled (or enchanted), to make pain an essential element of human actions. In a society marked by the triumph of pain and death, it is easy to understand that suffering was accepted as an inevitable element. The beginning of the process of expulsion of death, mourning, sickness, deformity, and violence from public spaces can be found in this collective recreation of misfortune, which is perceived in the context of calculated mockery and conscious irony.

Part of this form of enchantment derives from a Christological tradition that makes the *via crucis* the greatest form of misfortune, teaching that there is no consolation without pain, no rose without thorns, no writing without blood. Faced with the Spanish mysticism that, in the words of Teresa of Ávila, forces us to choose between suffering and death, Don Quixote nonetheless chooses life. Not an easy nor a contemplative life, but rather a life in which suffering does not operate according to a proportion between rupture and conquest or expiation and blame. The evaluative context in which Don Quixote understands his pain is not a part of the ethics of salvation or renunciation, but rather the struggle for freedom. What motivates Don Quixote to repudiate pain is not resignation but freedom: freedom as opposed to vileness; freedom as opposed to envy; freedom as opposed to ignorance, stupidity, and slander. The knight proclaims his absolute freedom not only to contemplate the world as he wishes, but also to contribute to its elaboration, even its perceptual fabrication; the freedom to leave his own story, denying the opposition between literary fiction and lived reality. Freedom at the moment of evading the empire of need and for pain, to such a point that the body feels relieved and thus better for its breaking, which even comes to be felt as healthy. For Don Quixote, freedom "is one of the most precious gifts heaven gave to men; the treasures under the earth and beneath the sea cannot compare to it; for freedom, as well as for honor, one can and should risk one's life, while captivity, on the other hand, is the greatest evil that can befall men."[43] Most of Don Quixote's actions, like the episode with the galley slaves, or with Dueña Dolorida, are aimed at the granting of freedom through "the strength of his arm and the intrepid resolve of his courageous spirit."[44] Freedom is the quintessence of what Don Quixote sees as his mission, as he thus rebuked a member of the Holy Brotherhood: "lowborn and filthy creatures, you call it highway robbery to free those in chains, to give liberty to the imprisoned, to assist the wretched, raise up the fallen, succor the needy?"[45] It is this freedom that he longs for when he is imprisoned, because someone who "is enchanted, as I am, is not free to do with his person what he might wish."[46] Above all else, his desire to free his beloved Dulcinea from her enchantment persists – the authentic tragedy of the Second Part.

Roger Bartra was right when he wrote that in "Don Quixote, melancholy itself is a choice, an act of will and an affirmation of freedom."[47] Bakhtin was also right when he commented that the humor in the novel is a source of liberation: "Laughter purifies from dogmatism, from the intolerant and the petrified; it liberates from fanaticism and pedantry, from fear and intimidation, from didacticism, naïvete and illusion, from the single meaning, the single level, from sentimentality."[48] Those writers who attribute this sublime source of freedom to the book rather than to its protagonist are mistaken. Or, better yet, they are wrong when they defend the freedom that inspired Cervantes' book, based on forgetting the pain of that freedom's main witness.

Religious uses of pain

The uses of pain have nothing to do with truth, but rather with drama; they cannot be explained by logic, but from the collective fabrication of personal experiences. The appropriate place for visualizing harm is not the world, but the theater; it is not identity, but performance.[49] In the framework of the theater, the same punitive gesture, the lacerating of the body through the age-old practice of flagellation, for example, may be interpreted as a necessity or an abuse, as a form of punishment or a way to salvation. Behind the expressive gestures there is no unchanging reality, but a detachable stage where the same blows may be fought as an unnecessary violation of bodily integrity, or on the contrary, be vindicated as an instrument of liberation. Neither is there exactly an individual who exists prior to the experience. Cervantes' protagonist, the archetype of the modern consciousness, is obsessed with the rigorous fulfilling of *his role*, with the vehement desire to convince *others*. As later in Descartes, his identity does not precede his experience, but rather is a culmination thereof.

In one of his first adventures, Don Quixote tries to prevent the beating of a mule driver. In the Second Part, however, he persuades his squire to deliver himself 3300 lashes with the intention of freeing his master's beloved Dulcinea, a martyrdom that the good Sancho is not willing to accept without resistance. In his proverbial simple-mindedness, Sancho understands that his Master intends to follow the saying "If you have a headache, put some ointment on your knees."[50] But he does not wish to be "the cow at the wedding," the animal that attends important events in the form of food, nor does he wish, even worse, to be "the friar's ass."[51] Without making any connection whatsoever between the mortification of his flesh and breaking the enchantment upon his Master's beloved, Sancho decides instead to beat the trees, crying out so loudly that it seems his soul is being torn out with each blow. His attitude questions the positive evaluation of self-inflicted pain in the context of religious asceticism and contrasts with the words Don Quixote addresses to him upon hearing his laments: "since you are so well-disposed, then may heaven help you; go on with your whipping and I shall move away."[52] Both the scene of the beating of the mule driver and this one explore the significant dichotomies of modern thinking. On the one hand, there is the public and the corporeal, on the other, the private and the spiritual. Whether as a form of punishment or as an instrument of liberation, pain arouses the religious and the punitive, the sacred and the secular, the physiological and the mental. Sacrifice, renunciation, expiation, purification, catharsis, and salvation are practiced within an evaluative framework in which personal disposition is imposed upon mere physiology in such a way that it is not only possible to extract positive consequences from bodily torments, it is also possible to develop the idea that redemption or liberation depends on the mortification of the flesh.[53]

The understanding of these experiences is not well suited to the language of juridical philosophy, where a beating only hurts as a beating. The degree of pain's voluntary nature, its simultaneously private and public character, natural and cultural character, all mean it cannot be captured by the philosophical jargon of sub-determined categories. On the contrary, the experience is built in a dramatic space that also includes a scenic backdrop. Cervantes can make fun of ascetic practices because his knight-errant shares rhetorical tactics and persuasive arts with the religious world. Religious asceticism and knight-errantry both emerge in a space that is neither entirely public nor completely private; that is neither totally visible nor radically opaque; that is not marked by necessity, but rather by the iron will and unbreakable determination to live and feel as others. In this place that is at once real and fictitious, literary and extra-literary, neither things nor people are what they seem.

To begin with, Don Quixote had already passed through a "Purgatory," according to Sancho, or a "Hell," in his own words, when he made the decision to isolate himself in the mountains to punish his body by living as a hermit. His *spiritual exercises* consisted of renouncing the world, courtesy, and modesty, and included the deliberate production of pain.[54] Although he was not seeking a mystical communion with God, but rather the conquest of his beloved, the dramatization of violence is unchanged, surpassing categories like external and internal, body and soul, private and public. Nuns, on the other hand, also formulate their conduct through rigorous imitation of a literary model. Just like Alonso Quijano, who lost his mind reading books on chivalry, the nuns of Counter-Reformation Spain discovered their vocation and the guidelines for their actions in the pages of sacred texts and, more specifically, in the martyrologies and the lives of the saints. Both mold their experiences using an imitative model. They do not live; they copy.[55] They do not feel, they imitate; they reproduce schemas and behaviors that they have learned from the pages of their bedside reading, either in hours of solitude or moments of group devotion.[56] The knight wishes to relive the feats of Roland, of Amadis of Gaul, and of other knights-errant. The devout women long for the early Christian martyrs; they wish they had lived in those happy times when they could have been martyred. Many of these texts were shared in the refectory or in the workrooms; there "they read of the atrocious torments suffered by the unvanquished martyrs," while longing, with fervent zeal "to join them in their fate, until spilling the last drop of their blood for the Catholic faith."[57]

These penitent practices, linked to what Esther Cohen has called *philopassianism* – the search for pain as an instrument for the *imitatio Christi* – reached a notable level of intensity after the fourteenth century and they were spread through the hagiographic reconstruction of the lives of the saints, written directly or indirectly by their protagonists.[58] The *Life* of the pious Suso, the *Autobiography* of Margery Kempe at the beginning of the fifteenth century, the lives of Catherine of Siena or Dorothy of Montau set the models. These are the names mentioned by Teresa of Avila in her autobiography, and they would lead to the formation of an imagined community that was built through "imitative chains:" from Catherine of Siena to Maddalena Pazzi; from Maddalena to Rose of Lima or Teresa of Avila; from Teresa of Avila to Isabel of Jesus or María Vela. Even when Esther Cohen applies the term to the Low Middle Ages, the deliberate search for pain as a form of theatrically recreating the Passion of Christ lasts well into the early modern period. And it concerns men as well as women. Giuseppe di Copertino [1603–1668], for example, famous for his providential clumsiness and tendency to levitate, managed to reduce his body to a skeleton through penance. His rigorous sense of existence led him to a systematic and bloody destruction of his body, flagellating himself to the bone at times.[59] Likewise, Francesco di Girolamo [1642–1716] beat himself with such force and holy vehemence that he always ended up losing a great deal of blood.[60] In the context of this "holy vehemence," an expression that is replaced at times by "*holy extravagance*," blows could be administered using whips, bars, sticks, or iron chains. Some burned their skin with boiling water or oil. The intensity of the examples varies, but not their intention. Dorothy of Montau, for example, made her injuries even worse by rubbing stinging nettles and bitter herbs into them.[61] The pious Suso fabricated his own bedclothes with barbs on the inside. For Catherine of Siena, who ended her days eating only consecrated communion wafers, nuns should actively look for suffering through the punishment of the flesh.[62] For the Italian historian Camporesi, asceticism turned the monasteries into torture chambers and seminaries into places for training in suffering and misfortune: "It was in truth an object of much amazement to see those dispirited young men, some crowned with thorns, others with ashes upon their heads, others with their arms tied to a piece of wood."[63]

In Spain, where there is an abundance of works dedicated to penance, sinners' guides, and treatises on the vanity of the world, the first mystics of the sixteenth century described earthly existence in terms of torment.[64] This is the message contained in the *Agony of the Passage to Death* by Alejo de Venegas in 1537, where life is interpreted as a "long martyrdom," a theme expressly pointed out in the *Third Spiritual Alphabet* by Francisco de Osuna. Eagerness for pain can also be found in the *Spiritual Exercises* of Ignatius of Loyola, who recommends combining "interior" penance, the experience of blame, and three forms of exterior penance: fasting, staying awake, and the punishing of the flesh. The last of these should produce considerable damage, such that "pain should reach the flesh without touching the bones, so that it gives only pain and not illness."[65] In all these cases, the imitative exercise begins with the systematic humiliation of the senses. Touch, sight, smell, taste should first be restricted and then punished. The experience limited sensorial capacity, creating a closed, cloistered world which was not exactly *senseless*, but *without senses*. Josefa María García [1673–1743], for example, forbade herself to look upon a man for her entire life, never listened to anything other than prayer, and subjected herself to rigorous abstinence and fasting. The few times that she ate, she added bitter herbs to her food so that it would be austere and unpleasant. She subjected herself to intense cold, suffered constant thirst and for some time she would not touch any part of her body other than her hands and feet.[66] Although Josefa moved through time and space, had visions in which Christ, her spouse, offered her blood, and the Virgin, her mother, offered her milk, and although her heart seemed so large that her ribs managed to open out from her chest, what most worried her spiritual director was "the penal exercise of their horrible and bloody disciplines."[67]

This "sweet creature" beat her flesh as though it were marble; she made and used all kinds of instruments for mortification, always preferring those that could reduce her body to contemptible remains. As in other cases, her spiritual life needed to use her body as a weapon of salvation. There was no communion with the divine nor liberation from earthly constrictions that did not pass through the flesh. Redemption could not be achieved through denial of the body, but rather through its continuous use and its all-embracing presence.[68]

Josefa was not alone in her eagerness to feel pain: "Every week on Mondays, Wednesdays and Fridays, once prayers were over, half an hour of discipline follows; such is the fervor of those incarnate angels that there are no words to describe this exercise, nor valor to think about it. It is a horrible spectacle to record that Choir stained with virginal blood."[69] Penance, scorn, poverty, or sickness were all regulated by this unrestricted passion to imitate and feel the sufferings of others: "this anxiety [to suffer] grew with the example of some nuns who lived in the convent at that time, and who greatly excelled in all kinds of internal and external mortification."[70] In the case of María Vela, a woman who did not speak, and who could easily be found crying from the affliction of not suffering enough, the need for mortification was so great that when it was denied her, she requested that God grant her the miracle of pain:

> the Lord heard her request and the next day He gave her an illness which she had to suffer for the whole of Lent. Because, apart from the continuous fever she suffered from with difficult accidents, every day for two, sometimes four hours, she felt as though she were being squashed in a press; other times, as though she were on a torture rack whose cords were being fiercely tightened.[71]

She was not the only nun that accepted this willingness to turn (natural) illness into its (supernatural) sign. Like the knight from La Mancha, who constructed reality according to his expectations, Josefa María García also prayed to God to reward her with illnesses and terrible pain, about which she never complained. After all, in the heart of religious communities where martyrdom seemed to be a condition of divine election, sickness provided an opportunity for martyrdom *by other means.*[72]

Theatricality does not eliminate the pain, but it renders it partially invisible, relegating the spectacle of cruelty to the intimate sphere. As in the case of Don Quixote, whose pain has gone unnoticed for entire generations of readers, physical suffering can be experienced and expressed in different ways depending on whether it is a pain that happens in the private sphere or whether, on the other hand, it is the result of public suffering. Lisa Silverman, a historian of torture in the early modern period, examines these two forms of manifestation of physical suffering by relating them to gender; in this reading, the brotherhoods of self-flagellation are the legacy of men, while asceticism and mysticism constitute key examples of women's appropriation of suffering.[73] In her view, although the exaltation of pain resulting from illness occurred inside convents, it corresponds to the public exhibition of self-punitive practices taking place in phratries and brotherhoods consisting mainly of men. According to Silverman, women flagellated themselves in private, because, for them, pain was not a matter of choice and consequently it could not be an object of public exhibition.

Although this argument is supported in the case of communities of flagellants, it confronts serious difficulties with regard to asceticism and mysticism. To begin with, in this context, it is difficult to know what is meant by "private" or "public" within the interior of the convents. In some cases, penitence took place before everyone's eyes. On occasions, fellow-nuns and monks castigated one other with vehemence, either on their own initiative or by order of the confessor.[74] The biographer of Josefa Vela, for example, felt notable admiration on seeing the nuns of Castellón, "innocent creatures, behaving so cruelly to one another."[75] The biographies suggest that penitence was practiced in secret, with the excuse that pride should not spoil the holy penitence. This is the case of María Vela, who, despite her delicate health, prayed for six hours a day, especially on her knees, disciplined herself three times a day, slept only four hours a night and, most importantly, did all of this in secret – a secret of which, however, we have all been informed. In all cases, penitence occurs in the indeterminate category of a well-known secret, of the partially private dwelling, of the happiness that, against all logic, can only be experienced *post-mortem*. The drama does not follow the logic of adaptation, but rather of concealment. The pain may be a secret but, sooner or later, a hand will lift the veil and will look beneath the habits. Then humility can appear without pride or vainglory. An entire life of austerity will have its small moment of reward when the sisters discover on the dead body the remnants of a penance borne in solitude and often in silence, revealing the atrocities she suffered during her life.[76]

Scarcely one year before the posthumous publication in 1664 of *The Treatise of Man* by René Descartes, for whom the heart was, at the same time, an organ and little more than a machine, the Jesuit Piergili published the official biography of the young abbess Clare of the Cross.[77] One night in August 1308 four holy sisters headed to the chapel, carrying the body of the abbess, who had just died. They undressed the corpse. Sister Francesca cut the body open with a knife. The others began to take out her intestines. The bladder retained a whitish color and when they touched it, it seemed to contain three small round stones in the shape of a triangle. As they continued to remove her insides, they reached the heart, whose large size surprised them. They placed it to one side in a wooden receptacle, along with the stones from the bladder, and put the receptacle into a cupboard. The disproportionately large heart became the subject of rumors and speculations among the other sisters, not just among the four who had taken part in the operation. It was remembered that the abbess used to say that "she carried Christ crucified in her heart." Furthermore, sister Marina recounted that Clare had told her about a vision in which Christ, disguised as a pilgrim, told her that he wanted to plant the enormous cross that he was carrying on his shoulder in her heart. It was a few days before they decided to look further at the abbess' heart. One Sunday night they took it from the cupboard, then removed it from the urn and knelt before it. Francesca said: "Lord, I believe that in this heart there lies your holy Cross, although I believe my sins to be so many that make me unworthy to find it."[78] And while she spoke she made an incision at the top of the organ. The excessive blood made it impossible to see anything at first. They knew very well, wrote Piergili, that the heart is concave and divided into two parts, it being a unit only in its circumference.[79] Francesca felt a nerve with her finger that formed a cross on the flesh, within a cavity that was also cruciform. Margarita began to call out: "a miracle, a miracle." Sister Giovanna, for her part, instructed Francesca to continue with her anatomical inquisition. The nun then observed another small nerve standing upright in the heart. When looking at it more carefully, they understood that it represented the whip with which Christ had been beaten. When this news got out, the Franciscan friars suspected that the sisters had been fooled as a result of their inexperience or excess of credulity. They contacted the bishop of Spoleto, Berengario Donadei, to denounce the women's credulity, rumor, and fantasies. Without further ado, Berengario left for Montefalco. His initial intention, wrote Piergilii, was to bury this scandalous news and severely punish the women. Once he was there, and standing before a congregation of theologians, judges, doctors, and men of the Church, Berengario asked to be brought the heart. He took it in his hand with a mocking gesture and opened it disdainfully. Then he saw in great detail both the cross and the whip. He also observed an even greater miracle. Both he and the other doctors discovered that when they touched the heart and examined it carefully, other mysteries of the Passion appeared: the crown of thorns, the whipping column, the three nails, the lance, and the sponge, all represented in such a vivid way that when he touched the tips of the lance and the three nails, Berengario pricked his finger as though they had been made of iron.

This story of the nuns entertained by the corpse of one of their sisters does not belong to the fourteenth century. The narrative structure and the nature of the plot, which rests on the direct evidence of anatomical structure depending on visual testimony, shows us that it is a modern recreation of a medieval heart. The biographer, Piergili, even allows himself to explain the operations carried out on the three stones found in the bladder, which always weighed the same amount whether they were weighed together or separately: a recreation of the Holy Trinity along the lines of experimental philosophy. What happened in the convent of Montefalco only comes down to us in a deferred way, through the self-interests of Counter-Reformation worship, with its exacerbation of pain and trafficking in relics. The abbess' heart only takes on cultural meaning in the context of the worship of the Passion Christ. Its symbolic value derives from the *Ecce Homo*, the Insulted Christ, the beaten Christ, the Christ of Pain. Faith not only leads to the acceptance of the Passion, but to its tools and instruments. The flesh folds into the so-called *Arma Christi* – the arms used by the Savior in his fight against evil. The cross, the lance, the whip, the crown of thorns, and the nails are the basic elements of the torture of the flesh. Likewise, the story of the abbess is inscribed within the context of the devotion to the so-called *quinquepartium vulnus*, or five wounds, which has a clear antecedent in the appearance of Francis of Assisi's [1182–1226] stigmata in the thirteenth century, but whose dissemination would take place toward the end of the fourteenth.

The moral superiority of the abbess, as with many other devout people, is achieved by identifying sickness and suffering as a sign of divine election, but also the self-imposed need to keep these signs a secret, so that the spirit does not succumb to vanity nor arouse suspicions of vainglory. Pain is experienced in silence and life goes by in pain. The cloister accepts both. Within the walls of convents, suffering does not happen in the light of day, but rather at nightfall, or at dawn; amidst shadows.[80] Sooner or later, the secret will become public; light will penetrate darkness. With death's liberation, the terrible ulcers, signs of mortification, or tumor that grew during years or decades of selfless subjection, are discovered.[81] If it was not inscribed on the body or made part of the organs, it will appear in the pages of a diary. Books, like the skin, also reveal scars, exposing past suffering. Obliged, even by their confessors, to leave testimony of their experience, the slaves of God – the nuns – not only read, they also wrote. In this, they resemble the knight-errant, who knows he is the protagonist of a new story that will, in turn, serve as an imitative model. The diary confesses pain to the reader in the same way that the cadaver speaks to the anatomist. In the pages of the biographies of Spanish nuns of the seventeenth century, visions, ecstasy, levitations, and imaginary journeys all join together with the inexhaustible desire for suffering. In the biographies of Mariana de Jesús, or María del Santísimo Sacramento, known as *La Quintana*,[82] María de Pol, or María de Vela y Cueto, there is nothing worse, no greater torment than the mere passage through the world, a constant reminder of Christ's Passion: "to suffer [wrote Saint Theresa]…or to die."[83] Its mere existence preaches a correspondence between suffering and earthly bliss, as though future retribution depended on a proportional relationship between happiness and suffering: "Blessed are those who mourn, for they will be comforted," is written in Gospel of Matthew.[84]

Let us take, for example, the autobiography of Isabel de Jesús [1586–1648]. This 38-year-old widow had already begun to tell her neighbors about her many visions before she entered, as a lay sister, the convent of *San Juan Bautista de las Agustinianas recoletas* in the town of Arenas de San Pedro, Ávila province, in 1626.[85] From the moment she entered the order, she did everything in her power to make her life as painful as possible. She restricted her use of light, avoided sleep whenever possible and, like many women before and after her, avoided food. Its mere presence caused her to retch, although Isabel, unlike some of the other sisters, did not only vomit when she ate but also, above all, when she wrote. Thus, her most terrible mortification was writing her own autobiography.[86] Each of the 758 pages of her book constitutes a triumph of self-denial, an immortal testimony of her misfortune.[87] The suffering is there, as inscribed on the pages of the book as on the geography of the body. The Passion is mimicked in bodies and expressed in books. In some cases, like that of Don Quixote, a face will also be left marked: not by the hand of God, but by the claws of a cat.

Like the line that separates the private from the public, the boundary between voluntary and involuntary acts also becomes blurred. What leads Don Quixote to bash his head against the stones? What makes Isabel de Jesús write her autobiography? Did these acts not constitute a desire to do away with free will, with self-love, with that "bloody sword that slits the throat of and puts an end to all virtues"?[88] What obliges the chastising of the body and its reduction to servitude? Silverman's argument rests on the idea that the pain and humiliation of women were not voluntary, in the sense that she who had been born to suffer pain could not choose it.[89] At least in seventeenth-century Spain, however, this natural predisposition to suffer has many counter-examples.[90] In the case of Lady María Vela y Cueto, a Cistercian mystic, suffering took on such varied forms that it often bordered on the extravagant. On many occasions her jaws remained shut for days as though held by clamps. Her determination was so great that not even a doctor, using all his force, could part them.[91] For this devout woman, holiness could be measured by austerity and by the most harsh and inhumane penance. Her daily practices included mortifying her sense of touch and depriving herself of sleep; on the few occasions that she got into bed, she placed a coarse cloth on it so that she would be unable to feel the sheets. She beat her hands, which some of her fellow sisters considered to be beautiful, with rope until the fingers swelled up and turned black. For many years, she customarily put chickpeas, "which were, by no means, small," under her feet.[92] Self-flagellation, of course, was part of her routine, as was silence and fasting. She built and made all kinds of cilices that, according to her confessor, "were horrifying:"[93] chains with spikes, others made of iron and barbed wire, wooden crosses filled with nails, wide belts made of tin. For her the greatest mortification was to be prohibited to practice this penance, and her greatest desire was to do so in front of the other sisters. Her greatest happiness consisted of "everyone despising her."[94] The prelate of the convent discovered that María practiced public constriction and, to serve as an example, kissed the feet of her sisters. Many of them could not bear the expression of happiness on the face of the nun who, in humiliating herself, extolled herself.[95] The capacity to bear pain is not completely voluntary, but rather a drive based on the greater conviction that our lives are not our own. Jesus himself had been the first to accept a will other than his own. During the early modern period, the Biblical verse "Let Thy will be done, not mine" was taken literally. When Vaquero rechristened the delicate María Vela as "the strong woman," he could not have been referring to her physical constitution, but rather to a will that was not in her own hands. After all, "the first and fundamental step of a perfect spiritual life is the mortification and negation of one's own will."[96]

The will to accept pain depends on God's will or, more frequently, the confessor's instructions. Such is the case of Catalina García Fernández, a widow from Castile, who entered a Franciscan community in 1661, adopting the religious name of Catalina de Jesús y San Francisco. Her confessor decided to subject her to most rigorous penances. He frequently made her undress to the waist and had others lash her back. He forced her to sleep on the floor, with only a block of wood for a pillow; he fed her with water and a little bread; and, on occasions, prior to the publication of some of the most emblematic similar scenes from Clarín's *La Regenta*, he forced her to walk through the streets of Madrid, barefoot and dressed in the way the authorities had laid down for heretics. While Catalina complied with the instructions of her confessor, many other nuns directly obeyed the will of their "Spouse." The deliberate desire to suffer was subordinate to the iron will to obey: "the venerable Mother was very ingenuous in looking for other voluntary and serious [pain]; and her husband was very vigilant in giving suffering to her, so that her virginal body would be reduced to perfect slavery."[97] In all of this, the words of Saint Paul resonate: "*castigo corpus meum & in servitudinem redigo*": I chastise my body and bring it into servitude.[98]

The imitation we have seen in this chapter and the representation we saw in the previous one are related in different ways. The theater of cruelty adapts itself to the theater of emulation not only because the representation is itself a form of imitation, as Erich Auerbach asserted in 1946, but also because the reproduction of appearances necessarily leads to a visible reflection of their effects. Even if it is not expressed through what today we would consider "the universe of the arts," imitation does not lack plasticity or material consequences. Like the carved heart of Clare of the Cross, the stigmata of Catherine of Siena, or the defeated bodies of Don Quixote and Sancho, the body, if not the canvas or the stage or the engraving, modulates and contents itself with the appearances of its model or the directives of its rule. However, the visibility, and consequently the evaluation, of these visible features depends on the confluence of a set of rhetorical elements that Aristotle already described in his *Poetics*. First of all, the quality of the imitation does not depend on the *dramatic move*, on this element susceptible to incite emotion through taking part in the spectacle. On the contrary, pain is expressed through the succession of scenes and, more particularly, through the concealment of that suffering that results from the will for servitude. Only in specific circumstances, marked by vicissitude or recognition, does the wound become visible and the suffering public. As in the case of the portrait of Catherine of Siena, the imitator shares with her model the instruments of mortification and signs of torture (see Figure 10). The verisimilitude of her portrait, as well as the conviction of the image, depends on the form in which the marks refer back to the original or conform to the model. The consideration of the harm itself lacks importance. The account should be coherent before it is referential. We are not faced with a body that suffers, but rather with a drama that is constructed in accordance with imitative elements and symbolic affinities. From this point of view, pain's visibility or invisibility depends on the adaptation of the imitator to her model, as well as the form in which experience is constructed in accordance with the accounts of others. This requires a more thorough explanation.

In the first place, neither Don Quixote's story nor Tiepolo's canvas initially refer to the experience of harm itself. The saint's stark gesture, for example, her extreme pallor or her cadaverous features do not concern her pain, but rather her imitative passion. It is difficult not to see in this painting the figuration of some other's expressions and experiences that the artist could have taken from the regulated representation of the Man of Sorrows and, especially, of the different figurations made by Guido Reni on the subject of Christ crowned with thorns. In a trivial sense, the painting does not represent suffering, but mimetic desire, the way in which the body resembles – in its composition, its tonality or even its gestures – the suffering of another. The misfortunes of Alonso Quijano are of the same kind. The imitative anxiety of our knight does not avoid pain, but it does relocate it in an emotional framework on which experience is built. Like the twentieth-century soldiers that Professor Joanna Bourke describes, who go to war thinking that the confrontation will be "like a film," Don Quixote also heads to his battle under the hope of the many heroic deeds he knows through books. However, unlike our soldiers that, with the first casualties, protest that defeat was not part of the script of "their film," Don Quixote always finds a way of avoiding adversity and rewriting his experience.[99] His misfortune is hatched under the spell of his tenacity, of the force with which he clings to his undertaking, and of the conviction with which he pulls himself together in the face of constant refutation (see Figure 11).

In the second place, and more importantly, the imitative element refers less to a physical or expressive result than to a dramatic experience.[100] Although from classical antiquity mimesis was related to the merely passive copy of objects and, more particularly, of their visible appearances, the early modern period transformed it into an interpretative activity.[101] As opposed to the Platonic version, which made imitation a merely pictorial reflection of nature, many humanists considered it, following Aristotle, a poetic recreation of human activities. Tragedy did not imitate things, but actions. In the decade of the 1970s, the French philosopher René Girard understood that it did not only affect visible gestures, but also invisible desires. He considered a structure of mimetic desire that included a mediator, an intermediate model that would allow for the satisfaction of desire.[102] Given that we do not know what we should desire, reasoned Girard, we end up craving what others desire. Like children who always want someone else's toy, human beings do not fight with one another to realize their own dreams, but rather to satisfy the yearnings of others. Like Don Quixote, who wants to be like Amadis of Gaul, or the strong woman who wants to be like Catherine of Siena, imitation is a voluntary act that, nonetheless, crushes the will; it is an act of visible consequences that, however, remain hidden; it is an act pertaining to a desire for identity and recognition that, nonetheless, does not precede experience but rather accompanies it. The theater of envy, as Girard denominated it, has three acts. In the first, the actors desire the same thing and are trivially identical. In the second, violence surfaces as a consequence of mimetic desire and the lack of distinction. In the third and final act, the fight of all against all is transformed into a conflict of all against one. Stigmatization (to use Goffman's expression) converts the scapegoat (to use Girard's expression) into a key element in the legitimization of violence. Here we are only interested in the first act, the moment in which the actors are still no one in particular and their actions are guided by the iron will of submitting to the imitation of others. The point of interest falls on recognition, on that rhetorical figure that Aristotle considers, along with peripeteia, one of the means used by tragedy to move souls. In the same way that the characters of the tragedy are deployed in the plot, identity does not precede but accompanies experience. In the same way that Alonso Quijano wants to be (but never ends up being) like Amadis of Gaul, and that María de Vela y Cueto wants to be (but never ends up being) like Rose of Lima. For a while, which may be his or her whole lifetime, the imitator lives in a world of experiences with no subject – just like Descartes, who before his first philosophical peripeteia lived in a world of doubts without certainties. The first thing is experience: to imitate, to doubt. Identity and consciousness will come later.

3
Sympathy

"We sympathize even with the dead"[1]

Cartography of misery

In the drama of pain, the spectator also plays a role, and not a small one at that. Although we assume too quickly the impossibility of sharing sensorial experiences, there is no scene of excruciating suffering that leaves us indifferent. On the contrary, we can only react to brutality and barbarism through the sensations of others. Our feelings of compassion, impotence, indignation, shame, or lewdness always come from vicarious emotions. At the base of the humanitarian gaze and philanthropic consciousness, compassion toward the suffering of another configures our experience of harm. In the eighteenth century, the philosopher David Hume defined sympathy as the means of sharing the pain or the pleasure of a third person. Edmund Burke, in a similar way, considered it as a "form of substitution by which we are put in the place of another man, and affected in many respects as he is affected."[2] When seeing the defendant in the dock, Adam Smith argued, we "place ourselves in his situation, conceive ourselves enduring all the same torments, we enter, as it were, into his body, and become in some measure the same person with him."[3]

Philosophy, so prone to questioning the veracity of others' testimonies, tends often to forget that this harmony of mutual sensibility requires no further demonstration.[4] The imitative practices and visual artifices we saw in the first two chapters could mold our sensorial experiences or our expressive forms; representation, imitation, correspondence, trust, narrativity, objectivity, coherence, or reiteration – the argumentative schemes used to bestow collective meaning on physical suffering or emotional ailments – may not be present, but sympathy is always obligatory. Whatever its nature or the way it is manifested, there is no human form of confronting the experience of harm other than through the spectator's gaze. The appraising reaction of the witnesses to tragedy may vary greatly, but there is no suffering that does not entail a social appraisal and, by extension, a form of expression linked to cultural guidelines and expectations. The most obvious implication of this theatrical circumstance, through which the victim not only feels pain but also senses that he is observed, is that it obliges us to conclude that where there is no observer, pain cannot be considered human. And on the contrary: new dramatic dispositions may bestow on entire groups of animate or inanimate beings emotional properties that they either do not initially possess or, as in the case of the dead, no longer belong to them.

Although the conformity of humors, ideas, and temperaments does not constitute a prerogative of the enlightened world, it was then that this agreement acquired a clear theoretical formulation and a no less extensive collective materialization. Mutual sympathy would provide the foundation of modern philanthropy and of beneficence, but also the basis of our aesthetic experience and political theory. Cultural history, including the history of literature or art, but also of medicine and science, aesthetics, and moral philosophy have all explored the passional and affective elements of the collective forms of tragedy. In all cases, studies begin with the (obvious) empirical finding that the misfortunes and dangers of the world do not affect all beings at the same moment or in the same proportion. Given that pain, like wealth or property, is not distributed in a homogeneous way, the Enlightenment promoted not only a logic of taste that permitted the ordering of the labyrinth of personal preferences, but also an emotional pact between persons with variable sensibilities and different affections. The foundations of this agreement lay upon the physiological disposition of organic tissues; for, contrary to how it might appear, humanitarianism never rested, at least initially, on moral sentiments, but rather on the physiology of sensitive fibers.

In France, the first explanation of this intersensorial capacity through which some people could suffer the misfortunes of others was broached in the work of Nicolas Malebranche [1638–1715]. His examples, based on the supposed influence of maternal imagination on embryonic development, could not have been more bizarre. In one case, a woman gave birth to a child whose gestures and skin texture reminded the mother of a saint to whom she was devoted. In the strangest case, another baby was born with mutilated limbs after its mother had witnessed the public execution of a convict. For Malebranche, this capacity to transform ideas into cutaneous marks and signs, which guaranteed the continuity of species and lineages, was not homogeneously distributed among human beings. On the contrary, those with the most vivid imagination and the tenderest flesh, women and children, could not see the wounds inflicted upon their peers without feeling in their own bodies the equivalent pain, the *counterblow*, which irremediably triggered the feeling of compassion.[5] In Great Britain, the new sensualist philosophies also found a source of inspiration in

physiological studies. Given that sensation provided the basis of all intellectual activity, cognitive capacities depended on their corresponding anatomical
structures. In the same way that organs could communicate their particular
sensations from a distance, they could also arouse an active interest in favor of
the misfortunes of others. In its simplest form, sympathy sanctioned the well-
known relationship between the sensitive tissues, including the possibility of
there being sensations that could not refer back to any direct stimulus. In its
most extreme case – as in *The Man of Feeling* by Henry MacKenzie – it was even
possible to die through the transference of another's suffering.[6]

From a social point of view, behavior toward children, toward criminals
and, more generally, toward the new undifferentiated category of "our equals,"
transformed sensitivity into a sign of distinction. In the case of animals,
travelers from the North frequently criticized the cruel spectacles of Catholic
Europe. The Earl of Clarendon, for example, classified bullfighting as a *"brutal
and barbarous"* spectacle, and in 1787 the erudite William Beckford claimed to
have felt the same blows and cuts as the bull had received.[7] The English painter
William Hogarth also made some of his engravings in the hope of reducing,
to some extent, cruelty toward animals, "the mere description of which causes
pain," he wrote.[8] For Humphrey Primatt, an Anglican reverend, *pain* was *pain*
regardless of who felt it; whether it was a human being or a beast.[9] While visiting Fontenelle in the *Oratoire* in Paris, the aforementioned Malebranche kicked
a dog several times. To the astonishment of his companion, he replied in surprise: "And what does it matter? Don't you know they have no feelings?"[10]
His position, indebted to the Cartesian visions that considered animals to be
mere automata, was greatly contested during the eighteenth century. For many
philosophers,[11] the behavior of some men did not differ much from some
brutes and, inversely, there were animals that behaved in a manner as intel-
ligent or more so than humans did.[12] David Hume, for example, granted them
the capacity of experimental reasoning, whereas Charles Bonnet, in his *Contemplation of Nature*, insisted on the possible kinship between men and the higher
apes.[13] Neither was sympathy an exclusively human prerogative. One of the
examples discussed by Addison in the pages of *The Spectator* consisted of cutting open a pregnant dog and taking some of the puppies out of her womb
while she was still alive. When introduced to a puppy, the mother began to lick
it, forgetting her own pain in favor of her instinct. According to testimonies, if
the puppy was taken away, the mother cried more at the loss of her little one
than for her own injuries.[14]

In its simplest and most idealized form, whether in punitive practices, on
the political stage, in aesthetic theory, in moral discourse, or in debates on the
souls of beasts, the experience of harm was built on an asymmetry between
the one who suffers and the one who watches.[15] On this everyone agreed. Both
for Rousseau – who conceived of piety as an instinct prior to all reflection and

philosophy – and for Hume – who defined fellow-feeling as the impression that the presence of another's suffering causes in our body – the world was divided, ideally at least, between the animal that suffers and the animal that watches.[16] In this we have not changed at all. Then, as now, our understanding of harm depends on this crude cartography of misery that divides humanity into those who consume pain and those who are consumed by it. The Enlightenment attributed differentiated features and defined characteristics to both groups; it placed the spectator and the actor, the audience and the victim, in an ideal space from which to describe their peculiarities and comprehend their mutual relations.

Unlike the imitator, whose pain slips away in the mimetic interpretation of its iconic model, we, the observers, do not experience harm in accordance with the logic of similarity, but of spectacle. We do not confront a universal form of suffering, but a particular event that does not affect us directly. Either through some technological means that open up a physical distance, or because the misfortune takes place in conditions alien to our own emotional situation, the adversity does not concern us. Before even knowing whether we can somehow contribute to find a remedy to the disgrace of others, we take up an intermediate space that allows us to see without being seen and judge without being judged. Our goal is not only to observe and consent, but also to value and discern. The misfortune, which does not have an exemplary or retributive character, confronts us with an isolated fact which may, however, be successively produced and reproduced. The spectacle demands our attention with a cry of "come and see," like in the circus. The accusation or reparation that follows the contemplation of the disgraceful fate of others is built, initially at least, on the logic of obscenity.

The victim, on the other hand, not only feels, he also feels observed. Far from the instinctive responses of the animal kingdom, his suffering is configured in accordance with our expectations and judgments. It does not matter that we, the spectator, remain hidden in the shadows; he knows we are there; behind the spotlight and further beyond, in the depths of his heart, within his breast.[17] Even in solitude, the person principally affected cannot feel or express himself outside of the rules and prerogatives of the scenic arts. This does not mean that his pain is feigned, but that only through this interpretative logic can he feel it *as pain*, as a culturally meaningful sensation that qualifies as precisely that. Given that sympathy and theatricality are mutually implicated, experience is configured once more in accordance with the principles of performative representation. On the one hand, the spectator can, against all logic, experience the sensations of another, enter into the body of another, and somehow be one being with him or her. On the other hand, the victim also modulates his or her experiences in accordance with outside evaluations and expectations. His way of feeling is not only natural, but also learned.

This shuffling back and forth in which the immediate sensations of some are related to the mediated sensations of others does not allow us to establish differences between emotions and judgments. Furthermore, given that feeling is also judging, the boundary between reality and fiction becomes very unclear, and further still: utterly diffuse. On the one hand, we can sympathize with imaginary beings. On the other, we can also ignore the suffering of real victims under the cover of their situation's dramatic qualities. Real pain can seem fictitious to us, and fictitious suffering may seem real. In the twenty-first century, we know a great deal about the theatricalized ways in which tragedy is informed or enjoyed. The contemporary experience of pain takes place on this imaginary stage surrounded by observers and sitters who enter and leave their bodies, shedding real tears for the death of imaginary beings or, on the contrary, selfishly confusing life with theater.

This is not the only conclusion of this dramatic circumstance. As we shall see below, sympathy also concerns the topology of distance, the qualitative forms of comparing more and less. Sympathy establishes scales, even before we can determine the empirical conditions of measurement. With regard to the relationship between observer and victim, ideas of contiguity or similarity combine with notions of distance and proximity. For David Hume, for example, family, tribal or national ties strengthen the relationship between their members such that peers of the same group hurt and feel for one other to a greater extent than they do for outsiders. Given that the closer the physical, emotional, historical, or cultural distance between the observer and the victim, the stronger the emotion will be, and moral feelings should contemplate the possibility of establishing a corrective procedure to reach a general agreement on the dissimilar emotions of others. In a recent text, Fonna Forman-Barzilai describes sympathy as a dramatic (i.e. theatrical) activity.[18] And she is not mistaken. The staging of mutual sensitivity configures an emotional topology in which the observer occupies an intermediate space that, neither too far nor too close to the victim, determines the structure that, from the eighteenth century onward, has been used to contemplate human tragedies.

Public sensibility

In his 1764 treatise *On Crimes and Punishments*, Cesare Beccaria [1738–1794] described pleasure and pain as the driving forces of all sensitive beings. Although this Italian philosopher accepted that human actions depended on physiological conditions, he refused to accept the determinist implications that emerged from the new "physics of the soul" proliferating in Europe at the time. Should the will be governed by the passions, he argued, we would have to postulate a sensibility that could serve as tegument of social stability. Far from vindicating self-indulgence, human nature opened the doors on a new social space governed by collective sentiments and not by personal passions.[19] His treatise, which initially proposed to disrupt the use of force in judicial practices, widened its scope until it came to include the most important subjects of Enlightenment philosophy. The search for well-being and progress led to the desire to increase the happiness of as many people as possible. In this it had much in common with some of the considerations of the *Preliminary Discourse*, a text that the mathematician Jean d'Alembert wrote as an introduction to Diderot's *Encyclopedia* in 1751 and which openly recognized that the ultimate reason for the search for knowledge was the need to preserve the body from pain and death.[20]

Born on 15 March 1738, Beccaria was the youngest son of a prominent Milan aristocratic family. His studies in philosophy began with reading the great luminaries of the French Enlightenment. The works of Montesquieu, Diderot, Helvetius, d'Holbach, or Voltaire pushed the young man toward the philosophy of the *salonnière*, which predominated in Parisian philosophical circles. A year before the publication of *On Crimes and Punishments* – the text that made him truly famous – Beccaria's cousin, Pietro Verri, had published his *Meditations on Happiness* in which this promoter of the Italian Enlightenment circle known as the *Society of the Fist* maintained that the search for well-being depended on a rational fight against the impediments to pleasure. It is quite probable that Beccaria became interested in the works of the Enlightenment through the society's periodic meetings, and that he then first conceived of writing a treatise against torture, like those that were appearing elsewhere in Europe. The second of the Verri brothers, for example, had also published a brief text denouncing the use of pain as tool to produce confessions under interrogation. Following the publication of *On Crimes*, the mathematician d'Alembert prepared a French edition of the work, which appeared in 1766. Voltaire published a commentary on the book and the Empress Catherine II asked Beccaria to contribute to the reform of the Russian legal system. In Spain, the first translation of Beccaria's work was by Juan Antonio de Casas in 1774. His version of the text gave way to the *Treatise against Torture* written by the Enlightenment writer Juan Pablo Forner in 1793.[21] In the German States, Frederick II also undertook a radical reform of penal law. Given that the aim of punishment was no longer to torment the criminal, but rather to make an example of him, it was even suggested that the prisoner secretly be strangled before being tortured.[22]

Beccaria's treatise took off from the prior assumption that it was not only the convict who suffered the agony of the body, but also whoever was observing the application of the punishment. For this reason, the pain should be administered using criteria, of a rigorously economic nature, related to public sensibility rather than to the magnitude of the crime. The intensity of the torment ought to be regulated through the impression that the scene produced in the imagination of the witnesses, without depending at any point on the convict's gestures or signs of suffering. The sentence had to produce "the most efficient and lasting impression in the minds of the men with the least possible torment to the body of the condemned person."[23] If this were not the case, that is, if the administration of justice were to take place in private or in secret, or if the pain were out of proportion with the goal of the punishment – which should never be revenge, but rather the prevention of the crime – we would be faced with an act of flagrant violence, injustice and tyranny. Whether through Hume's concept of emotional contagion, through the counter-blow described by Malebranche, or through the natural instinct of compassion designated by Rousseau, only by means of a vindication of mutual sensibility could Beccaria suggest that the intensity of the punishment had to depend on an emotional agreement between those who, farther from the gallows, could not feel the cuts or blows upon their own flesh.

Beccaria's proposal is not without difficulties. To begin with, the book never explains how the witnesses manage to experience sensations at a distance. It does not tell us either how the impression that the scene of torture produces on the public can be accepted as a measurement of the pain required for the administration of the penalty. Although the relationship between the crime and the punishment may have been established with a mathematical precision, there is no indication of how such a measurement is to be provided. Neither does Beccaria reveal the physiological mechanism through which we might vindicate compassion, *Mitleid*. The treatise does not offer any notion of measurement and tells us nothing regarding the possibility of collective pains. The speed of the judicial process may imply that the punishment suited the crime or the pain suited the offense, like the effect and the cause – in such a way that there can be no doubt regarding the juridical and physical necessity of the law – but Beccaria never says how to establish a relationship between the crime and the punishment using an unspecific proportion between the passion of the condemned criminal and the compassion of the impartial spectator. The paradox is even more noticeable when we realize that, for this Milanese aristocrat, civil society rested on an imaginary agreement regarding the collective capacity of suffering from a pain which cannot be strictly felt. Perhaps his silence was deliberate. After all, his treatise never intended to contribute to the development of anatomy or natural philosophy. Neither was it a treatise on the universality of sensations or moral sentiments. What we do find on reading it, however, is a conceptual clarification of the kind of problems we are confronting here. In the first instance, the reform of the penal system implied the establishing of a functional correspondence between a type of experience (in principle private) and a kind of sensibility (in principle public). In the second place, we need to know how we could experience pain at a distance. More importantly for our purposes, we should be able to determine to what degree the response of the audience in the face of the deliberate infliction of pain can be established as an indicator of the intensity of corporal punishment that should be applied to the criminal.

The appearance of what the historian Michael Ignatieff so aptly called "the just measure of pain" has been explained by a wide variety of arguments.[24] On the one hand, the new social reforms, while attempting to liberate citizens from the disproportionate sufferings of the past, triggered a progressive reduction of judicial procedures that involved a disproportionate production of pain. The garrote, the noose, burning at the stake, stoning, or the wheel gave way to much more refined punitive systems. The scenes of immense brutality that had accompanied the judicial executions or interrogations during the Middle Ages or the early modern period were gradually replaced by coercive measures or less brutal punitive practices. Rejecting the extensive use of muscular articulations, sensory receptors, and innervated tissues during judicial interrogations, the Enlightenment endeavored to force confessions "without pain or chains."[25] Likewise, techniques of confinement began to be linked with both productive and educational criteria. This decline of physical violence took place at the same time that philosophers began to call into question cruelty to animals, slaves, the insane, children, or the destitute.[26] Following this line of reasoning, so often denied by the facts, the scenes of immense brutality that accompanied judicial executions and interrogations began to disappear from the public scene at the heart of an increasingly enlightened society.[27]

Other historians have also debated whether the reform of the penal system that began in the seventeenth century and gave rise to new penitentiary institutions was merely a more effective form of political coercion. From the standpoint of the influential text written by the French historian and philosopher Michel Foucault, between the end of the eighteenth and the beginning of the nineteenth centuries there was no restriction in the art of punishment, but rather a transition from the punishment of the body to the oppression of the spirit. The book in which Foucault proposed these ideas – *Discipline and Punish* – begins with a long quote describing the 1757 execution of a man accused of attempted regicide. Damiens, as was his name, was condemned to be dismembered by four horses tied to his legs and arms. But Foucault was not interested in the obscene repetition of corporal punishment, but rather in its transformation into new social policies, which would lead to the "birth of the prison." Only a few pages after his detailed description, Foucault quotes a code from 1838 defining the prison system and, by extension, regulating and restricting the behavior of prisoners. The superimposition of these two texts could not be more dramatic: first the punishing of the body, then the loss of freedom, the enforcement of labor, and the regulation of behavior. In both cases, personal identity is replaced by the mark of political power, but the second form of punishment implies a greater capacity for social control and does not suggest, as the first does, the need to maintain the law's predominance through the abuse of force.

There are various reasons that make this interpretation unsatisfactory. In the first place, the birth of the prison and the formation of the new penitentiary system did not take place at the same time in different regions of Europe. Historical evidence does not allow elimination of the dissimilar pace at which the system of corporal punishment was replaced by a form of political coercion based on the deprivation of freedom. In the second place, the regulation of the penitentiary system and, consequently, the replacement of the spectacle of suffering with the solitude of the cell, forced labor, and the silence of the prison are part of a process that Foucault does not explain but merely describes. The French historian shows us two successive ways to confront crime in the early modern period, without providing the reasons that caused one scene to follow another.[28] On the one hand, we have the brutality of the *Ancien Régime*; on the other, the penitentiary system. What we miss is the nexus that connects both events and, if possible, explains them in the context of their own historical development. If what differentiates the penal system in the *Ancien* and the New Regime is the object of execution itself – the body in the first case and the soul in the second – then what we lack is the connection between the body and the soul; that is, as long as we are not willing to argue that these punishments are not mutually exclusive and that the merciless use of violence or the police regulation of conduct does not imply, in either case, losses of moral identity or corporal dignity. Perhaps after all the dichotomy between the punishing of the body and the suffering of the soul is supported by a false dualism that does not understand, for example, that the mutilation and the exposure of the body is already a punishment for the soul and, likewise, that the very restriction of movements defined by the prison system brings with it a significant amount of pain for the body. The disdain that this archeology – Foucault's particular historiography – shows for a history built on terms of origins and causes is very well known. It begs the question, however, whether the elimination of a causal connection also allows for dispensing with any attempt at historical explanation. Even more so when, curiously, Foucault explicitly denies the most plausible reading: that penal reform is inscribed within the new culture of sensibility.[29] In this case, as we will see below, what is at stake is not a dichotomy between the body and the soul, but between the private and the public. The restriction of punitive practices produced not just a variation in the object on which violence was inscribed, but also in the punishment's intention. To put it another way: repression no longer aspired to political control through an abuse of force, but rather to the sustaining of a social pact through the education of the citizenry. Given that the safest but also the most complicated way of preventing crime was by improving education, punishment could no longer be tied just to the body of the criminal, but mainly to the imagination of the witnesses.[30]

Along the lines of this last interpretation, we could inscribe the transformation of the penal system adhered to by Beccaria within the context of the process of civilization described by the German sociologist Norbert Elias. In this case, we would have to explain the emergence and consolidation of a form of sensibility which was expressed primarily by means of self-repressive behaviors:[31] an internalization of the norm which allowed citizens to establish nexuses of identification with their peers rather than forms of subjection to the Absolute State.[32] Although Elias' sources were etiquette books, the references to this new moral economy of the body may be very easily multiplied. They range from the care of the body to treatises on anatomy. Given that "we were born for one another," as wrote the naturalist Andry in his *Orthopédie* of 1741, "we should avoid possessing features that may surprise or cause rejection among our fellows."[33] While beggars were prohibited from showing their malformations at the doors of churches,[34] the use of makeup spread as a means of concealment more than a way to accentuate beauty.[35] In a world usually described as a mass of more or less physically deformed individuals, the covering up of signs of illness became a requirement for sociability. Physical disproportion and moral vice should be hidden by means of a coercive behavior, by a norm of aesthetic and ethical decorum. Consider, for example, the social death that accompanied Madame de Merteuil – the protagonist, along with Viscount Valmont, of *Dangerous Liaisons*. At the end of the novel, her enemies are unsure whether to favor the indignation that her behavior deserves or to succumb to the pity inspired by her state. She has not only lost an eye, but, as a result of smallpox, her sinister figure serves as the most visible result of the decomposition of her soul.[36] Her flight to Holland constitutes yet another sign of concealment from someone who, in a simple *tour de tête*, has simultaneously lost her elegance, her distinction, and her presence.

In the new culture of sensibility, the signs of pain must avoid any excess of expressivity. The norm that regulates conduct no longer needs to come from the State; on the contrary, civility, understood as an internalization of the law, denies the private character of our human nature and its functions. Distinction and decorum take on a more dramatic tenor in the absence of features or attitudes that leave much to be done or much to be said. What Castiglione had called *sprezzatura*, a kind of dissimulation in the face of the limits of human nature, a concealment of the bodily needs and, consequently, an appearance of social lightheartedness, became more widespread. Public life rested on marks of distinction able to hide the body's anatomy and organic functions. The philosopher David Hume, for example, states that when the wife of Carlos III was presented with some gloves and tights, her butler replied haughtily: "You should know, Sir, that a queen of Spain has no legs."[37] In *Traité de l'Education des Filles*, the French writer Fénelon [1651–1715] had also proposed a policy for restricting expressiveness. Woman should be silent, submissive, economical and fertile.[38] Almost 100 years later, Adam Smith insisted on the same idea:

> we are disgusted with the clamorous grief, which, without any delicacy, calls upon our compassion with sighs and tears and importune lamentations. But we reverence that reserved, that silent and majestic sorrow, which discovers itself only in the swelling of the eyes, in the quivering of the lips and cheeks, and in the distant, but affecting, coldness of the whole behavior.[39]

Very far from a politics of compassion, sympathy requires a well-apprehended and internalized norm through which the victim could step outside of herself, contemplate her situation as an impartial observer would, and accept that to sink under the weight of pain and despondency will always seem in some way mean and despicable;[40] thus "as nature teaches the spectators to assume the circumstances of the persons principally concerned, so that she teaches this last to assume those of the spectators, so as to be able to evaluate their situation in this candid and impartial light."[41] We can never establish any judgment about our feelings unless we displace ourselves and try to focus on them from a certain distance, that is, as long as we examine our own behavior "as we think any other fair and impartial spectator would do."[42] While mutual company gives human beings a mirror allowing them to comprehend the propriety or impropriety of their own passions, the beauty or ugliness of their ideas, social sympathy consists of a splitting up by which "I divide myself into two persons; the I, the examiner and judge represents a different character from that other I, the person whose conduct is examined into and judged of."[43] Social harmony depends on an emotional pact through which these two groups of human beings, those who suffer and those who watch, can reach agreements. The unequal distribution of pain produces a problem that is at once moral, political, and aesthetic. On the one hand, the observer takes on the circumstances of the protagonists and identifies with them as far as possible; in other words, he or she appropriates them. On the other hand, the person principally affected internalizes the position of the spectator, seeking that their expressions be in concordance not with the cause that generates them, but rather with the disinterested perspective of an impartial judge. This is why the virtues of sensitivity agree with the requirements of (self-) restraint.

The control of passions makes possible a philosophy of decorum and, consequently, a standard of conduct derived from the restriction and limitation of gestures. At the same time that death, mourning, illness, deformation, or violence were expelled from public places, punishment was also subjected to this new courtesy toward the pain of the condemned person and, above all, to the sensibility of the witnesses. The three old companions of Western culture – pain, sexuality, and death – disappeared from the new spaces created for the enjoyment of the new urban bourgeoisie. This is the part of the argument that was taken up by Elias' disciple, the Dutch historian Pieter Spierenburg, with regard to the birth of the prison.[44] Given that the cruelty of punishment that had prevailed during the Renaissance depended on unstable and uncertain political organization, as greater levels of control over the population were achieved the spectacle of violence could become dispensable. As the distance between physical pain and moral suffering decreased, the space that separated the private and the public widened; or, better yet, the capacity of experiencing sensations from a distance or of showing emotions without cause was expanded. The measurement of pain did not rest as much on its physiological seat as it did on an inter-sensory and, more strictly, an inter-subjective notion.[45] Given that harm was no longer the intrinsic goal of punishment, but rather an instrument of political education, punishment should produce a longer-lasting impression in the imagination of the witnesses by means of the minimum use of violence on the body of the condemned criminal. As Spierenburg explains, "the death and suffering of fellow human beings were increasingly experienced as painful, just because other people were increasingly perceived as fellow human beings."[46]

One of the elements of the new culture of sensibility was consolidated through the emotional reaction generated by the reading of novels. Authors like Samuel Richardson in England or Jean-Jacques Rousseau in France benefited from the ways in which their readers identified with the protagonists of their imaginary worlds. Submerged in an altered state of consciousness, the reader found pleasure in this form of identification with these literary victims.[47] Not for nothing has the rise of the novel been placed in relation to the appearance of a form of literary realism that shares with moral philosophy its interest in the same human experiences.[48] The examples that appear in the treatises of moral philosophy reappear in the *The Spectator* by Joseph Addison, fill the pages of Henry Fielding's novels, and shape the masses in Hogarth's engravings. Sympathy, which affected all social strata, was particularly cast toward criminals, slaves, children, and animals. Whether in the theater, in poetry, in painting, in opera, or in the novel, virtue was revealed through the public expression of private emotions.[49] From a narrative point of view, the literary genre termed *factual fiction*, or literary realism, rested on the proliferation of diaries and novels which, written in the epistolary genre, made possible the readers' identification with the victims, to the extent that they could adopt the position of the other "with all its minutest incidents."[50] Sociability was interpreted as a sentiment aimed at the suffering and pain of others. "What is generosity, clemency, humanity, if not pity applied to the weak, the guilty or the human race in general?" wrote Rousseau in his *Discourse on the Origin and Basis of Inequality among Men*.[51] Benevolence, or, in its most refined form, philanthropy, became one of the new pleasures of the nascent bourgeoisie.[52] The *sensorium comune* was transformed; not into an anatomical position of the physiological body, but rather into a space of association of the body politic. The *locus affectis* that receives and combines sensations did not form a part of the brain, but was located instead at the very nucleus of civil society. Common sense – which Thomas Paine [1737–1809] wrote about in one of the great pamphlets of the American Revolution – went further than the brain and the nervous system and reached the imaginary tissues of the physiology of the body politic.

It is true that the connection between the culture of sensibility and the reform of the penal system has a significant number of historical refutations. To begin with, this period that called for social sympathy, sensitivity, and compassion also saw, within the context of what the French historian Labrousse called "the history of resistances," a considerable increase in public executions.[53] The events of the end of the century would suffice to call into question a progressive elimination of the public spectacle of capital punishment. The point I want to emphasize here, however, is that beginning in 1750, the measure of pain no longer depended on any connection between stimulus and response.[54] On the contrary, the constant correlation between crimes and punishments could only be established through the appeal to vicarious pains, for, as Beccaria defends, "as souls soften, sensitivity grows, and as this occurs, the severity of the punishment will have to decrease for the relation between the object and the sensation to remain constant."[55] Examining further the equation between private punishment and public response, Beccaria eliminates the causal connection between the lesion inflicted upon the body and the way the sensation is presented to the spirit. The minimum pain necessary that is inflicted on the criminal has nothing to do with the perception of pain, but with the moral disposition of the witnesses and, finally, with their capacity to experience sensations at a distance.

By placing the emphasis on the public character of private suffering, Beccaria has modified the object of torment's application, which can no longer be the body nor, as Foucault argued, the soul of the condemned criminal, but exclusively the imagination of the witnesses. For this reason, the observer's response can provide a constant measurement of the violence that should be administered to the criminal. Given that education has taken the place of vengeance, pain can no longer be regarded as a private event, but as a public and vicarious sensation. The fact that we ignore how to assign values to the terms of this equation does not call into question the permanent nature of its proportionality. On the contrary, this constant is the only element of judgment that permits us to establish a relationship between private pain and public sensibility.

Counterfactual pain

Beccaria was not the first to assert that civil society was based on public sympathy toward private pain. The study of the connection between one's own sensations and the emotions of others can be found in two great works from the end of the 1750s: the *Theory of Moral Sentiments* by the Scottish philosopher Adam Smith [1723–1790] and the *Philosophical Inquiry into the Origin of our Ideas of the Sublime and the Beautiful* by the Irish thinker Edmund Burke [1729–1797]. Although these authors have passed into history for contributing to the consolidation of two new fields of research, the almost unanimous agreement that connects their works to political economics or empirical aesthetics should not prevent us from considering their works from a different perspective. To begin with, both philosophers aspired to establish universally applicable rules and norms in such elusive areas as aesthetic judgments and moral sentiments. Of no less importance, their investigations rest upon pain as the cornerstone on which to defend a logic of taste or a moral theory freed from personal circumstances or intimate desires. In both political theory and the philosophy of art, the emphasis falls upon an observer capable of recognizing him- or herself in the actors of the theater, the protagonists of novels, or in the condemned upon the gallows. The Enlightenment, which did not invent voyeurism, nonetheless theorized like never before on the figure of the critic, the public, the reader, or the chronicler.

The historian Lynn Hunt is right to connect the invention of human rights with the cultural processes of empathic identification that proliferated during the second half of the eighteenth century.[56] Many of these processes are framed within a "politics of pity:" the result of compassion toward the wretched of the world, understood *en masse*, with no distinction among them and with no reference to the reason that initially turned them into victims. She is wrong, however, to consider that the impartiality of the observer – with which moral theory, empirical psychology, and also political philosophy are concerned – depends only on identification or mimesis. In the works of Burke or Smith, sympathy is not given under the form of empathy or emotional contagion, but through an imagination that is at the same time performative and reflexive. The observer not only dreams, but also judges; she does not only look, but also determines the propriety or impropriety of the conduct of others. More important still, she does not only reflexively identify with what she sees, but also with what might have happened, or with that which, against all evidence, cannot happen nor will ever happen. It is only through this fantasy that mimesis is transformed into a potentially universal and virtually just emotion; only in this counterfactual way of experiencing the pain of others can the observer reach sufficient distance to construct a universal position – one that is just in its evaluation and general in its sphere of application.

Unlike a politics of pity, based on immediate identification with the person who suffers, the "politics of justice" cannot do without the enunciation of tragedy. Here, observation is linked to verbal expression because the observer is not there only to look, but also to report. The observer's expository capacity transcends his/her (subjective) emotion and explains his/her (objective) desire to provide a historical record. In his detailed study of distant suffering, the sociologist Luc Boltanski identifies three expository forms that, with all their historical variations, serve to account for the spectacle of violence. The first two, he tells us, may take the form of accusation or philanthropy. The first, accusation, stems from the idea, as old as humanity itself, that it is easier to construct a moral system when an agreement is reached as to who is directly responsible for the evil being denounced. In this case, the observer not only looks on but also condemns. In the second, on the other hand, where sympathy toward benefactors is greater than hatred toward executioners, the action is directed toward philanthropy rather than toward revenge. Although the Enlightenment considered both strategies, the critique of sentimentality and the denunciation of resentment have no place there. The history of sentimentalism forms part of Victorian culture, whereas resentment – linked not so much to the imputation that the philosopher Nietzsche aimed at Christianity, but rather to the history of political action – was during the eighteenth century only beginning to be written.

There is a final possibility, however. In this third *aesthetic form*, the observer cannot be drawn toward denouncement nor does s/he succumb to sentimentality. On the contrary, s/he keeps his/her gaze steady in the face of horror and does not blink in the face of truth.[57] In the world in which we live, nothing seems stranger than this connection between what we call today the sphere of aesthetics and the world of politics. In the eighteenth century, however, the relationship between both of these elements was not merely episodic. It came from a concept of justice that, defined as an individual virtue rather than a system of laws, was based on a gaze that was not located in a specific place, that had no point of reference or perspective, and that, therefore, could at least in principle be universal, objective, and disinterested.[58] The works of Beccaria, Smith, or Burke sought a way to go beyond one's own perspective so as to acquire a universal norm related to the application of law, the acceptance of virtue, or the recognition of beauty. We are no longer dealing, as we saw in Chapter 1, with the construction of an ideal model – for in this case the forms of objectivizing pain have nothing to do with the production of an archetype – but with the agreement or disagreement of our affections. In the absence of a mechanical procedure to clarify the validity of our judgments or the justice of our sentiments, the Enlightenment, using the homogeneity of the physiological constitution of human beings as a point of departure, establishes a topology, a parceling out of the moral ground and of the logic of taste. This division is inexorably accompanied by an imaginative exercise through which we cannot only put ourselves in the place of another, but in the place of *any* other who is not tied to us in any way and with whom we feel no relationship at all. In the most extreme case, which was the basis of both Smith's and Burke's work, it is necessary to imagine a (non-existent) context with which to clarify the virtue of our feelings or the validity of our judgments.

None of this is present in the politics of pity. Its forms of social sensibilization or moralization, responsible for the creation of emotional communities, do not permit the identification with a third party that, against all logic, has not been the victim of any tragedy. Neither do these forms permit sympathy toward a suffering that might have happened but that, against all evidence, has not occurred nor ever will occur. Whereas compassion feeds on what it sees, sympathy pertaining to moral sentiments and aesthetic judgments requires the imaginary representation of a strange and distant scene – from a physical, emotional, and cognitive point of view. The impartial observer, the figure that governs this semi-fiction, is based upon the maximum distancing and the maximum disproportion, as only through this loss of scale can a general model be constructed that permits the establishment of a logic of taste and a jurisprudence of passions. The legacy of this counterfactual pain is manifest nowadays in all the forms of tragedy's enunciation: from journalistic visualization to cinematographic culture. You, who missed the plane that just crashed, how do you feel? You, who did not go to work the day your colleagues were blown up, what can you tell us? However, the loss of references between what is really lived and what is merely imagined is not a prerogative of the twenty-first century, but rather a consequence of the theatricality of harmful experience. This harmful experience, in turn, stems from a single source: an imagination capable of depicting the absent, that which might have happened but has never occurred. This dramatization owes a great deal to this form of altered experience through which, far from feeling sorry for victims and far from using their pain to encourage our own feeling of security, we build a supposedly universal scale that permits the aesthetic and ethical evaluation of the experience of harm.

The construction of this experience stems from a demand for impartiality that extends to human actions as a whole. We should look without interfering, analyze without meddling, let nature operate without modifying its effects. As observers, we may be more or less attentive, but like the astronomer who contemplates the spectacle of the Universe from a distance, nothing binds us to what we are looking at. Given that our passing through misfortune is caused by chance circumstances, our activity should not and cannot be governed by the logic of necessity. Unlike the martyr, whose function is to serve as a witness, we, as spectators, do not participate directly in the drama of experience; we do not form part of any family or emotional community; we are invisible, impartial, independent, free, and, above all, disinterested, neutral. Suffering and pain do not affect or concern us. Nothing connects us in any way to the spectacle of violence. As in the chronicles of *The Spectator*, which frequently begin with the story of someone who was just passing by, who happened to be there and, by the same principle, who easily could not have been, the figure of the observer is built upon the chimera of our concealment. Our cultural legacy, which can no longer do without this symbolic imagining or without the emotive characteristics of the fourth wall, has not only made the public a protagonist, it has also made it a privileged element of the cartography of tragedy.[59]

The distance that separates the observer from the victim also has implications for the latter. If the former behaves like a Newtonian astronomer who can only contemplate the universe without interfering in its processes, the victim also seems to act as though there were no audience. Both in the real world and its fictional counterpart, feelings do not seem to be mediated by technique nor manipulated by rhetorical artifices. In epistolary novels, for instance, the fabrication maximizes immediacy so that the reader may believe themselves to be the direct recipient of the letters written by the characters. Reading takes them to an imaginary space where they can strengthen their social ties.[60] The author vanishes, leaving the impression that the spectacle has no intermediaries. Those who write, who speak, *are speaking to me*, *writing to me*, the reader seems to say. Likewise, in visual art, the artist seems to capture the absent gaze and involuntary gesture of someone who acts as though they were not being observed. The sitter transmits a false sensation of intimacy with the conviction that his or her acts are being carried out behind closed doors and without the presence of witnesses. Absorbed in his or her solitude, the sitter's comedy requires the maximum concentration. Diderot's writing on art stresses the same idea. For the editor of the *Encyclopédie*, actors, like artist's models, should act as though no one can see them, given that "although a dramatic work is written to be acted, both the author and the actor should forget the spectator."[61]

The constitution of an agreement between different persons requires the staging of a projective imagination that not only imitates the gestures of those who accompany us, but can also be triggered in the absence of direct facial knowledge.[62] Smith's work would not have come to be a short treatise of what we call today "empirical psychology" were it not for the fact that it does not limit its scope of application to face-to-face contact, but endeavors to clarify the terms and conditions of an emotional agreement between observers and victims who have never met or seen each other. This simulation, which transcends the narrow frontiers of the present situation, permits the establishment of a judgment on the propriety or impropriety of another's passions and, therefore, also permits the reaching of universal agreements on moral sentiments and aesthetic judgments. For what principles regulate the logic of taste other than those that affect the imagination? And what is the imagination if not the capacity to represent images of things at will, whether in the manner and the order that they were received by the senses or combined in a new way and in a different order?

Both Smith's and Burke's works were written a little after the execution of Damiens in 1757, but neither of them dwells on the minor context of punitive practices. The reason for this is simple enough. Even though the Enlightenment public participated less and less in penal violence, the scene of the gallows was still too close to the spectator. Neither did the abolition of torture that spread throughout Europe allow the enunciation of a universal form of distant suffering for it is one thing to internalize juridical norms, and quite another to understand the ways in which the law becomes a means of regulating conflicts or, as Foucault put it, a "ritual form of war."[63] The equation anticipated by Beccaria between the pain of the condemned criminal and the sensibility of the public should be valid, but its proportions cannot be resolved within the transformation of punitive practices. In *A Vindication of Natural Society* – a pamphlet published in 1757 – Edmund Burke had also shown himself to be in favor of eliminating any manifestation of positive pain. His ideas were taken up again in England by the utilitarian philosopher Jeremy Bentham [1748–1832], who proposed a modification of the penitentiary institution in accordance with economic criteria. Given that the purpose of punishment was no longer revenge but the prevention of crime, the sentence should become longer rather than more intense. The new economy of pain began, undoubtedly, with the way in which the men and women of the *Ancien Régime* began to look on convicts as their "fellowmen" or even as their "equals" – with the same passions, feelings, affections, and organs – but this egalitarian policy was not followed by the proposed reform in either the purpose or the goal of the punishment. The modification of the punitive system required a broader agreement on suffering at a distance; an agreement that should include both the theory of art and the regulation of moral sentiments. Once established that the punishment should not be directed to the body but to the imagination of the witnesses, as Beccaria suggested, any reform of the legal system should set up the ideal conditions under which persons affected differently could reach agreements on their unequal emotional sensations and affections.

For the politics of justice to replace the politics of pity, the contemplation of immediate tragedy had to give way to the representation of universal disasters. The victims no longer matter! Neither face-to-face pain, nor emotional contagion, nor imitative logic was sufficient. The logic of taste and the theory of justice required the constitution of a new intermediate space for those who watch, and not just for those who suffer. As observers, we should distance ourselves from all community ties and all spurious interests. We must begin by turning our eyes toward the strange underworld of global disaster, not only because of the disproportionate nature of all natural catastrophes, but also because of the infinite distance that all apocalyptic representations entail. As opposed to the affection that is shown here and now – either as a result of illness, punishment, or war – universal catastrophe is expressed as a conglomerate of experiences, like a visual painting capable of capturing the entire history of human suffering in a single instant. Contemplation of the catastrophe amplifies the sensation of distance or, to use Burke's own definition, of "astonishment without danger." In this it is similar to other forms of the theatricality of harm. No matter how "exquisite" the evils that affect us directly are, what makes them unbearable – and for this reason also worthy of merit – is their anticipation of other even more extreme sufferings. Only from a distance, through an imaginary projection toward possible circumstances and accidents sensed beforehand, can we turn illness or defeat into an object of fear or delight.

Along with distancing, the observer must lead his or her imagination toward the radical absence of logic and measurement. This space where the dead exist alongside the living, where all moral rules have been broken, and where all logic is suspended, is no longer hell – or the forest, desert, or sea – but rather the naturalized version of the inferno: the natural catastrophe still described in the eighteenth century, or even in the twenty-first, in apocalyptic terms. As surprising and unexpected events, these "visitations" – for this was the name by which they were known – interrupted the rationality of the Enlightenment just as monsters had done in the Renaissance. The emphasis could fall on the immorality of the damned or on their logical and just deserving fate, but the episode as a whole questioned, above all, the regularity of nature and its processes. For some, like Mandeville or Hobbes – like Lucretius' spectator who contemplates a shipwreck from the tranquility of the shore – the misfortune of others bolsters our own sensation of safety. Visualizing the ills of others strengthens our position, and reaffirms our (false) conviction of the firmness of the ground on which we stand. For Adam Smith or for Burke, on the other hand, the contemplation of misfortune never had the purpose of increasing our feeling of safety, but rather of acquiring the rule that permits us to evaluate and judge the passions and emotions of others. In the same way that the contemplation of beauty guarantees the perpetuation of our species, delight in the face of misfortune also contributes to the maintaining of our social order.

Both the *Theory of Moral Sentiments* and *The Philosophical Investigations* share with some other Enlightenment books an interest for the way in which natural catastrophes should be faced and understood. Each one of them, which appeared shortly after the Lisbon earthquake of 1755, reflects on this tremendous disaster. They do not do so, however, in the usual way. Our philosophers do not discuss the rational circumstances of a phenomenon that called into question blind faith in optimism. They do not, as did Voltaire, for example, take pleasure in the fact that the earthquake took the lives of a number of inquisitors, nor do they argue, like Rousseau, that the magnitude of the misfortune was due to the abusive effects of civilization and progress. The emphasis is neither on the dead nor the injured, but on the rules that govern the imagination of those that, from the most distant and remote corners of Europe, purchased the images and listened to the testimonies, converting the pain of others into a bottomless source of consumption.

The earthquakes in Sicily in 1693, Lima in 1746, or Port-au-Prince in 1751 were still fresh in the memory when some 60,000 of the 250,000 people living in the capital city of Portugal lost their lives. Some perished crushed beneath the churches where they had congregated to celebrate All Saints Day. Others drowned. Fires devastated the city for the following five days. The effects of the tidal wave that accompanied the tremor led to floods in Morocco and the coasts of Cadiz and Huelva in Spain, and caused the flooding of the Guadalquivir River as it passed through Seville.[64] It was not the first time that the Enlightenment would confront catastrophe. In 1720, the plague annihilated the population of Marseilles and, on a much larger scale, 10,000,000 people died in 1770 during the famine that devastated Bengal.[65] After Lisbon, it seemed evident that danger did not only come from the Orient, nor was nature only wild in the virgin territories of the Americas. On the contrary, the magnitude of the tragedy questioned the uniformity of natural processes on all fronts. "The city that had ceased to exist," to use an expression from the time, not only had the third busiest port in Europe, it was also the capital of an Empire that extended as far as Brazil and Paraguay, Mozambique, and Angola, as well as the cities of Macao and Malacca. Inheritors of an inveterate tradition of explorers and conquistadors, linked to merchant traffic but also to the slave trade, port business, and the Catholic religion, Lisbon's catastrophe was unparalleled and, to a certain extent, unprecedented. Not even the fire that destroyed London in 1666 could compete in the magnitude of the devastation.[66] The capital of the cartographers' empire had been, literally, wiped off the map. Along with perplexity, astonishment, and even incredulity in the face of the news of the earthquake, an avalanche of humanitarian aid arrived from all over Europe. Ships sailed from Hamburg and economic aid was sent from France, England, and Spain. Such compassion was not always determined by emotional contagion but also by economic interest. After all, along with the loss of human life, the earthquake caused a financial disaster with implications for many British, Spanish, and German merchants.

Unlike the application of penal law, the earthquake did not obey any retributive logic – not even a disproportionate logic like that which led to the quartering of Damiens. The earthquake's absence of necessity and its lack of prediction, which did not differentiate it from other violations of the natural or social order, led to different intellectual and emotional reactions. Historians have written accounts of many of these, especially those linked to the debates on the justification of evil, frequently forgetting that the first reaction was the desire to domesticate the sensation of novelty that accompanied the tragedy. Edmund Burke himself had begun his text with a reflection on the curiosity produced by singular events. Some years later, Adam Smith would distinguish, in his *History of Astronomy*, between the admiration incited by the unexpected, the surprise caused by the grandiose, and the wonder provoked by the novel.[67] On the other side of the Channel, Count Buffon had also begun his influential *Preliminary Discourse on Natural History* with a reflection on the way in which the study of the extraordinary contributed to the passion for knowledge. To the alleged impossibility of building a science of accidents – as Aristotle had declared in Book VI of his *Metaphysics* – the Enlightenment offered an interpretation of the unforeseen event as an instance of a natural regularity.[68] Once the symbolic character of suffering had been abandoned, the philosophers launched themselves *en masse* to account for pain without referring to the intervention of supernatural forces or hidden powers. It was not until 1760 that the Royal Society of London sought to clarify the nature of the earthquake in terms of the exclusive interaction of secondary causes. (See Figure 12).

The Lisbon earthquake was not only a devastating event, but also a propitious occasion for aesthetic contemplation and compulsive consumption. Burke's own statement that "we find a certain and not small delight in the misfortunes and pain of others" seems to sanction, aesthetically, the spectacle of blood.[69] The tragedy began to be described or depicted with all the rhetorical forms of literary exercises or iconic models, just as literature had endowed its novels with all the mechanisms required to make apparent the absence of intermediaries. Suffering at a distance was placed under the alibi of a spectacle "based on real events," whereas the "real events" were described using the rhetorical vocabulary of fabled stories.[70] As material for consumption, pain was also marked by two different forms of disproportion. On the one hand, the victims of the earthquake, who had committed no prior crime, lost in a single instant their health, their family, and their patrimony. They had been left with nothing but the internal conviction of their innocence. In this sense they were like the wise Job. On the other hand, the dimension of the tragedy produced apocalyptic reactions, ruptures in the social order and in the moral array of things: mothers abandoned their children, kings their subjects, and God his herds. For some, the earthquake was a penalty that God had inflicted on a nation of traders and speculators separated in their customs and moral precepts from the Church's commandments. For others, including among them many free-thinkers and philosophers, one had to look with disdain on any attempt to include God in understanding the suffering of Lisbon's people. One would have to end up admitting *His impotence* or *His ill will*, wrote Diderot. Impotence if He had wanted to avoid the disaster and was unable to, ill will if He had been able to avoid it and had not wanted to.[71]

Unlike these two contending positions, for Burke or Smith, sympathy did not have to point to this or to that particular accident, but to the circumstances that could have occurred or to those that would never happen. Commiseration with the dead, for example, can only be understood by means of this imaginary recreation of the emotions that we, in their circumstances, think that we might feel but which we have never felt and never will be able to feel. Compassion toward animal pain forms part of the same category. Although Smith was not, like Bentham, a clear opponent of cruelty to animals, his concept of sympathy allows us to consider it irrelevant whether or not animals feel as we do. The physiological disposition of animals is much less interesting than the (human) capacity to recreate their circumstances. In the extreme, both Smith and Burke propose an example idealizing all elements. Let us imagine, they claim, a collective misfortune, dramatic and disproportionate, that, as a matter of fact, has not taken place. Let us also imagine that the observer were the archetype of a humanitarian man. The question is: What would this man feel?[72]

Smith, who obviously knew about the Lisbon earthquake, uses a similar, but imaginary, scene that he locates in distant China. The final reason for this simulation is very simple: that which allows the establishing of a rule, the principle of all proportionality, cannot be subject to any limitation whatsoever. The pattern that should serve to establish the measurement cannot be limited by the conditions of measurement that it itself will help to strengthen. The secularized version of the measure of pain requires that we place our experience beyond any possible distance, in remote spaces and distant territories. The Orient, not the hereafter, will allow the configuration of the milestone, the scale on which to build the proportionality of sentiments and the homogeneity of affections. This is a form of imaginary recreation that would later be used by Diderot, in 1773. As opposed to the assassination of a single Mandarin, which is the example employed by the encyclopedist, it is not enough for Smith to deliberately finish the life of a single man.[73] We must imagine a massacre of apocalyptic proportions to ponder the magnitude of the catastrophe. Let us envision, he writes, that a horrible earthquake devastates China. As the humanitarian man has no family members among the dead nor friends among the injured, his distance from the disaster will be both physical and emotional. What does the tragedy mean to this imaginary and well-intentioned spectator? What might he think? What actions would he take? Smith considers that he would probably feel a deep sense of pity; that he would make numerous reflections on the precarious nature of life; that, if he were analytical, perhaps he would also enter into disquisitions on the effects on the economy or on trade. Once this beautiful philosophy and these philanthropic sentiments had been expressed, he would continue with his affairs as if nothing had happened. However, "If he was to lose his little finger tomorrow, he would not sleep to-night; but, provided he never saw them, he will snore with the most profound security over the ruin of a hundred million of his brethren."[74] Smith then asks himself who, to avoid his own misery, would be able to sacrifice the lives of a hundred million of his brothers, provided he had never seen them. Would the humanitarian man be willing to sacrifice the lives of millions of people if by doing so he could keep his little finger? No, he answers. But he would not be motivated by either his humanity or his benevolence, but by his reason and his conscience; in other words, by his capacity to internalize a norm that allows him to sympathize even with those with whom he has no relationship or ties. The "inhabitant of the breast," the impartial observer corrects the confusions of self-interest, indicates and points out the deformity of injustice, establishes the exact proportion of our sentiments and our sensations.

Whereas Smith constructs an imaginary earthquake that devastates China, Burke imagines a tremor capable of destroying the city of London.[75] The effect is the same in moral philosophy and the theory of art. Proximity, which permits an empathetic identification with victims, also limits the logic of taste, for whenever pain is too close, it cannot become a source for aesthetic experience. If the principles of the imagination are the same in all human beings, their differences of criteria cannot depend on either physiological constitution or the causes of affections, but on the level of natural sensitivity and, above all, on the proximity or distance with which they contemplate their object."Terror is a passion that always produces delight when it does not press too close," wrote Burke.[76] If the origin of the tragedy were too imminent, the fear would also be too intense and the only desire would be to escape. In sum, proximity would limit sympathy to its most elementary form of contagion.

Both in moral philosophy and in the logic of taste, the measurement of pain does not depend on a relationship between sensorial stimuli and one's own sensations, but rather on the physical, emotional, and cognitive distance that separates the spectator and the victim. The rhetorical relation between (hidden) observers and actors who pretend there is no audience permits the construction of an ethical, political, and aesthetic stage on which to enact the drama of tragedy.[77] The administration of the punishment should be economical; the expression of pain must be proportioned; the aesthetic judgment has to be just. In all three cases, this can only be achieved by gaining *distance*, given that only this position of privilege permits the maintaining of the gaze, avoiding imitation, resentment, or benevolence. It does not matter whether this equation is described in terms of the relationship between crimes and punishments, as in Beccaria, in terms of the norms of taste, as in Edmund Burke, or in terms of social sympathy, as in Adam Smith. This plurality of senses suggests, firstly, that the forms of objectification of pain were marked from their beginnings by a reflection on the witnesses and, with regard to conscious sensorial experiences, by the emotional agreements between them. The homogeneity of spectators makes possible an intersubjective conception of one's own sensations; but it still requires an ulterior condition. Together with the physiology of proximity and the recognition that others are our equals, there ought to open up an aesthetics and politics of distance; for only by renouncing what is near, immediate, familiar, or present can the passions and expressions of others be considered just or proportioned.

4
Correspondence

How much farther does anguish penetrate in psychology than psychology itself?[1]

The century of pain

"I was born in the century of pain," the American philosopher and scholar Charles S. Peirce [1839–1914] wrote toward the end of the nineteenth century. Compared with the violent events of the twentieth century, the periodic wars and famines that swept through Europe in the early modern period, or the fear and defenselessness of medieval life, the nineteenth century seemed rather a monotonous period marked by the sacrosanct and tedious principles of bourgeois morals. In light of the significant transformations of the previous century, we could consider the Victorian era as a time suited to the order and progress that positivism turned into a political proclamation, one even fit for exportation to the colonies. Economic development, trade, and new social relations based on consumption brought about large-scale events for the masses and universal exhibitions. The novel without heroes, the new form of narrative, extended the passions to the landowners of Jane Austen's novels, the shady citizens in the impersonal apartments of Tolstoy's Russia, the morally decadent *beaus* depicted in the books of the Italian Alexandro Manzoni, the mediocre soldiers and proprietors of Chekhov's stories, and the inhabitants of the stifling Vetusta, the imaginary and oppressive city Leopoldo Alas Clarín depicted in his novel *La Regenta*. And yet, in the nineteenth century pain took on a leading role within the social, political, and scientific arenas as never before. Physical anguish and psychological suffering became progressively more central both in private life and the public sphere. Men, women, and animals experienced a renewal of the harmful uses of the body, linked to colonial exploitation and new working conditions as well as the technological developments of medicine and science.[2]

First of all, the devastating military events of the twentieth century could cause us to lose sight of the degree to which the previous century was marked from its very outset by incidents of extraordinary physical violence. In the Iberian Peninsula, the nineteenth century began with the War of Independence and ended with a military defeat in the Spanish–American War of 1898. In the intervening period between these two conflicts, the Spaniards also had to endure the pressures of the Carlist Wars, along with the news that arrived of military campaigns in the former colonies. French contemporary history began with the revolutionary Terror, and continued with the Napoleonic campaigns and the countless executions that took place during the reign of Charles X, between 1824 and 1830. The urban uprisings of 1830 and 1848 also had a devastating effect, for only from these bloody barricades can we understand how Napoleon III could found the Second Empire, a political regime that ended in yet another conflict, the Franco-Prussian War of 1870. To this the French would still have to add the events of the "Terrible Year," as Victor Hugo termed the repression of the Paris Commune in 1871.

Along with the spices and exotic objects that poured into shopping centers of Northern European countries, news also arrived of the most cruel forms of colonization. The Opium Wars between England and China from 1839 to 1842, the Abyssinian War, the Boer War, and the Crimean War in 1853 between Tsarist Russia and Turkey and its western allies, made cities like Sebastopol – whose names had previously only evoked distant exotic paradises – fashionable. In the United States, the mere memory of the Civil War would have been enough to convince Peirce of the truth of his statement. Beyond this, however, slavery, the living conditions of the thousands of immigrants arriving from the East, or those found on the Western frontier, the genocide of the Native Americans, and the fear and uncertainty of immigrants' and colonists' lives helped to forge a national identity which depended to a large extent on the logic of a violence democratized through the use of two new technological tools: the rifle and the revolver.

War has always occupied a significant place in the history of pain, and not only during the nineteenth century. As in the times of Marcus Aurelius, direct contact with the annihilation of bodies may lead to meditation, but it may also suggest means of treatment or care. Most considerations on the nature and use of physical suffering focused on military surgeons, whose proximity to the battlefield anticipated much of the knowledge that would later be obtained in the wars of the twentieth century by other doctors and anesthetists. The cases of Baron Larrey in the Napoleonic Wars or Silas Weir Mitchell in the American Civil War are two magnificent examples among many others we could mention.[3] At the same time, the nineteenth was the first century in which the pain of military violence was transmitted using mechanical means of reproduction. While the daguerreotype appeared in the Mexican Wars, graphic news correspondents first worked during the Crimean War. Their photographs aimed to show the soldiers' suffering using photographic plates that they distributed in cities as objects of information and consumption.[4]

The history of pain in the nineteenth century also concerns suicide and murder. Great novels such as Dostoyevsky's *Crime and Punishment* or *The Brothers Karamazov*, as well as Émile Zola's *Thérèse Raquin*, turned murder into an object of public entertainment. Sir Arthur Conan Doyle's *The Adventures of Sherlock Holmes* made it a logical pastime. Charles Peirce is in debt to these stories for his formulation of different ways of thinking, including the inference of the best explanation or *abductive* reasoning. Domestic violence, as well, with permissive laws and customs regarding rape and child abuse, turned European cities into hotbeds of assault and rancor. Beatings formed part of an educational system that used vigilance and compulsive work as a coercive system, like in a prison regime. Pupils in educational institutions were also subject to exercises of physical and moral discipline. Both forms can be observed in the fragile bodies and sad eyes described by Dickens in his novels, including *David Copperfield*, the most autobiographical of his works, or in the resentful perspective of many of the characters portrayed in the Russian novels of the time, from Chekhov's *The Steppe* to Turgenev's *Fathers and Sons*. The cane, the rod, and the staff were widely used in the penal context, but also in the educational and family spheres.[5] They could be legitimately applied to women and children to ensure their submission and obedience. In the South of the United States, these instruments were joined by the whip, which beat the black population into submission. Harriet Beecher Stowe's novel *Uncle Tom's Cabin* gave a good account of the misfortunes of Southern slaves in a book that would serve as a lesson against the unjust distribution of pain in the former colonies. After all, not even those who had signed the Declaration of Independence of the United States, like Thomas Jefferson, thought that slaves shared the same feelings as the white man:

> Their griefs are transient. Those numberless afflictions, which render it doubtful whether heaven has given life to us in mercy or in wrath, are less felt, and sooner forgotten with them. In general, their existence appears to participate more of sensation than reflection. To this must be ascribed their disposition to sleep when abstracted from their diversions, and unemployed in labor. An animal whose body is at rest, and who does not reflect, must be disposed to sleep of course.[6]

Both in the military arena and in the colonial landscape, physical suffering appears as a terrible but inevitable circumstance. The same applies to the working world. Pain was no longer vindicated as a sign of divine election, but was rather interpreted as part of the inexorable laws governing historical progress.[7]

At the turn of the century, Thomas Malthus [1766–1834] had already defended the abolition of social benefits on the basis that unemployment, poverty, and hunger would allegedly act as an incentive to improve the most underprivileged classes. The publication in 1859 of Charles Darwin's *Origin of Species* discussed in great detail this trend of converting the fight for survival (of all against all) into a necessary condition for natural selection (of the fittest) and economic progress (of a few). In the natural order as well as the social arena, the relationship between evolution and violence was essential and not accidental. Hidden but real, pain and suffering were pulling the strings of civilization and history. Fear, an emotion that we now associate with uncertainty, then referred to the anticipation of pain and death.[8] The Victorians did not worry about the unknown, but about the invisible beings and forces that hid behind phenomena: from those forces governing the behavior of bodies to the recently discovered microscopic organisms. Emotional states were the result of hidden forces and uncontrolled instincts: colonial exploitation lived on under the cover of commerce in the same way that surplus value made economic profit possible; beneath moral virtues there lay confusion and resentment; the variety and beauty of the natural world covered up the fight for survival. Within the social world, at least in Herbert Spencer's vision, the survival of the fittest was at work. Childhood traumas, unconscious memories, or fixed ideas lived on in personal and collective identities. Below the surface of model Victorian families, sexual instinct flowered. The merits of Marx, Nietzsche, or Freud depended to a large extent on looking into the shadowy world that made economics, ethics, and customs possible. Each one of these thinkers, in his way, suggested that the new bourgeoisie lived surrounded by technological developments that they could not control, by passions and instincts that were beyond their comprehension, and by organisms that threatened their health. In all three cases, harm contaminated appearances, whether we spoke of the pain of exploitation, false morals, or unconscious trauma.

Everyday coexistence with suffering did not turn pain into an object of study, as would happen in the twentieth century. It was rather an instrument for cognitive investigation. The discovery of chemical anesthesia, research into organ functions supported by vivisection, the emergence of experimental psychology, as well as the advance of clinical medicine all modified the way in which harmful experiences were evaluated. The new physiology, for example, replaced old speculative hypotheses with an empirical program that depended to a large extent on animal experimentation and, consequently, on the deliberate production of pain. In France, the three most representative authors in the formation of this new physiological science – Bichat, Magendie, and Bernard – justified this new form of violence with the conviction that the same laws governed the nervous systems of all mammals. As experimental models, animals could replace the saints of Christianity, becoming "martyrs of truth," as Albrecht von Haller called them. The creation of the first professorship in physiology at University College London in 1821 has only relative importance compared with the experimental laboratories that were springing up throughout Europe, or with the generalized use of vivisection. The new theories on the vital functions, which defined health as "the silence of the organs," were supported by invasive practices. Animals could, and can, replace human beings because the most characteristic elements of our experience, such as, for example, articulated language, lacked cognitive relevance. Organ functions could only become an objective fact if science were able to replace the shades of subjective nuances with the ugliness of merely true statements.[9]

Medicine also established a link between the symptoms of an illness and organic damage. Given that the former depended on the latter, hospitals were drained of patients as they filled up with diseases.[10] This replacement of the patient with their illness fostered practices linked to the objectification of symptoms, the anatomical location of the injury, and the intersubjective measurements of conscious feelings. Whether in medicine, physiology, or psychology, the development of new observational instruments cannot be separated from these attempts to replace the patient's narrative with the clinical history of his or her symptoms. As in Flaubert's or Zola's works, inspired by Claude Bernard's thinking, the physician aspired to describe the illness from the point of view of nowhere. The stethoscope, the thermometer, the taking of blood pressure and, as of 1895, X-rays, were added to more invasive procedures. Every cavity or orifice of the body corresponded to a device that amplified the senses as a source for the appropriation of data. Thermometers, sphygmomanometers, and galvanometers not only increased observational accuracy, they also replaced a science supported by the (private) language of the experimenter with an objective measurement.[11] Most *self-recording* instruments fall into this context. One of these apparatuses was the myograph, designed for visualizing muscular contraction. Equally significant was the kymograph, able to measures changes in arterial pressure. In the same vein, the graphic methods developed by Etienne-Jules Marey sought to replace the plurality of languages with a unified language of natural phenomena.[12] For Marey, the inventor of the sphygmomanometer and the polygraph, predecessors of "lie detectors," wherever objective relationships between phenomena – like the pulse or the heartbeat – could be represented visually, there was no need to make the patient's private languages take part in the evaluation.[13] Psychology and, as a last resort, psychometry, appeared as the most suitable scientific responses for combating solipsism.[14]

Medicine and physiology were not the only areas that vindicated the goodness of suffering. Philosophy also played its part. Romanticism had already consolidated a cultural tradition that sought to convert pain into a vehicle for aesthetic greatness, an element of education, or an inalienable quality of history. In its most spiritualized forms, philosophy had begun by pointing out the connection between beauty and pain, or even better, stating the need for "a world of pain that educates our intelligence," as Keats wrote.[15] The historian Steven Bruhn was quite correct when he considered that the question should not be how the end of the eighteenth century articulated the experience of pain, but rather the opposite: how pain articulated experience at the end of the Enlightenment.[16] The works of Lichtenberg, Winckelmann, Schopenhauer, and Hegel have no dearth of references to the meaning and utility of pain for life, art, education, or history.[17] We can situate along the same lines Goethe's *Sorrows of Young Werther*, a melancholy story of amorous disenchantment, which would have enormous social repercussions. Whether we think of the work of Schiller or Hölderlin, suffering took on new meanings when seen from the standpoint of one who knows the mechanisms of tragedy. At the end of the century, in a chapter entitled "The Enjoyment of Pain," the Finnish professor Yrjö Hirn explained this in the following terms:

> If we take into account the powerful stimulating effect which is produced by acute pain, we may easily understand why people submit to momentary unpleasantness for the sake of enjoying the subsequent excitement [...] The creation of pain-sensations may be explained as a desperate device for enhancing the intensity of the emotional state.[18]

No other definition of masochism, even in psychiatry, so faithfully summarizes the elevation and modification of experience. The key word of this definition is "desperate:" a "desperate device for enhancing the intensity of the emotional state." And Hirns was not alone in this thinking. Some years previously, the philosopher Frederick Nietzsche had also built his perspectivist epistemology on a re-evaluation of suffering. In his view, how deeply we can suffer determines our rank and authority. In *Schopenhauer as Educator*, he even quoted the teachings of the mystic, Eckhart: "the beast that bears you fastest to perfection is suffering," he wrote.[19] In the framework of his philosophy, the experience of pain and pleasure could no longer be seen as opposing terms. On the contrary, there was pleasure in pain and not only metaphorically. In *The Will to Power*, he illustrated this idea with the emotional impact that tickling had in the moment of coitus. His example was aimed at affirming displeasure as an ingredient of pleasure. Given that pleasure and pain were not conflicting realities, the presence of the latter was not an impediment to happiness. Rather, between pleasure and pain there arises a game of excesses, resistances, and victories.

The instrumental use of pain in the realms of science, education, economics, and punishment – along with the daily presence of physical suffering, the introduction of chemical anesthesia, and the development of new pharmaceuticals – produced a general re-evaluation of the experience of harm. The nineteenth century saw a change in the conditions of pain's theatricality – the way in which suffering was presented as a spectacle. It also saw a crisis of trust in private testimonies, and more generally, a new appreciation of suffering in relation to pragmatic considerations. Unlike the late Middle Ages, where pain was interpreted as a sign of election, and unlike our contemporary world, which has elevated the quest for a painless society to the level of dogma, the nineteenth century considered animal or human pain as a necessary part of economic progress, cultural heritage, or scientific needs. Far from turning the maximum amount of pain into a mnemonic device, the nineteenth century defended the *least pain necessary* in all cases, whether in a medical, surgical, scientific, political, or social context. This culture and economy of the "least pain necessary" extended from punitive practices to colonial politics and wars; from the philosophy of teaching to surgical and therapeutic innovations; from the treatment of slaves on Southern plantations to work management in industrial centers, mining exploitations, and agrarian societies; from the pain inflicted on animals in experimental physiology to the cries and fainting that accompanied surgery, obstetrics, and odontology. In all cases, physical suffering stood as a means of obtaining a punitive example, an educational model, an epistemic consequence, or a financial profit. What the philosophers of the twentieth century pompously called "the problem of other minds," in other words, the difficulty of knowing whether and how we can access the consciousness of others – including among them not only men and women, but also children and animals – merely makes us reconsider in analytical terms the dysfunction produced by this instrumental use of pain in the Victorian imaginary. Even before the subjectivity of consciousness could be considered an "objective fact of science," as the philosopher of the mind John Searle wrote, and even before pain could achieve a supposed independent and intersubjective measure, science, including the most common surgical practices, rewrote private experience in terms of supposedly universal categories and gestures. In this move, pain did not renounce its temporal dimension but did reject its personal character – everything that seems most intimate and private. This is what objectivity is all about: in order for facts to flourish, people must be expelled; procedures must be sought to render their words superfluous and their gestures unnecessary.

This chapter and the following one, centered on the Victorian experience, examine the ways in which pain was objectified, particularly in surgical practices, including the new spheres of odontology and obstetrics. They also consider these means of objectification in light of the introduction of chemical anesthesia. Along with representation, imitation, and sympathy, correspondence (*adaequatio*) is yet another sub-determined category, another *topic* (understood in the Aristotelian way) – like those commonplaces that allow reasoning to the point of generating conviction – historically employed to articulate and modulate the experience of harm. Pain, in this case, is not learned through visual representation or mimetic recreation. Neither is it aroused through the distancing that aesthetic experience or the politics of justice allow, but rather through the iconographic and, later, mechanical capturing of its common elements. The question is no longer "how can we", people affected differently by the same sensations, agree in the face of the suffering of others, but rather to what extent can we establish a scale, a standard that is the result of a monotonous function between the physical injury and the experience of pain. The transformation of the subjective experience of harm into an "objective fact" not only concerns the history of experimental psychology, but also another set of practices linked to the formation of a semiotics of suffering. Before becoming a fact, pain became a sign; a natural sign that, connected to other visual elements, allowed for the elimination of subjective elements from the practice of medicine.

The signs of pain

The French Revolution did not do away with all tyranny. Louis XVI's death by the guillotine did not distance citizens from either pain or death. Quite the contrary, the transition between the *Ancien* and the New Regime turned fear into a form of suffering shared by witnesses and victims alike. The new order did not benefit some at the expense of others; it did not make distinctions between social strata or human classes; it did not safeguard the nobles or the Church; it did not discriminate between the strong and the weak, the bourgeoisie and the peasants, the rich and the poor, or men, women, and children. On the contrary, suffering equaled and deformed their faces; it modified their gestures and expressions; it turned their public presence into a theater of uniform masks, cries, and gestures. Given that pain effectively behaved like a wild animal, there were many pens ready to write its story; not a political or civil chronicle of collective suffering, but rather its natural history – the way in which harm was expressed as a natural phenomenon and, in the extreme, as the cry of life itself. Of all these accounts, that of Marc-Antoine Petit [1766–1811] is particularly significant.[20] In 1799, this doctor and surgeon from Lyon produced a text that, in subject and appearance, resembled the old tradition of political diatribe.[21] Its style still oozed with the prose of the enlightened Buffon's famous *Discourse* for his *Natural History*. He was then 33 years old:

> Citizens: I have come to speak to you about your enemy, the eternal enemy of mankind, a tyrant that with the same cruelty strikes the young and the old, the weak and the strong, who does not respect either talent or rank, never pauses even before sex or age; who has no friends to pardon nor slaves to favor, who afflicts his victims in front of their friends, at the heart of their pleasures; who does not fear the brightness of the day more than the silence of the night; against whom anticipation is vain and the defense is more uncertain as the enemy seems to take up arms against us with all the forces of its nature.[22]

Some years previously, in 1793, the Convention had ordered the destruction of Lyon, a city that the Jacobins considered a focus of royal resistance. Under the slogan *"Lyon no longer exists,"* around 1800 people were assassinated by the so-called *mitraillades*, musket shots fired against the civilian population, while the guillotine executed many others.[23] Their bodies fell to the ground as easily as the buildings of the second most important city in France. Or the opposite: the walls yielded like the breaking bones of an anatomical structure. Although the comparison came from the theorists of the New Regime, it did not go unnoticed by the surgeon Petit. In 1796, a mere three years after the massacres, he gave a new speech at the opening of the course on Anatomy and Surgery of the Hôtel Dieu, on the influence of the Revolution on public health: "Revolutions are to the political bodies upon which they act the same as medicine to the ailing human bodies over which they should re-establish harmony."[24] Both in the physiological organism and the body politic, a feeling of harm must always precede the reestablishment of health. In his view, the same physical or political suffering that gripped humanity was not only a sign of illness but also the first manifestation of its cure.

Many other voices joined in with this proposal. In 1823, Jacques-Alexandre Salgues, a medical doctor of the University of Paris and a member of the Academy of Sciences, wrote a treatise *On Pain Considered from the Point of View of its Usefulness*.[25] Prior to that, in 1803, François Marie Hippolyte Bilon [1780–1824] had published his *Dissertation on Pain*. In some cases, specific pains were examined, like J. Ph. Hamel's doctoral thesis on facial neuralgia, but for the most part they were small texts that appeared, especially in France, following the thread of the new physiology.[26] They also had imitators and followers in the rest of Europe. The Italian Benedetto Mojon [1781–1849], for example, following Bilon's text and the reflections of Pietro Verri, published a small essay *On the Usefulness of Pain* in 1818.[27] Eight years later in 1826, William Griffin [1794–1848], a member of the Royal College of Surgeons of Edinburgh, printed his *Essay on the Nature of Pain*, a translation of his dissertation *De dolore*, which would become the first text on this subject published in English.[28] As with Petit, all of these treatises interpreted and justified physical suffering, no longer in accordance with supernatural recompense, but rather with mundane needs. Life was sufficient to account for pain because pain was fully identified with life. The presence of physical suffering was an evil only for those who lacked medical knowledge or political standing. Apologists vindicated it as an intermediate state that did not seek the salvation of the soul but rather the survival of the physiological body and the constitutive improvement of the body politic. From his point of view, individuals as well as the general public perceived with horror that which, to the trained eye, was no more than the very expression of natural politics. "Pain is no evil," Griffin declared.[29] This absolute harm that could only be learned with fear and only borne with impatience was a gift from providence or, as Salgues put it, "a faithful friend." Whether at birth, in infancy or in old age, pain tells us uncomfortable truths, without a care for our laments or moans.

Immersed in a naturalist principle, which searched for a function for each and every one of the sensations and emotions of the body, these treatises drew a well-defined border between sufferers and doctors. Only the latter make an adequate judgment on our pain experiences. We, who do not know the actual cause of our ailment, also see our intellectual capabilities limited. Confronted by a situation always perceived as negative, the same feelings that trigger our suffering make us incapable of proper judgment. Pain increases our ignorance in at least three different ways. First of all, we, the patients, suffer perceptual dysfunctions so as to "feel that our ailments grow in comparison with those who have no sorrows."[30] In a sense, suffering increases or decreases our personal identity, depending on our present situation and our hopes for the future. Secondly, we, the patients, can incorrectly identify the cause of our ailment and trace the origin of our pain to the wrong place, or even to a non-existent location. Finally, our body may have an ailment that does not reach our consciousness: we may be ill, and feel nothing. Our vision may be limited, wrong, or clearly insufficient. From a medical standpoint, pain, however, produces signs that are not necessarily negative, not necessarily conscious, which point toward a morphological ailment or an organic illness.

For these new apologists, Mahon's entry in Diderot's *Encyclopédie* proved completely wrong in writing that no harmful experience could be considered healthy.[31] This encyclopedia had also been largely unable to recognize pain as a sign which, correctly interpreted, could offer the first step toward a remedy. Given that the pain is expressed, at least initially, by means of expressions and gestures, accurate knowledge of morbid states allows for a distinction between the way in which patients complain and the way in which they ought to do so. The uterus, for example, which can be cut and cauterized without pain, causes unbearable suffering when affected by cancer.[32] The same applies to the stomach, the intestines, the gallbladder or the bladder. Even if we do not react from contact with a probe, we may suffer considerably in the presence of a stone. Signs of pain cannot, and should not, be interpreted by means of the incorrect way in which we transmit our emotions, but rather through experimental observation and etiological explanation. The testimony, the more-or-less articulate way in which we explain our ailments, has scarcely any cognitive relevance at all. On the contrary, the correct evaluation of our illness depends merely on an anatomical examination; on geography and not on history.

The framework of the new life-science interpreted patients' gestures and words through a semiotics that lacked all reference to empty hypotheses, popular expressions, or private evaluations. For the new physicians, the way in which patients evaluate and describe their pain was only of relative interest, and how they classify it had absolutely no scientific interest. Most of these evaluations came from old humoral theories, popular wisdom, or merely subjective experiences. The former differences between *heavy, tight, pulsating,* and *sharp* pain made no sense at all.[33] It would be the same, ridiculed Bilon, to divide suffering into sweet, bitter, or sour. Given that all these pains were associated with a specific ailment, which in turn depended on a morphological injury, the distinction could only be made through a correct identification of their place of residence, their *siège* (seat). Put another way, the classification depended on the localization of the ailment regardless of the patient's often-incorrect opinion.

Whereas the clinical history must compensate, modify, and interpret the subjective evaluation of the ailment, physiological knowledge aspires to build an unvarying connection between the (visible) sign of the disease and its (anatomical) lesion. This must be done through an observational and experimental exercise. The first concerns the eyes and the second the hands. Before getting to the patient, the new *"physiology of reasoning,"* as Bichat called it, rests on the manipulation and, ultimately, the experimental destruction of the organisms of other species. On the one hand, this exercise treats human beings as though they were animals. On the other, it rests on the conviction that animals should behave like human beings on the dissection table.[34] Whether through compression, contusion, inflammation, burns, stings, fractures, dislocations, or the destruction of the organs, true knowledge has nothing to do with compassion or sentimentality.[35] Humans and animals may be compared once it is agreed that the distinctive features of the latter are nothing but an obstacle for the study of their organic functions. Though experiments were not carried out on the patients, at least not directly, the way in which humans were treated depended on knowledge obtained in another place, at another time, and with another species. It was not the first time in history that the search for truth depended on the bodily torment of an other. On the contrary, the new physiology was based on a long tradition that, as in the case of judicial torture, always preferred the testimony of a body to the confusing words of a witness. From a cognitive standpoint, only the latter may lie. The organism, which only follows its natural development and has no interest other than its own survival, neither cheats nor makes mistakes. Its story cannot be transcribed by means of any linguistic articulation but rather through a potentially infinite set of expressive elements, such as color, movement, texture, or even taste. If we could just overcome our repugnance toward experiments with live animals, wrote François Magendie [1783–1855], studies of the vital functions would have the same status as the exact sciences; their laws would seem as universal as the axioms of mechanics.[36] For him, as for other physiologists, the deliberate causing of pain would serve to separate facts from fables, to set truth against prejudice. Emile-Edouard Mouchy depicted him carrying out an anatomical lesson in 1832. The number of observers, 12, recalls another similar transmutation. However, unlike the endlessly represented scene of the Last Supper, knowledge here replaces Salvation atop an operating table. Even more heretically, a dog has taken the place of the lamb. In this new form of exploring the body, the patient's contradictions could be counteracted by the organs' argumentative solvency (see Figure 13).[37]

Emotion, including its quality and intensity, is reinterpreted within the context of a developed theory of signs. Physiology did not dispute the presence of harm, but re-evaluated the cultural meaning of pain by studying organic ailments through a semiotics of the patient's complaints, based on a philosophy of correspondence: "perhaps it would not be impossible to recognize that this or that organ may be affected by a painful ailment, carefully studying the kind of complaint that goes with it," wrote Bilon.[38] As an instrument for prognosis, pain allowed establishing a distinction between different sensitivities, including those that depended on social extraction or sexual differences. The doctor had to learn to interpret the patients' expressions, gestures, and attitudes, the intensity and modulation of their cries, the grimaces on their faces, the color of their cheeks, the look in their eyes, or the movement of their hands or limbs. Private experience was reinterpreted through a phenomenology of the ailment, where the sign comes about as an involuntary response to an injury: "it will be seen that a man who is operated on for the hip gives out different cries from one who is operated on for a tumor,"[39] wrote Bilon. For Doctor Cartier, of the Hôtel Dieu, the cries emitted as a response to the surgeon's saw were sharp, whereas those caused by cauterization had a deeper tone. The patient emitted them involuntarily. Gestures, even those that differentiated holding tightly and pulling violently, were regarded as just as automatic as sweating, breathing, or blushing.[40] Richet, a doctor in a Paris hospital, would still refer to and debate the work of Dupuytren, who held that some especially sensitive patients suffered from nervous accidents following painful surgery, and of Brown-Séquard, who had supposedly proven that both the animals and men of the New World could better bear traumas and operations than those of the Old Continent. Although will and courage could be important in the presence of acute pain, most physiologists agreed that the same causes universally produced more or less the same effects, in accordance with reflexes and automatic mechanisms, even when the patient was etherized.[41]

In 1876, the Italian doctor and anthropologist Paolo Mantegazza [1831–1910] published an illustrated atlas of the expressions of pain. His *Atlante delle espressioni del dolore* contained 123 illustrations of both real subjects and works of art.[42] For this prolific intellectual and founder of Italy's first professorship in Anthropology, in Florence, it was possible to establish a geography of pain, a repository of acts and gestures related to harmful experiences. His catalog ranged from muscular contractions, paralysis, respiratory problems, secretion, and peripheral vasomotor movements to psychic expressions such as muteness, unusual eloquence, and delirium. Muscular contractions, for example, could affect the face, the trunk, or the limbs; they could produce partial or general convulsions as well as tremors. The set of illustrations made up a veritable catalog of expressive signs. Sighing, weeping, screams, moaning, and also tears, salivation, urinating, vomiting, sweating, diarrhea, paleness, skin rashes, erections, blushing, anger and hatred, erythema, and religious feelings all formed a part of this tableau of physical and psychic expressions. His *Physiology of Pain*, published in 1880, constituted only one part of these phenomena of mimicry, such as expressions of sensitive experiences like hunger, of passions like envy, or of intellectual experiences like doubt. They could also include elementary feelings such as anger or composite feelings, such as the mixture of pleasure and pain in sexuality and childbirth.[43]

Although pain was recognized, along with fever, inflammation, or other sets of symptoms, to have a clear diagnostic value, it also appeared to have a therapeutic function.[44] Even if it no longer guaranteed salvation in the next world, suffering could help to stay alive in this one. Frequently considered a tyrant, a *"proteiform monster,"* pain was also the best of physicians and the origin of all remedies, "the most vigilant of doctors," according to Griffin, the "sentinel of life," as Bilon put it.[45] The most explicit and uncomfortable sign of illness already formed part of the treatment. Its appearance, which obliged the affected parts to be immobilized or required the patient to rest, was regarded as the first therapeutic element and, in appropriate doses, helped to rid the muscles of numbness, revitalize the tissues, and, more generally, strengthen the body's energy.[46] Given that nature was gifted with reparative faculties and had the capacity to heal wounds, at least when these were the result of fatigue, an accident, or an inflammation, it seemed logical to act by means of mimetic procedures which, in adequate doses, were able to bring about the same effects.[47]

These methods, used especially during the first half of the nineteenth century, made up a repository of a new form of pain: *iatrogenic* pain, which was deliberately induced by a doctor. The surgeon John James, for example, wrote that a compress with half a pint of boiling water applied to an inflamed area was an instantaneous remedy.[48] The same results were expected from dry cuppings, the application of caustic chemicals to the skin, such as silver nitrate, ammonia, or cantharides (Spanish fly), used both internally and externally, or tartar emetic, a compound of potassium with numerous adverse effects, which was only recommended in nauseating doses.[49] Along with traditional remedies, where bleeding still held a privileged place, other "evacuating" therapies began to appear, such as diuretics, expectorants, sudorifics, as well as purgatives and enemas, which were combined with hot baths. Topical remedies – made of oil, milk, or animal blood – were administered in the form of baths, vapors, fumigations, cataplasms, or compresses. Therapeutic methods included chemical agents that produced blisters, fluid removal, and other so-called counter-irritants, which caused considerable physical and moral suffering for the patient.[50] The most radical remedies, known as "rubefacients," destroyed the epidermis and ate up the tissues through some form of friction, sometimes even using nettles. Petit considered flagellation to be a remedy as efficacious as Japanese acupuncture, whether it was carried out using "ropes or tied leather strips, or lead or iron bars." The latter, he tells us, "on being armed with sharp points produce, through the spilling of blood, the same beneficial effects as Japanese acupuncture."[51] Along the same lines, Jean-Baptiste Bonnefoy, an attaché at the Royal College of Surgery in Lyon, considered that the use of electricity and the application of the sea torpedo, a cartilaginous fish that could produce currents of more than 200 volts, could eliminate, or at least temporarily alleviate, rheumatic pain, gout, sciatica, migraine, tumors, hemorrhoids, toothache, dizziness, or insomnia.[52]

At the most extreme end of this catalog, some physicians even argued that pain could be used to alleviate pain by means of artificially producing an even more intense sensation. The use of cauterization, blister plasters, and highly harmful fluid draining took on a newly central role.[53] Cauterization, for example, was attempted in treating paralysis, apoplexy, cerebral epilepsy, rickets, cancerous tumors, gout, and neuralgia. For Louis-François Gondret, fire was the tonic par excellence, a remedy whose application had the advantage of rehabilitating moral and physical faculties with a single application.[54] His doctrine, known as "pyrotechnics," included the cauterization of all kinds of patients, a remedy that was "less cruel than it seemed" and whose only drawback was a vivid and intense pain that was, however, short in duration.[55] Quoting different sources, Dunglison also considered that the benefits of cauterization should not be belittled by the false belief that it caused an unbearable amount of pain: "we see many persons bear it, for the first time, without giving signs of very acute pain," he wrote.[56] The arrival of the *moxas*, a cure imported from the Orient that consisted of the application, as close as possible to the ailment, of a cylinder of cotton that was then burned, may be considered along the same lines.[57] At the beginning of the nineteenth century, Baron Larrey wrote a treatise on the matter and included it in his *Recueil de Mémoires de Chirurgie*: "One of the most common objections that have been adduced against it, is the great degree of pain which it occasions, but even this has been greatly exaggerated" he wrote.[58] For this military surgeon, *moxa* could be used successfully for abdominal pain, in cases of asthma, paralysis, and chronic pain like painful tics, hemiplegia, or rheumatism, rachialgia or *Tabes Dorsalis*, the degeneration of the nerves of the spine – on which the author Conan Doyle wrote his doctoral thesis – as well as different tumors and scar tissues. For many other doctors, this counter-irritant was especially recommended for chronic illnesses, while the tartar emetic was administered in chronic as well as acute cases of pneumonia, in fractures, chest pain, colds, backache, inflammations of the lungs, and in gout pains.[59]

These recommendations are better judged in the context of the more or less unsuccessful fight to find palliative remedies for different kinds of physical suffering throughout the entirety of human history. Iatrogenic pain – produced by the healing process itself – although related to a particular understanding of the organism in connection to old humoral theories, was also a response to the difficulty of finding appropriate and universal forms of treatment. We must keep in mind that, at least until the middle of the nineteenth century, and even later, the history of pain relief gets confused with the history of the placebo effect. As late as 1826, the Scottish surgeon William Griffin wrote laconically that in the face of the most harrowing suffering and chronic and lasting pains, one could only prescribe "a balanced diet, fresh air, moderate exercise, a change of residence and an optimistic spirit."[60] In view of some of the remedies used at the time, he was not entirely wrong. In the mid-nineteenth century, the procedures for palliating acute pain consisted either of the ingestion of some substance likely to dull the consciousness or of an attempt to block the nervous system surgically.[61] Certain narcotic and hypnotic substances had been known since antiquity. Mandrake leaves, for example, were boiled in milk and used as a sedative, and mandrake root, whose form was visibly anthropomorphic, was ingested to alleviate pain during surgery. Belladonna, so called because it made the eyes of women shine more brightly, was also employed in the Middle Ages. In the thirteenth century, Teodorico Borgognoni [1206–1298], spoke in his *Surgery* of a soporific sponge soaked in opium and henbane, which was perhaps the most popular anesthetic in the medieval world.[62] At the beginning of the early modern period four or five substances with narcotic properties were known: the aforementioned mandrake, cannabis, opium or opium tincture (known as laudanum), and, of course, alcohol. Along with these, a plethora of popular remedies began to accumulate, based in equal parts on oral tradition, ingenuity, and desperation.

In the case of toothache, for example, some of the palliative procedures – such as the ingestion of cooked mouse skin, already recommended by Dioscorides in the first century in his *Farmacopea* – had been integrated into popular culture and were used alongside ointments and spices, principally cinnamon, cloves, laudanum, hot brandy, and opium.[63] For the same kind of ailment, in the sixteenth century the French surgeon Ambroise Paré recommended that the patient gargle with his own urine. This will not seem strange at all if we remember that the essence of urine – which the refined Marchioness of Sévigné [1626–1696] applied internally as an effective remedy against vapors – was also employed to combat epilepsy and apoplexy. The anonymous author of the *Pious Surgeon* suggested applying a filling made of cantharides, a vesicant substance extracted from a coleopterous insect that was known as "Spanish fly" until well into the twentieth century.[64] A popular remedy for teething children consisted in rubbing their gums twice a day with blood from a rooster's crest.[65] Nicolas Lemery, in his *Universal Dictionary of Simple Drugs*, proposed a dry powdered compound made of human excrement for inflammations of the mouth.[66] Bloodletting was also practiced frequently, and, according to many patients, with moderate success.

The methods of tooth extraction were not much more benign. On the contrary, the popular Romance-language expression "to lie like a tooth-puller" derived from the almost always un-kept promise that it was possible to pull teeth without pain.[67] To alleviate suffering, the surgeon Baptiste Martin recommended "wild cat excrement," while the first edition of the *Medicine of the Poor* considered nicotine spirit or dog earwax to be almost miraculous remedies.[68] The French doctor and surgeon Ambroise Paré pointed out that extractions should not be performed too violently, given the risk of dislocating the jaw, causing a cerebral or ocular concussion, or even ripping part of the jawbone away with the tooth.[69] In the eighteenth century, the English surgeon John Hunter, in coherence with his own system and anticipating the proposals of many apologists, suggested that in those cases where there was no symptom other than toothache, the treatments could act by derivation; in other words, through a stimulus applied to some other part of the body. Thus, "burning the ear with hot irons has on occasions been an effective remedy against toothache," he wrote.[70]

In both medicine and physiological experimentation, the utility of pain was always subject to various restrictions. First of all, its clinical value depended on its intensity, and in order to be considered useful, pain ought to be moderate. There was no justification whatsoever for the anguish and anxiety that accompanied suffering when it was too acute or too continuous. The "faithful friend" was never well received when it crushed all hope of being eliminated without the destruction of one's very being.[71] No one ever doubted that pain offered no recompense or benefit to those who suffered from gout, neuralgias, or muscular contractions, whose effects were as atrocious as their causes were unknown. Neither did it produce the desired effect when it attacked the body in the form of cancer or other incurable illnesses. Secondly, to be favorable for medical knowledge, apologists understood that pain should particularly be felt in the limbs and external parts of the body. It lacked justification when it affected the internal organs. Thirdly, it should affect only a limited number of body parts. Finally, the pain's duration should be brief. The apologists never defended the use of the merciless pain of cancer or other diseases of the organs, which, after annihilating the instruments of life by a slow and insidious process, make sufferers consider death the most desirable of solutions.

The same limitations also applied to experimental practices. Although in debt to the old materialist philosophers, most physiologists promoted the use of animal experimentation in order to obtain the most knowledge with the minimum amount of pain.[72] "We must try to subject the animal to the least painful situation possible; pulling or squeezing its ligaments to the necessary point, but without separating them from the flesh," Albrecht von Haller wrote in the eighteenth century.[73] In both the surgical context and the experimental sphere, a state of ataraxia should precede the production of pain. In one case, "it is necessary [following the incision], to allow the animal to calm down [...] observing the animal's rest, silence, relaxation and suffering expression."[74] In another, the surgical preparation that sought to avoid any unnecessary suffering (where it was possible) was as important as the surgical operation itself.

All these considerations foretell the later distinction between chronic and acute pain, as well as between clinical and surgical pain. Pain's apologists defended the usefulness of a harmful experience in the case of acute pain resulting from an organ lesion, but they almost never defended the advantages of surgical pain and were never in favor of chronic suffering. In this last case, they argued, continued pain and pleasure seemed to lead naturally to their own destruction.[75] Given that sensations always entailed a comparison between different states, Bichat argued that even those pains considered *absolute* and that would seem not to depend on our judgment or emotional state only affect us while we are not accustomed to them. For him as for others, pains and pleasures tended to become relative once they became routine: "eight days following the introduction of a probe through the urethra the patient no longer felt any pain."[76] In more extreme but no less frequent circumstances, all sensations, painful and agreeable alike, are wiped out, eventually becoming imperceptible, whether they be pessaries in the vagina, posts in the rectum, or catheters in the tear ducts. If all this sensorial experience is accompanied by a relative judgment on the current and prior state of the organism, the greater the (subjective) impression, the greater the (objective) difference between the two states. This is why those sensations we have never experienced before are those that affect us the most. And, on the other hand, the organism naturally tends to lose interest in everyday experiences, including, according to Bichat, the sexual interest aroused by one's partner. Given that pain and pleasure are nothing more than compared emotions, which only exist in reference to a prior and a posterior state, we must therefore conclude that just as there are no infinite pleasures, neither can there be perpetual sufferings. In a remarkable refutation of the Church's sanctification of pain, physiology contradicts in a single argument both conjugal fidelity and the late medieval imaginary, which painted Hell as a place of eternal suffering.[77]

Finally, the possibility of using pain as a cognitive tool depended on the existence of a proportional relationship between the intensity of the pain and the gravity of the lesion, as well as a correspondence between experience and expression. Although it was not difficult to find exceptions to this general rule, such as different forms of dental pain or a painful tic, this apparent lack of logic could always be explained by indicating that either these pains did not endanger the patient's life, such as pain in childbirth, or that it was the very patient who broke the equation, introducing subjective elements. The proportion between pain and "real" danger – not apparent danger as perceived by an ill person – was always constant, such that a whole cognitive system, based on the mere observation of the symptoms, could rest on this uniformity. When the time came to establish a semiology of pain, Griffin, for example, considered that one should not only examine the pain's intensity, but also its constancy, its location, or the symptoms to which it was connected.[78]

The pain of childbirth

"What you call the pain of childbirth has no other name than agony," wrote Doctor Charles Meigs [1792–1869].[79] For this doctor from Philadelphia, the nature and intensity of the pain of childbirth were totally indescribable and incomparable with any other kind of physical suffering.[80] The severity of this pain had already been described in many manuals on obstetrics, including that of the Enlightenment surgeon William Osborn, who considered it the most inhumane of all suffering.[81] The discrepancies concerning the mortality rate of women during childbirth and their own expectancy of survival contrasted with the certainty of an inevitable experience. At the moment of childbirth, the death of the mother was probable, but her suffering was assured. The relationship between the forms of suffering and the forms of giving birth was so close that uterine contractions were often generically referred to as "the pains," while the moment of childbirth was known as "the scream."[82] The most natural birth occurred when the baby was born "through the force of the pain," as the surgeon Brudenell Exton wrote.[83]

As in the case of premenstrual pain or the symptoms that accompany menopause, childbirth constituted yet another painful experience that women experienced as a result of their gender, and for which there scarcely existed palliative remedies.[84] In the case of menstrual pain – especially pressing in educated women – bloodletting, hot baths, enemas, and sedatives were frequently administered, combined with large doses of patience and resignation. Popular remedies abounded as far as the pains of childbirth were concerned. In some cases, relics and reliquaries were arranged in the room. In others, a concoction was prepared using the head of a deer. While some women asked for holy water, the most unfortunate drank large quantities of alcohol. In the seventeenth century, the French surgeon Pierre Dionis had already recommended wines and liqueurs from the Canary Isles, which were shared equally between the woman giving birth and the midwives.[85] Many women made different kinds of promises: to free a prisoner, recite a novena, or obtain the belt of Saint Margaret. Others, the most religious, asked for masses to be performed. Women did not react the same way to the same symptoms. While some of them screamed from the beginning of their contractions until they destroyed their throats, others remained calm for most of the process. Before the arrival of chloroform – a substance that had already been described in the 1830s by Liebig, and which the doctor Guillot prescribed as an antispasmodic without anyone at the time realizing its anesthetic properties – and even afterwards, pain appeared not only as a consequence of a natural action, but also as a punishment imposed on women after the Fall.[86] This could explain why, in 1591, a woman named Eufame Macalyne was condemned and burned at the stake, accused of asking for relief before the birth.[87] Although this is an extreme case, the idea that maternity was inextricably linked to pain determined the mythology of procreation during the Middle Ages and the Renaissance. Even after the first births carried out with the assistance of chloroform, arguments were still made against its use under the pretext that it was against the divine mandate, as laid down in the Book of Genesis: *in pain you will bring forth children.*

Around the year 1800, an anonymous painter depicted the moment of delivery in a markedly naturalist painting (see Figure 14). The scene takes place in a closed room with no ventilation or natural light. The woman gives birth seated on a piece of furniture covered with a cloth and which she uses as a birthing stool. Her gaze stares off into infinity. A basket and a bottle lie on a table beside her – probably *caudle*, a broth prepared with wine and spices, which the mother used to sip during childbirth. An old midwife is waiting to receive the child, whose head is already emerging, and another woman is tipping water into a dish, taking up a secondary position. While the presence of these female assistants is very well documented, the masculine figure seems to break the homogeneity of an event in which the presence of men was limited until well into the eighteenth century, and even then only to those cases when a surgeon's intervention was required; this only happened with premature births or when the position of the fetus made it advisable.[88] What historians have called the "obstetric revolution" was linked to better knowledge of anatomy, the generalized use of forceps, and a professional quarrel related to financial demands. At the same time, the arrival of surgeons at the birthing stool to attend to those births where there were no obvious complications also brought about a modification in the evaluation of this painful experience both before and after the introduction of chloroform.[89] In this sense, obstetrics was no different from other professional activities, such as surgery or odontology, which were likewise developed under the threat of professional intrusion and the dissemination of new surgical instruments.

In the seventeenth century some obstetrics manuals still classified births into natural, preternatural, and *contra natura* (anti-natural). This taxonomy did not depend on anatomical considerations, but on a specific theological measurement of the time of the pregnancy and the length of delivery.[90] To be considered natural, a birth had to fulfill two conditions completely unrelated to the position of the fetus or the technical difficulties of labor. First, birth should occur following the complete gestation period. Secondly, it should last no longer than the time taken to recite a *Miserere*. Prayer number 52 of the *Book of Psalms*, the foundation of the baroque mythology of procreation, gave a new meaning to the Latin expression *Ora et labora* (*be at prayer and be in labor*).[91] Although during the Enlightenment and the early nineteenth century childbirth progressively lost its religious connotations, it could still be divided into periods and measured in units. From Pierre Dionis, in the seventeenth century, who considered that labor should take a "reasonable" time, to William Tyler Smith, in the nineteenth, who judged that first births should last 24 hours, the technical modifications brought about by surgical practices included a clinical re-evaluation of the subjective elements involved in the process.[92] The emphasis on the historical nature of birth never limited its dramatic nature. On the contrary, it permitted its manifestation in accordance with a theatricalized logic in which the surgeons came to take over the lead role from the midwife and the woman giving birth. The arrival of surgery to the birthing chair brought about a conceptual re-evaluation of pain's expressions, which were now interpreted in correspondence with a set of signs, like elements that only take on relevance in the context of a codified system.

From the beginning of gestation until after the birth, the entire process of pregnancy and delivery was framed by signs and inscriptions. Inspired by the new physiology, obstetricians began to look for indications, isolate symptoms, and, no less importantly, eliminate prejudices. Birth, which ought to end with the emergence of the baby, always began with the dismissal of popular knowledge. There was no room for excuses; the woman had to expel her child as well as her ignorance. The surgeon, on the other hand, had to disregard the mother. The process ought to shine light into the darkness and combat credulity and fanaticism in equal measure. Unlike the mother, who was frequently wrong, the clinical gaze and the expert hand did not allow for mistakes. The appearance of obstetric surgery was not only linked to anatomical knowledge or the use of new instruments which required appropriate training, but also to a professional practice that put subjective elements on hold, including the way in which the mothers complained or interpreted their symptoms. According to the new men-midwives, the appearance of the mother's face, the position of the baby's head, the inclination of the womb, or the phase of the moon at the moment of gestation were of no use in knowing the sex or number of the unborn. On the contrary, they relied on the ceasing of menstruation, the swelling of the breasts, and the growth of the belly. In some cases, backache, hardening of the muscles, vomiting and nausea, difficulty urinating, intermittent dizziness, and the presence of varicose veins were sufficient signs for identifying the beginning of gestation.[93]

The study of these signs served to trace a dividing line between "true" and "false" pregnancies. The distinction was clear: for whereas the first ones ended in the birth of a child, the second ones put an end to the surgeon's reputation.[94] In either case, the practice was based on an interpretive semiotics of the woman's gestures. Thus, when the doctor finds out what time the labor pains began, their frequency, intensity, and duration, he does so with the sole intention of establishing their nature and determining their cause, in such a way as to favor those sufferings that help the birth along and fight against the others.[95] The "true" pains caused by contractions would be sufficient to give birth to the child.[96] "False" pains, on the other hand – not only imaginary or exaggerated pains, but also those caused by some intestinal or abdominal problem – would have to be combated by using preparations of opium.

In 1853, Doctor Cazeaux, of the faculty of medicine in Paris, attempted to establish a correct identification of women's expressive signs and their other physiological circumstances. He was only interested in "real" pregnancies and "true" pains. As part of a cartography of sensation, these true pains could be classified as keen, frequent, dreadful, elevated, excessive, violent, or "mosquito" pains – so called due to a "comparison with the pain caused by a bite from that insect."[97] On the other hand, those pains denominated *precursor*, *preparatory*, *expelling*, or *corrupt* were tied to the development of the birth like a physiological guide, allowing an evaluation of each movement or the circumstances of each contraction. The presence of each one of them determined a precise emotional reaction. Under the influence of *precursor* pains, for example, future mothers took on a melancholic air that grew progressively more violent. As birth progressed, the pains became more frequent and, coinciding with the dilation of the neck of the uterus, keener and closer. Each new sensation arrived with a slight shiver, which quickened and intensified the pulse. The woman's face became redder, she grew hotter, her tongue dried, and she often felt nauseous and vomited. The future mother became upset, cried, and grew desperate and irritable. At the end of the contraction, the sufferings did not completely disappear; rather, while she was still under the power of the last pain, she began to dread the one that would come next to take its place. At the moment of the birth itself, when the abdominal muscles seemed to come to the uterus's aid, her efforts increased, and just as the baby's head emerged from the womb and the contractions became more energetic, she would cry out. The baby's transit produced a horrible pain, made up of sensations of varying intensity and transmitted through the parietal protuberances at the level of the ischium. Soon after, the head would emerge.

Throughout the process of delivery, the mother finds herself subject to a force much greater than her will. Her cries and laments do not belong to her. It is not she who screams, but her pain that rends the screams from her; not she who is crying but rather the contractions that pull out her tears. A natural force opposes her desire to express her emotions – a force that modulates her expression and limits her gestures. The pain produces a set of expressions that, from her first convulsions onward, she can neither hide nor control. They are as involuntary and automatic as the dilation of the neck of the uterus or the contractions of the abdominal muscles. Her will, like the rest of her intellectual faculties, lacks practical relevance or cognitive interest. It does not matter what she feels or what she says. On the other hand, the expressive signs inscribed on her body are of interest, and very much so. For the obstetrician Meigs, for example, the way in which the mother squeezed the hands of those she held onto should be enough to determine whether or not the birth had entered the expulsion phase or if she was still dilating. For him, as for others, if the duration, intensity, or frequency of the contractions were not equal to the duration, intensity, or frequency of the pain, it was only due to differences in the age, temperament, or education of the mother. Some will protest in excess for slight sensations whereas others will hardly complain from very strong contractions.

Cazeaux, for example, describes the case of a woman in labor who, following prolonged efforts and interminable suffering, suddenly changed her facial expression and began to sing the great aria from *Lucia di Lammermoor* at the top of her lungs.[98] In the third act of Donizetti's opera, which premiered in 1839, the main character loses her mind and, minutes before fainting, sings *Il dolce suono*, an aria with some of the highest notes ever written for a soprano. This is not the only documented case of pain altering the nervous system to such an extent that the sufferer's behavior borders on the irrational, the criminal, or the ridiculous. Some doctors put forth that, with their intellectual capacities diminished, the future mothers said the most extravagant things in their delirium. According to Doctor Montgomery, this outbreak of irrationality occurred especially when the child's head emerged from the womb. And even following the birth, he argued, there might be a kind of shuddering or nervous shock similar to that experienced by workers whose limbs were amputated in accidents.[99]

Just like electricity, which when passed through the nervous system produces contractions and grimaces quite independent from the will or the consciousness, the cries and laments of the mother make up a puzzle that only the doctor was able to interpret with probity. Unfortunately, the mother frequently contaminates the natural expression of her pain, either due to her sensitivity, education, or prejudices. If these spurious elements could be eliminated, her physical reactions would correspond to those of any other superior mammal; for, as a mere physiological being, nothing should distinguish a woman from a beast. In *The Expression of Emotion in Man and Animals*, published in 1872, Darwin also considered the expressive signs to be invariable elements that neither depended on the person nor the species. The same gestures could cross over biological borders and manifest themselves in animals with equivalent morphological structures: "The female hippopotamus in the Zoological Gardens when she produced her young, suffered greatly; she incessantly walked about, or rolled on her sides, opening and closing her jaws, and clattering her teeth together."[100] Following Bichat, who claimed that to distinguish between true and false pain it was only necessary to take the patient's pulse, Edmund Chapman claimed that pain that caused a reddening of the face and a rapid pulse should be maintained, or even increased, to facilitate the birth.[101] With regard to false pain, which Cazeaux called "neuralgic," there was no doubt about its hysterical nature. A woman becomes violent under its effects, and unlike the hippopotamus in Regents Park who suffers in silence, she cries out and invokes death, begging to be killed or put out of her misery.[102]

The mother's ability to subvert the equation between the physiological stimulus and her expressive gestures was subject to two significant restrictions. The first, purely biological, depends entirely on anatomical conditions, for the mother's will is not able to bend the course of nature in all circumstances. The second, artificial, would take place after the introduction of anesthesia, and would allow the elimination of the subjective elements from childbirth. Once put to sleep, the woman's body could be manipulated without her incidental perceptions, changes in mood, or the incomprehensible modifications of her states of consciousness. Ever since James Young Simpson [1811–1870], a Scottish obstetrician, administered ether to a woman in 1847, it became perfectly clear that the elimination of the mother's suffering, as long as it did not eliminate muscular contractions, did not interfere with the development of the birth. On the contrary, the labor could continue its course even when the sensations of pain had disappeared completely.[103] The advantages of chemical anesthesia in the battles to legitimize obstetrics are beyond doubt. The possibility of avoiding a type of suffering that even some doctors considered agonizing, and of doing so not only in laborious births but in any birth, at will, and without interfering with nature, could only have advantages. Since chemical anesthetics only eliminated consciousness, the subjective modulations of the experience, along with all the elements that prevented the relationship between the contractions and the expression from remaining constant of pain, also vanished.[104] Anesthesia did not turn the body into a corpse, but it did allow the physiological processes to act without the presence of witnesses. Its employment inevitably modified the uses of pain, for even when Simpson himself understood suffering as a sign of uterine contractions, he also recognized that it was not a trustworthy indicator. There could be both painless contractions, those that took place with the mother under anesthetic, and pain without contractions, namely "false" or "spurious" pains.[105]

Between January 1847 and September 1848, Simpson operated on 150 patients under the effects of ether. In November, he began to use chloroform.

Administering both of these substances he was able to prove that not only did physical suffering disappear, there was also a liberation from *"unnecessary mental anguish,"* a decrease in the fear of agony, as well as, in his own words, the disappearance of the nervous shock that often accompanied childbirth.[106] Resistance to using both substances came from many sources and acted on different fronts. Some objections were based on technical reasons, but others had ideological motivations. For Doctor Meigs, for example, annulling the pain of childbirth through the inhalation of narcotics was little more than "a questionable attempt to abolish one of the general conditions of man."[107] The use of ether was not only an affront to natural morals, it also spread as a consequence of excessive and exaggerated complaints which Doctor Merriman, among others, considered non-existent in the primitive world and amongst savage peoples.[108] In other words, Western women succumbed to the sensitivity of their own education before accepting the natural provision of their suffering. If they were not troubled by fantastical readings, poorly informed comments, an inappropriate education, or inadequate social conventions, the future mothers would take on the pain of birth naturally and with wise resignation. It is not barbarism, but rather the excess of civilization, that has modified the pain threshold, turning a natural event into a nervous crisis. What's more, assuming that there were 50 contractions lasting some 30 seconds each during a birth of 4 hours, he reasoned, the woman would not suffer for more than 15 or 16 minutes distributed over the 4 hours, which to Merriman seemed insignificant.[109] In his view, there would also be no difference between losing consciousness as a result of inhaling gases or of excessively ingesting alcohol. In both cases, women reached the same state of stupefaction, without the ability, in this chemical drunkenness, to either control their pain, or in more sinister consequences, to control their pleasure.[110] On this point, Doctor Isaac Ray, a member of the English society of obstetrics, considered that the surgeon should always be especially vigilant during those moments in which women seemed more given to display *instinctive behavior.* During sexual activity, pregnancy, or breastfeeding, strange thoughts, extraordinary feelings, uncontrolled appetites, or criminal impulses could take over their innocent minds. But the same also happened in the moment of birth. Tyler Smith, for example, one of the founders of obstetrics, commented that sexual excitation was very visible during childbirth; on occasions reaching a state of erotomania.[111] What's more, the signs of an orgasm frequently replaced the pain of contractions and birth, which constituted a moral objection that could increase still more if these facts were known by parents and husbands. Many years before, Pierre Dionis had explained that there were even some women who wanted to feel the *accoucher's* hand in their vagina at all times, which the surgeon considered had to be accepted with patience and "with all decency," more for the benefit of her imagination than the aid of her body.[112]

Freed from her volatile temperament and the ability to speak, the anesthetized woman left not only her bodily integrity but also her moral decency in the doctor's hands. The generalized entrance of surgical practices as well as chemical anesthetics into natural childbirth led to a series of dilemmas. On the one hand, the elimination of subjective elements allowed the surgeon to concentrate on the objective functions of the organism, without the distractions and accompanying elements of the female condition. On the other hand, however, chloroform eliminated not only consciousness but also morality. The idealizing of the birth conditions of women in so-called "primitive" peoples or "savage" societies led to the same quandary. Even if we were to accept that hypersensitivity is a characteristic of civilization, the brute and inert body, subject to the arbitration of its own instincts, guarantees neither decorum nor decency. For Simpson, nevertheless, the impure thoughts that some attributed to the etherized women in labor only came from colleagues who had bad information or worse intentions: "Never in my life," he wrote, "have I glimpsed the least sign of indecency in either words or actions in any patient anaesthetized with chloroform."[113] Doctor Miller was of the same opinion; he considered that even though hysteria could be easily induced by an incorrect administration of chloroform, this should not be considered a counter-indication of the procedure. For his part, Simpson argued that if anesthesia supposed an interruption and modification in the natural course of childbirth, the same could be said of any other activity in the art of medicine; likewise, the progress of civilization, which permitted the use of footwear or modes of transport, should be considered equally anti-natural.

Although cases of abuse against anesthetized women were not unheard of, one need not turn to criminal conduct to understand the place occupied by the inert body of an anesthetized woman in the Victorian imaginary. The history of painting in the second half of the nineteenth century abounds in representations of old, bearded scientists contemplating, either alone or in a group, a young woman who has fainted, fallen unconscious, or died.[114] The most well-known of these scenes is the 1887 painting by the French artist Pierre André Brouillet, which has the fascinating title *A Clinical Lesson at the Salpetrière*; that is, the mental hospital for women in Paris. We find a similar representation in Gabriel Max's *The Anatomist*, painted in 1869, where an anatomist melancholically contemplates the breast of a young female corpse. In Henri Gervex's 1887 painting *Before the Operation*, a group of wise men crowd around an unconscious and half-naked woman. In all these cases, the person on the dissection or operating table is a woman who possesses the sacrosanct virtues of bourgeois morals; at least while she is asleep, more so if she is dead, she is good, silent, and sexually available.[115] The Spanish painter Enrique Simonet y Lombardo, in the last year of the nineteenth century, also produced an admirable canvas showing the anatomical exploration of a woman's body. Inspired by other paintings of the time – and also probably by the frontispiece of *Madame Bovary,* which depicted its author, Flaubert, as an anatomist – an old man holds in his hand the heart he has just extracted from the cadaver. The professor gazes at it admiringly, as though he might be able to discover in this mass of muscles and blood a trace of feeling, a last breath of life (see Figure 15). The pictorial argument rests on the opposition between the objective and the subjective; the civilized and the savage; the masculine and the feminine. Perhaps more than anything, the painting exemplifies an opposition between the brain, the organ responsible for knowledge, and the heart, the seat of the passions. The solitude of this figure in black, who contemplates with incredulity the trophy he has just ripped from the body, is more than slightly perturbing. The axis of the painting is the triangle formed by the heart in the anatomist's left hand, the scalpel in his right hand, and his sad, almost perplexed, ecstatic and incredulous expression as he contemplates the remains of the dead young woman. The painting's marked chiaroscuro, the contrast in light between scientific activity and the deathly passivity, the profile of the anatomist and the foreshortening of the corpse, along with the neutral background of the room, make up the basic themes of the work. The painting was initially called *And She Had a Heart!,* and only later came to be known as *Anatomy of the Heart.* The initial title, with its exclamation mark, tells us that an anatomical exploration has taken place as an efficient way of confirming, against all prior evidence, that the young woman lying on the dissecting table possessed an organ whose existence had been questioned. Hence the admiration in the face of proof that the ungrateful woman who rests on the dissecting table possessed at least the material possibility of having feelings; her probable indifference and wayward behavior could not be attributed to a morphological accident.

In the logic of this strange metonymy that compares the heart with the sexual organs, birth would be the moment of systole, whereas conception would be that of diastole. For Tyler Smith, one of the proponents of this rhetorical figure, "the living beings that flow in uncountable numbers through the uterus are as insignificant in the great torrent of life as the myriad globules we see in the circulation of the blood through the microscope."[116] In other words, the involuntary action of the heart also corresponds to the mechanical action of the uterus, whether in the moment of conception or birth. In both cases, the woman appears as a being that, through education or nature, is incapable of controlling either the beating of her heart or the throbbing of her sex. Outside the logic of correspondence, pain appears as the result of an incorrigible susceptibility, whose correct evaluation must be held above the woman's testimony, without attending to her cries and laments except to reinterpret them and place them in the cartography of systematic knowledge and in the semiotics of objective signs.

The measure of pain

Science is measurement, Nancy Cartwright wrote in 1989.[117] More than a criterion of demarcation, this philosopher was declaring her intentions regarding the reality of magnitudes and the difficulty of understanding scientific activity without them. For Cartwright, the scientific image of the world – the image originating from scientific theories themselves – requires the use of measurements in the same way that the manifest image of the world – that which depends on our daily knowledge of objects – has no need for such power to intervene. Writing in 1966, the German philosopher Rudolf Carnap had also defended the idea that the difference between commensurable and incommensurable capacities did not depend on anything intrinsic to nature itself. There was no natural frontier dividing the domain of objects into two disjointed classes: on the one hand, incommensurable properties and, on the other, magnitudes. Perhaps at first glance it might seem that there are immeasurable relationships but, according to Carnap, this does not depend on the relationships themselves. Quite the contrary, given that magnitudes are not a property of objects, but rather a consequence of the development of the sciences, we must conclude that only the most developed disciplines offer specific measurement systems, whereas the other disciplines are at a much poorer stage of development. In the case that concerns us, the difficulty lies in establishing whether and how it is possible to make a fundamental measurement of pain and, more generically, of conscious subjective experience.

The appropriate proportion, the exact measurement, or the economical distribution that we saw in the previous chapter may provide an approximate answer to the interpretation of another's emotions and sensations. The passions of others, including their harmful experiences, may seem to us to be comprehensible, well represented, fair in their origin, or economical in their means of expression, but none of these characterizations would seem to be sufficient, or *scientifically* sufficient. We can see, imitate, represent, understand, or even sympathize with another's pain, but at least on certain occasions, what we would want, above all, is to measure it; not just to establish a proportion or correspondence, but also to assign numerical values to a scale. Nor does the distribution of experience in accordance with terms like "mild," "moderate," "severe," or "unbearable" alone solve the problem of the sensation's intensity. As in the case of temperature, sometimes it is not enough to know that other people are cold or that the bath water is hot, but it is also necessary to find a procedure to determine how cold or how hot. Do we perhaps need a *thermometer* of the passions, a mechanical instrument that, working merely as a register, could substitute the opinions of others? The transformation of (subjective) experience into an (objective) fact responds affirmatively to this question, attempting, against Kant, to establish a science of subjectivity capable of rising above the semiotics of pain or the cartography of tragedy.

As we have just seen, the objectification of private experience began by replacing personal testimony with inscriptions of an intersubjective nature. In order to parcel out and measure the sensorial universe, one must begin by eliminating all unjustified complaints and disproportionate laments. As opposed to introspection and testimony, the new science of the intimate sense had to be rooted in physiology and physics.[118] Philosophy's own constrictions were gradually lost as the virtues of the science of consciousness, based on physical or physiological study of conscious sensations, were made public. When Wilhelm Wundt extolled the autonomy of psychology, he did no more than assume the position that had been consolidated during the 1840s, partly under the auspices of the physicist and physiologist Herman von Helmholtz.[119]

Like physiological research, psychological investigation, interested in establishing a correspondence between the magnitude of sensations and the intensity of stimuli, was also based on the artificial production of pain. Although the purpose of the research was never physical suffering itself, harmful experiences allowed establishing of functional correspondences between injuries and sensorial intensities. The struggle to find these correlations seemed all the more reasonable given that, under normal circumstances, a small prick with a needle in the finger causes tolerable pain, whereas a strong blow with hammer to the same place normally unleashes severe pain.[120] The instrumental use of pain began with two prior conditions. In the first place, it was necessary to assume the stability of the object under investigation, as numerical values could not be assigned to an unstable or unpredictable experience. As in the philosophy of taste, which had to presuppose a common physiology for all human beings, the psychology of experience likewise had to begin by accepting that the thresholds of sensation remained constant in the same person and more or less constant between different individuals. No less important was the pre-eminence given to the purely mechanical capturing of the values of the sensation. The distancing Adam Smith proposed in his concept of the impartial observer had to be replaced with the effect of a mere mechanism or, if this were not possible, by easily replicable responses, so that the same stimulus would produce the same reaction in the same individual in a sufficient number of cases.

The greatest effort to introduce a numerical function into the study of subjective sensation belonged to Gustav Theodor Fechner [1801–1887]. This physicist, educated at the University of Leipzig, has reached posterity for developing an empirical law according to which the intensity of the perception of a sensation is proportional to the stimulus that causes it.[121] As he explained in his *Elements of Psychophysics*, a work published in 1860, the motive that guided his research was an attempt to establish "the exact science of functional relations or relations of dependence between the body and the mind."[122] It was supposedly on the morning of 22 October 1850 that he decided to relate the increase of bodily energy to the corresponding rise of mental intensity.[123] He sought to demonstrate that a series of psychic intensities corresponded to a geometrical series of physical intensities. This was a supposedly objective relationship between physical phenomena and psychic states that Fechner attributed to the works of his fellow physiologist Ernst Heinrich Weber [1795–1878]. In 1846, Weber had published his *Tatsinn und Gemeingefühl* – a work that could be translated as "Sense of Touch and Synesthesia."[124] Some time before, Bourguer had attempted to establish a correlation between subjective sensation and the objective intensity of light, and even prior to that, the scientist Ohm had defended a logarithmic relationship between the force of a current and the length of the cable.[125] At least from the age of 23, Fechner was convinced that qualitative research had to replace the quantitative spirit that had guided Ohm's or Jean-Baptiste Biot's research. However, this did not prevent him from setting about, under the pseudonym Dr Mises, to promote the virtues of *Naturphilosophie* – a speculative philosophy of nature – writing on subjects as esoteric as the *Comparative Anatomy of Angels*. A student of medicine in Leipzig, translator, and professor of physics, in the last years of his life he dedicated himself to the theory of art, and between 1866 and 1872 he published 12 articles on the two *Madonnas* of Dresden and of Darmstadt, so as to determine, experimentally, the paintings' authorship.

Given that subjective sensations cannot be calculated by direct methods, Fechner began to consider an indirect procedure for measuring the capacity to feel sensations.[126] Thus he established a unit that he termed "barely noticeable difference" (*bnd*), which he defined as the (differential) threshold that separates two sensations. His reasoning suggests that if our sensations did not depend directly on the stimulus but on their relative differences (very much in harmony with the physiological knowledge of the time, which considered, as we have seen in Bichat, that all sensations are relative), then any increase in the stimulus would produce a similar increase in the sensation, such that the intensity of the perception of a sensation would be proportional to the stimulus that caused it.[127] In this way, Fechner arrived at the conclusion that he had discovered the procedure for measuring sensation, albeit indirectly, and therefore he had been able to establish a functional relation between the body and the soul.[128] Some researchers in the twentieth century accepted that Fechner's law was approximately valid for calibrating the intensity of pain. In the mid-twentieth century, Hardy, Wolff, and Goodell established a scale of 21 *bnds* or pain intensity units, between the scarcely perceptible prick to throbbing pain.[129] Each group of two *bnds* was given the name "*dol*," so that the complete scale for the intensity of pain consisted of 10.5 *dols*. Some *dolorimeters* were even designed based on this experimental framework. Despite all these efforts, there were nonetheless many questions that remained to be answered: What does it mean if someone's level of pain is three *dols* or five *dols*? Are two simultaneous pains measuring three *dols* equivalent to a single pain of six *dols*? And what to make of the difference between intensity and duration? What is the relation between a pain of three *dols* that continues for weeks and a momentary pain of seven *dols*?

Throughout the twentieth century, despite the evidence in its favor, the relationship between the intensity of pain and the magnitude of the lesion was progressively revealed to be incomplete for various reasons. In the first place, this occurred through studied cases of congenital anesthesia – a strange condition consisting of an innate inability to feel pain, which consequently completely calls into question the proportional correspondence between stimulus and response. People suffering from this illness must learn how not to injure themselves while chewing or walking with fractured bones. Sooner or later, bacteria enter injured areas, making their way to the marrow. Episodic anesthesia is much more common than this rare disease; this is a condition that eliminates pain from the consciousness for a few minutes or hours following an injury.[130] Finally, as we shall see later, there has always been pain that either cannot be associated with any known morphological lesion whatsoever, or pain that remains once the damaged area has been completely cured, as occurs in the well-documented phenomenon of phantom limbs: pain felt by amputees in limbs they no longer have. Even leaving aside the case of masochism, which we shall examine in Chapter 6, not all pain is accompanied by a lesion; nor is every lesion accompanied by suffering. At the end of the nineteenth century, Alfred Goldscheider harshly critiqued the idea that physical pain could be considered the effect of a specific sensation. This German neurologist considered that suffering could be generated by any kind of stimulus, provided that it also produced the adequate intensity. In this way, he developed the idea that pain had its origin in the central nervous system and depended not only on the intensity but also the summation of different impulses. The American psychologist Henry Rutgers Marshall and the German physiologist Ernst Heinrich Weber debated whether pain had its own networks of transmission. In their opinion, pain was not even a sensation; rather, it was an emotion that, unlike other sensations, could be provoked by an infinite combination of causes. The argument reached its culmination when, in all logic, Marshall recognized that pain could be imaginary. In 1894 he wrote in the *Journal of Nervous and Mental Diseases*: "neurologists are wasting a considerable part of their valuable time searching for transmitters of pain in the spinal cord and nerve endings."[131]

It was more problematic accounting for the supposed relationship between the intensity of the stimulus and its psychological or sensorial dimension. Countless experiments carried out in the field of psycho-physiology tended to establish that the quality and quantity of the pain perceived amounted to much more than a variable depending on sensorial stimulus, and that one had to take into account the psychological and cultural phenomena that did not depend on the nature or the quantity of the stimulus. One of the examples quoted during the 1950s and 1960s concerned the observations made by the anesthetist Beecher during the Second World War. A field surgeon who worked at the hospital set up on the beaches at the port of Benzio in 1944, Beecher was enormously surprised to find that, when he asked the injured soldiers admitted to the hospital whether they felt any pain, more than 70 percent said no. Beecher concluded that part of the response was due to the increased possibilities of survival, and more concretely to the expectation of being evacuated. In these circumstances, it was possible to think that the connection between the lesion and the pain was not uniform in all cases.[132] Much earlier, other surgeons had already been able to prove that the relationship between the intensity of pain and the gravity of the lesion did not always remain constant.[133]

These counter-examples have not impeded a profusion of attempts to safeguard an objective measurement of pain. The reasons for this insistence depend on considerations of a philosophical and pragmatic nature, which cannot and should not be ignored.[134] On the one hand, objectivity always appeared as the ontological corollary of truth, or as the result of the direct correspondence between words and things. Outside of journalism and politics, which generally consider objectivity in terms of distancing or disinterest, nineteenth-century science understood that the truth of our pronouncements on the world depended on their correspondence with the structure of nature. This means that pain, independently of its subjective perception, should be possible to investigate through purely mechanical procedures, especially in those cases involving children and animals, to whom we have no direct linguistic access.[135] At the same time that the ideology of scientific objectivity became freely accepted, clinical medicine had and has the need to establish a scale permitting, among other things, the administration of drugs not only suitable for different ailments, but also in proportion to the intensity of the pain. However, of the three methods developed since the end of the nineteenth century – psychophysical stimulation, standardized questionnaires, and responses from patients relating their pain to a scale of intensities – clinical medicine has opted for the latter two.[136]

In the history of other empirical sciences – and especially in the history of physics or natural philosophy – these processes of objectification are usually explained through the gradual introduction of metric concepts or the acceptance of an intersubjective use of private experiences.[137] It is not by chance that objectivity has been interpreted as a loss of perspective that, linked to a set of analogous terms, such as "disinterest," "impartiality," or "distancing," postulates an absence of subjectivity in the process of knowledge. The universality of science and its experimental practices seems to require the deliberate abandoning of all that is most ours to adopt, in a notable epistemological constriction, *the point of view from nowhere*.[138] At least in principle, anyone would be willing to recognize that objectivity is opposed to subjectivity in the same way that truth contradicts falsehood or that public facts represent a moral victory over private interests. In the history that concerns us, however, objectivity not only appears associated with a loss of subjective reference, but also with a considerable modification of perceptual capacity and, more particularly, with the susceptibility of accounting for a phenomenon that is invisible for the spectator and relatively ineffable for the person who suffers from it. Given that pain hides behind the physiological gesture and the anatomical structure, the escape from perspective does not consist of renouncing what is most ours in order to adopt the point of view of God, but rather accepting the point of view of others. The objectivity of pain, the inevitable conclusion of a theme of correspondence, was never a *less social* process but rather a *more social* one, which depended on the homogeneity of witnesses more than on the uniformity of the symptoms.[139] The objectivity of pain, to put it another way, never consisted of a mathematical modification or reformulation of a "non-observable entity" – or, as Edmund Burke put it following John Locke's terminology, a "simple idea" – but rather of the development of a set of experimental techniques linked to the unity of the subjects, and not the objects of knowledge.[140]

5
Trust

The drama of unconsciousness

The emergence of anesthesia is a well-known story. Two dentists, Horace Wells and William Thomas Green Morton, along with Charles Jackson, a scientist, disputed which of them deserved the glory of having "conquered pain."[1] The three men found themselves immersed in a confusing and bitter quarrel, which we could sum up as follows: Wells had the idea but didn't know how to apply it; Morton achieved the first experimental success but didn't know how to put it into practice. Jackson, who had neither the idea nor the opportunity of developing it, managed to patent the product, although no one ever paid anything for it. Each one of them sought to be the one and only discoverer of anesthesia; a term that was, incidentally, none of their idea. The dispute over the priority of the discoveries led Wells first to alcoholism and then to prison – after, for no apparent reason, sprinkling vitriolic acid on a group of women who were out for a walk in Brooklyn – and finally to suicide by cutting his femoral artery while in prison. Morton, for his part, died of a heart attack and Jackson ended his days in a psychiatric hospital.

Historians have written profusely about the circumstances in which these three gentlemen fought for the honor of having "defeated pain."[2] The dispute began when Horace Wells tried to apply the narcotic effects of nitrous oxide to dental surgery. In 1845, he proposed a public demonstration, which unfortunately ended amidst the screams of his patient. Wells's collaborator, William Morton, decided to conduct an experiment with ether vapor, a gas that the chemist Michael Faraday had described as having similar properties. He began his experiments with a goldfish, and then moved onto a hen. He cut off the hen's crest while it lay as though dead. On his next attempt, his dog Nig did not completely lose consciousness, but he was afraid of his owner from that moment on. Following a struggle, he also etherized two of his students, Spear and Leavitt. Both of them reached a state of over-excitement, which prevented the trial from producing conclusive proof. The dentist then decided to pay any-one who was willing to breathe in the gas voluntarily, because when he himself had inhaled it on repeated occasions he had never been able to remain con-scious long enough to describe the results. Finally, a man named Frost arrived at his surgical office. He was a healthy and corpulent musician who was suffer-ing from a severe toothache. When he awoke, on Morton's insistence, he wrote the following:

> This is to certify that I applied to Dr. Morton this evening at 8 o'clock, suffering under the most terrible toothache; that Dr. Morton took out his handkerchief, saturated it with a preparation of his, from which I breathed about half a minute, and then was lost in sleep. In an instant more I awoke, and saw my tooth lying on the floor. I did not experience the slightest pain whatever. I remained 20 minutes in his office afterward, and felt no unpleas-ant effects from the operation. Eben H. Frost. Boston, 42 Prince Street, Sept. 30, 1846.[3]

A few days later, Morton called John C. Warren, a surgeon from Massachusetts General Hospital, and asked him whether he could use his new substance on the operating table. The demonstration took place on 16 October 1846. A cer-tain Gilbert Abbot, 20 years old, was to have a vascular tumor cut out of his lower jaw. Morton questioned his patient before beginning. "Are you afraid?" he asked him. "No. I feel confident and will do precisely as you tell me," the young man replied.[4] A sepulchral silence hung over the theater throughout the operation. Gilbert moved his extremities from time to time; his face twitched, but, apart from that, he seemed entirely asleep. There were no screams, cries, or weeping. "I have seen something today which will go around the world," Doc-tor Bigelow, who was also present, apparently exclaimed.[5] The surgeon Holmes suggested the word "anesthesia" in a letter to Morton in November 1846, partly to replace the original word "*letheon*," coined in honor of the River Lethe of Greek mythology, making reference to oblivion.[6]

In the twentieth century, 100 years after the first application of anesthesia in surgical operations, History – with a capital H – echoed some of the rhetoric used to describe these events in the previous century. "The battle," "the con-quest," and "the victory" were some of the expressions employed to depict the use of narcotic substances during surgery. These words, taken from military rhetoric, suggested a point of inflection in the way that all human beings, from all periods, in all known time, had related to pain in the critical moment of surgery. The introduction of anesthesia was celebrated as a new "revelation" or "liberation" from slavery comparable to what had occurred in Tsarist Russia or the South of the United States. There were no relative victories or partial conquests. There was, simply, a *before* and an *after*, which replaced the medical practices governed by the "mind that never doubts and the hand that never trembles."[7] The screams and cries that had echoed in the operating theater throughout the history of humanity gave way to a new strange and disquieting silence. When Queen Victoria of England herself accepted treatment with chloroform for the birth of her fourth child, on 7 April 1853, the Hippocratic Oath, according to which it was up to the Gods to relieve pain – *divinum est opus sedare dolorem* – was fully incorporated into the art of medicine.

Despite the initial enthusiasm, the appearance of anesthesia had to face some resistance. The events of 1846, which spread like wildfire in the following three months and reached all of Europe by the end of the year, had to pave the way amid no shortage of reticence and criticism. Much of this resistance arose in the context of corporate struggles over the professionalization of surgical practices; other criticisms were framed within the broader spectrum of moral discourse, military opinions, and humanist arguments. Anesthesia obliged many surgeons to take a side with respect to the translation of certain excerpts of Genesis; and the other way around – many religious sectors had to make pronouncements concerning the possibility of subverting what had been understood as either the retributive element of the human condition after the Fall or a value linked to maternity or the military spirit. Given that pain was natural, it was reasoned, it must be necessary; it was a cross that human beings could merely learn to bear, either as a form of expiation, a means of salvation, or an instrument of physical or spiritual strengthening.

Anesthesia's detractors did not lack arguments. The editors of the magazine *Chelius*, for example, could not understand the advantages of a physical state that could hardly be distinguished from an ethylic intoxication. Any surgeon who refused to operate on patients who were unconscious as a result of a massive consumption of alcohol would not agree to do so, they reasoned, with patients who presented similar symptoms as a result of inhaling gas.[8] Some doctors, though not many, openly defended surgical pain, referring to the supposed benefits of suffering for the patient's recovery. For Pigorov, for example, it was repugnant to perform an operation on a person bereft of feeling and consciousness.[9] Contrary to the most popular opinion that the best surgical operation was the fastest one, for this Russian surgeon, as before him for the apologist François Bilon, the patient's cries guided the scalpel.[10] Pain, a certain Doctor Copland argued in 1842, was a wise provision of nature that should be suffered by patients to help the operation and improve their convalescence. Not without irony, Professor Elliotson wondered whether the history books would ever recall that such a stupid thing was ever uttered; for while the phrase would make a dent in history, its author would soon fall into oblivion.[11] In France, where most physiological research was carried out on live animals, some big names joined the fray. The physiologist Magendie, for example, declared to the French Academy of Science that surgical pain was trivial, and explained that any attempt to annul it was of very limited interest.[12] As late as 1847, the *Edinburgh Medical and Surgical Journal* considered physical suffering beneficial in most cases, given that preventing or eliminating it was very dangerous for the patient.[13] On the other hand, many surgeons felt that anesthesia could be unsafe and, although infrequent, death attributable to its use was sufficient to add practical problems to the existing ideological difficulties.[14]

Despite these opinions against anesthesia, most of the profession shared the conviction that the inhaling of gases was just another method for avoiding surgical pain. In an activity that depended to a great extent on public satisfaction, the only path was to encourage any procedure that permitted the recruitment of clients. Anesthesia formed part of the same battery of measures intended to banish the cruel and inhuman features that had been associated with the practice of surgery since time immemorial and which had irredeemably impregnated the collective imagination. "Physicians have been accused of a want of feeling for the distress of human nature and surgeons of actual cruelty," wrote James Moore, a member of the Surgeons' Company of London.[15] Enlightenment thinker Henry-François le Dran [1685–1770] thought along the same lines, considering his obligation to restore health whenever possible, and alleviate incurable suffering when not.[16] In order to cause only strictly necessary pain, he recommended evaluating the patient's age, strength, constitution, and emotional state so as to decide whether he or she was in a fit condition to put up with the fear, suffering, and danger of an operation. It was important to choose the right season and, if urgency did not allow, keep the room at the right temperature. The surgeon should have at least two sets of each instrument available and be sure to have enough candles. Equally important, the operation should be carried out expeditiously because even a single moment of agony would seem too long. Doctor Chapman [*c.* 1680–1756] also considered it important that pregnant women should not lay their eyes on any instrument that might upset them.[17] Gentleness of manner seemed to be as important as skill in the application of remedies. A surgeon should work with kind movements and behave calmly. Lack of gentleness, which would alarm both the patient and the family, should be replaced by a "*nature bien élevée*" and a "*raison cultivée*": the head should direct the hand and not the hand the head.[18]

This new form of surgery did not eliminate the theatrical nature of the harmful experience, but it did modify the elements used to build its drama. Although the gestures were regulated by social conventions and cultural expectations, professionalization would add new rules to the spectacle's economy. Silence replaced noise, courtesy replaced barbarity, and kindness replaced indifference. Sensitivity no longer depended on a (mass) public that vindicated brutality as a form of private expiation or collective identification. On the contrary, the new surgeons rejected the "puerile ceremonies" that, during the early modern period, had transformed suffering into a source of entertainment. Pain with a spectator, which still constituted a constant element of surgical operations and punitive practices even in the eighteenth century, was replaced by a professionalized comedy distanced as far as possible from ritualized celebrations of blood.[19]

This transition from noise to silence, present in surgical practices as a whole, was especially visible in the case of dental surgery. Far from the grand operations and birth scenes, the fights between the surgeon, the barber, and the tooth-drawer to obtain the monopoly over a guaranteed illness, which, especially as a result of changes in diet, was associated with large financial compensation, began at the end of the seventeenth century.[20] The tooth-drawer, whose practice rested almost exclusively on what had been learned through a repetition of cases and with no training other than oral tradition, began to compete with the new professionals, whose art rested, at least in principle, on anatomical knowledge. Histories of dentistry place the beginnings of this profession around the middle of the eighteenth century, especially following the publication of the works of Pierre Fauchard and John Hunter. Fauchard, the author of the monumental *The Surgical Dentist* published in 1728, first coined the word "dentist." John Hunter, for his part, published *The Natural History of the Human Teeth*, between 1771 and 1777, a book that the new professionals greeted as one of the great milestones of their new practice.[21]

While in the early modern period the loss of teeth was a part of the punishment inflicted by God after the Fall – which consequently required a (collective) purification – the new surgery did not recognize any connection between suffering and culpability, nor any other internalization of sin other than lack of hygiene, ignorance, and imprudence regarding the physiological functions of the jaw or the anatomical structure of the teeth, or an excessive liking for chocolate, which surgeons were already warning against. When necessary, extraction could be carried out in many different ways. In extreme circumstances, the tooth-drawer placed his sword in the patient's mouth from atop a horse; in other situations, he would pull on a string tied to the tooth while threatening the patient with a piece of burning coal (see Figure 16). In the anonymous canvas in Figure 17, the grimace of the patient, whose arms have been tied to his body by a rope, finds not even the slightest glimpse of commiseration from the official who looks at him with disdain. On the contrary, in a notable gesture of contempt, he uses his leg as a lever against his patient's body. The man's wrinkled, masculine, virile, bad-tempered countenance contrasts with the beseeching, feminine, and resigned face of the patient. What allows the tooth-drawer to be included in the history of theater and of the *commedia dell'arte* is not the fact that the members of itinerant theater companies were often dentists who also did theater or actors who also pulled teeth, but rather the festive and carnivalesque context of an operation that was increasingly carried out away from the public square.[22]

In the drawing made on an envelope, addressed to certain J. Chapman in 1894 by someone whose initials were C. E. H., all the expressive elements have been modified (see Figure 18). This new image suggests the replacement of manual skill by the work of a machine that, in carrying out the extraction automatically, transforms the scene into a supposedly painless event performed with a professional touch and mathematical certainty.[23] Long after the first operations carried out using clinical anesthesia, the caricature points out – even if to debate them – the advantages of technological development over manual procedures. As in the times of the guillotine, which supposedly replaced the skill of the executioner with the assured effect of a mere mechanism, tooth drawing could be carried out "painlessly" through recourse to technological developments. It was not the ability, but the technique, that freed Victorian men and women from their torments and fears. The use of new instruments, whether in odontology, obstetrics, or surgery, constituted a mark of distinction that placed the *ancients* on one side and the *moderns* on the other. The practices of the former were based on an artisanal tradition, whereas the latter had their roots in anatomical knowledge and technological innovation. The new instruments marked a point of inflection between informed knowledge and mere verbiage; they allowed the successful carrying out of more complex operations and the undertaking of others that had previously been impractical. Whereas the use of the dental pelican, the forceps, or the new scalpel demonstrated trust and confidence in the empire of reason, those who like Simpson defended the use of anesthesia also supported industrialization and progress. The fears caused by trains, stated this obstetrician, were no more logical than those caused by the inhalation of gases.

A new relationship of trust came to replace the values associated with the way in which pain should be withstood, either through bravery or stoicism. The arrival of anesthesia in the operating theater brought about unhurried dialogues and controlled gestures. Although the appearance of narcotic gases did not in itself change the scenery of experience, it did allow the protagonists to interpret a different comedy. The surgeon no longer behaved like an executioner, but like a gentleman. The patient, on the other hand, no longer endured the operation like a martyr, but like a corpse. Although the anesthetized body crossed border regions and intermediate spaces, its experience was no longer marked by an excess of feeling, but by a loss of consciousness. The experimental framework of this new life experience was not a fixed structure, but an unstable reality.[24] The arrival of anesthesia culminated the trend to weaken the body, limit its vitality, and restrict its strength, whether through the use of chemical substances or mechanical procedures. The Victorians were right when they spoke of freedom without palliatives and unconditional victory. The possibility of inducing sleep at will divided the entire history of humanity into two periods: the conscious and the unconscious. And yet, soporific gases did not prevent the surgical trance from continuing to exist, inscribed in a ritualized context where the patient had to give in to the uncertain and the unknown. Its appearance gave access to new ways of attending the body and forced the introduction of a new element into the evaluation of painful experience: consciousness. The relationship between geography and history, between the locus of the ailment and the patient's narrative, which the first modernity tried to understand in an automatic and proportioned way, gave way to an experience that, mediated by the will, could deliberately hide the perception of pain or, conversely, involuntarily perceive a sensation that the patient would never be able to remember. These two problems will be addressed in the last two sections of this chapter. Before doing so, however, we must relocate the history of anesthesia within the (varyingly successful) search for procedures to combat surgical pain; and second, within the necessity to reduce the patient to an inert and insensitive body.

The remedy

As late as 1846, the debate on suppressing surgical pain appeared somewhat hasty and even absurd. For Doctor Velpeau [1795–1867], for example, the mind could not understand cutting instruments and pain independently from one another.[25] The entire history of mankind confirmed this inviolable connection. Given that everything that cuts, hurts, he argues, what would be the point of discussing impossible cases? And he was right: until the middle of the nineteenth century, there was no universally effective procedure capable of removing physical suffering from the operating table. On the contrary, surgery prior to the inhalation of gases was governed by two principles: hold down and debilitate. The initial strength of the patient had to be restricted, either by using one's hands, mechanical utensils, or, better still, through an initial weakening of the body's capacity for resistance. Before the first cut was made, the patient, who would have been bled several times and given emetics, laxatives, and a light diet, already resembled a corpse. He would be as though dead, reduced further by a proliferation of hands; the less his initial vitality, the less the need to limit his movements through the use of force.

Before the arrival of ether, surgeons had only few palliative remedies at their reach. Opium, a plant known since the time of Celsus, was never used before the twelfth century, and later only employed as part of postoperative treatment. As late as 1796, the physiologist Benjamin Bell recommended administering it following the operation, and never before, to avoid the adverse effects that it produced on the organism.[26] Along with cinchona bark – used in treating malaria, and later for the extraction of quinine – antimonials were frequently employed to cause vomiting and thus contribute to a general weakening of the body. Equally popular was the so-called "Dover powder," a substance named after the English doctor Thomas Dover that was nothing more than a sudorific mixture of opium and potassium sulfate, plus another emetic, in this case ipecacuanha.[27] As far as alcohol is concerned, patients and surgeons drank it in equal proportions, and although Pierre Dionis recommended that the patient be given "half a glass of wine to better resist the pain," there are reasons to think that doses were frequently much larger. What some called the "nervous delirium of those operated on" was for others no more than an alcoholic rapture similar to that attributed to some pregnant women. According to Richet, far from drinking in moderation, patients "arrived for their operations drunk."[28]

Diderot and d'Alembert's *Encyclopédie* includes the illustration of a very revealing surgical chair. This fascinating object, which reminds us in all its details of a torture chair, seems to have been designed to restrict as effectively as possible the patient's movements of resistance. The shackles held the head firm, kept the neck straight, and limited the brusque movements of the trunk. Many nineteenth-century humorous illustrations of amputation share with this image the indirect representation of pain through the human or mechanical force necessary to restrict the violence of the body. Far from the cross of Biverus (see Figure 7), which measured all suffering in terms of the Passion of Christ, the right amount of pain, and the way in which it should now be interpreted, takes place now without the mediation of supernatural elements or values. On the contrary, the proliferation of hands seems enough to assess the proportion of the tragedy. Long before the arrival of other mechanical instruments of measurement, and outside of the refined reasoning of psycho-physics, surgical practices quantified pain in accordance with the force required to immobilize the patient. In a treatise in 1784, the surgeon James Moore sought not so much the immobilization of the body as limiting its sensitivity by cutting or compressing the nerves. His initial experiments were carried out using a tourniquet that put pressure on the sciatic nerve, the cural nerve, and the obturator nerves of the leg.[29] Years before, Hunter himself had tried to produce lethargy by interrupting the blood flow of the carotid arteries. However, what was more common for debilitating the body was bloodletting combined with hot baths and un-strenuous diet.[30] Moore knew that he needed to compress the nerve without interfering with the circulation of the blood. To this end, he designed an instrument that he called the *compressor*, and decided to test it for the first time in St George's Hospital, in London, on a leg amputation. During the circular incision through the skin, the patient did not scream or move a facial muscle. Only a few grimaces of discomfort appeared on his face during the sawing of the bone.[31] Used in France and the UK, the *compressor* didn't take long to fall first into disuse and later into oblivion. The patients complained excessively. Moore's colleague Griffin found their objections unfounded, for "as they had not experienced the pain of amputation without the compressor, it is difficult for any patient to estimate the comparative merits of the two forms of operation," he argued.[32] However, one patient in particular, who had already had one leg amputated without the compressor and was to be subject to a new operation, complained so loudly of the pain caused by the instrument that he declared that he would without a doubt much rather have the operation performed without it.[33]

Although some surgeons, like James Wardrop [1782–1869], bled their patients until they fainted, the greatest measure against surgical pain depended for a long time on the skill of the surgeon and, more specifically, on the speed of the operation.[34] There were two different methods for extracting bladder stones, for example: the French method, via the lower abdomen, or the English method, via the perineum. The latter technique began with the patient being tied down by the ankles and his movements impeded by the help of at least five assistants; the stones were extracted then using a finger, a spoon or forceps. In 1835, all this was carried out on a man from Gloucestershire in 2 minutes and 15 seconds. This might seem fast were it not that, according to the English writer Samuel Pepys, Doctor Hollier extracted a stone from him that was the size of a plum in a little under one minute. Doctor George Hayward – one of the first surgeons to operate on patients using anesthesia – took less than two minutes to amputate the leg of Alice Mohan, a 21 year-old young woman who had been treated with ether by Doctor Morton. Many surgical treatises gave descriptions of the operations followed by the time taken in carrying them out. "The gleam of the knife was followed so instantaneously by the sound of sawing as to make the two actions appear almost simultaneous," it was said of Robert Liston, who could perform an amputation in less than 25 seconds.[35]

Despite this brevity, the decision to subject oneself to the scalpel generally came after many tribulations. The patient had to choose between the torture of the illness and the torment of the operation. In some cases, surgery was demanded as a therapeutic procedure or as an extreme method of alleviating incurable and prolonged suffering. William Griffin, for example, explained that although he tended to avoid complicated operations, he always made exceptions for cancer, when he used the scalpel more out of compassion than efficiency. A patient attended by Alibert, who described his pain as akin to wild dogs biting and ripping his entrails, soon after hanged himself with a cord from the ceiling. The medical official at the center of *The Case of George Dedlow* said that he looked at the preparations for the operation with relief and trust, which would be inexplicable for anyone who had not experienced his six weeks of torture. Once his arm was amputated, he looked at it and happily exclaimed: "There is the pain and here I am. How queer!"[36] In other cases, however, the decision was exactly the opposite. In 1837, for example, a 25-year-old woman, who was suffering unbearable pain from a tumor and whose life was in serious danger, did not consent to an operation.[37]

Of course, this strange anticipation of what we call today "informed consent" was not generally applied to accidents at work or in battle. On the battlefield the decision to operate did not depend on the patient's preferences, but on the surgeon's opinion. For John Hunter, who had served in the Seven Years' War, military conditions made any form of foresight impossible. His non-operation philosophy, which considered that it was better to do nothing than to do something badly, led him to suggest an anti-surgical practice. In the case of bullet wounds, it was best not to try to find the bullet. With wounds to limbs that required amputation, it was best not to carry out the operation on the battlefield. With gunshot wounds to the abdomen or thorax, it was generally best to do nothing at all.[38] The surgeon Larrey, on the other hand, claimed that as a consequence of these measures, humanity had been deprived of expeditious cures for their ailments.[39] In his opinion, the surgeon should decide whether it was preferable to save a life, save a leg (if this was the affected limb), or eliminate pain. Unlike for Hunter, who preferred not to operate if it put life at risk, Larrey considered it advisable to delay the operation when, without loss of life, the leg could also be saved.

The arrival of anesthetics modified surgical practice in many different ways. In the first place, operations could last longer. Lack of bodily movement and gestures of resistance meant that more attention and precision could be used in cutting into delicate areas. The impossibility of carrying out urgent operations on overexcited patients no longer existed. Previously, the necessary lengthy preparations had made it almost impossible to the save the lives of many accident victims; now, chloroform eliminated physical movement and nervous shock with the first inhalation. Of course, the advantages for patients seemed immediate. Given that they no longer had to confront the pain of surgery, their previous state of alarm and excitation was greatly reduced. Faced with the possibility of surgery without suffering, patients showed themselves more willing to go under the knife without waiting for the pain from tumors, aneurisms, or kidney stones to become unbearable. For the surgeons, the possibility of avoiding unnecessary torment was also received with pleasure. In 1848, Doctor James Miller, professor at the University of Edinburgh, had no qualms about affirming that anesthesia afforded great relief to the surgeon as well as to the patient. An opinion that, in his view, did not require justification: "to no ordinarily constituted man is pain otherwise than repugnant whether it occurs in himself or in another."[40] Before every operation, Doctor Abernethy commented that he felt as though he were about to be hanged that very moment. His case was similar to that of the famous Doctor Liston, who lost many hours and missed many a meal as a result of the anxiety brought on by thinking of an imminent operation.

Last, but not least, anesthesia opened up a new form of minor surgical operations and diagnostic procedures. Unlike previous times, where the surgeon was only called when things were going very badly – when the midwife had not been able to deliver the baby, the *dentatore* had not managed to extract a tooth, or when an amputation seemed to be inevitable – the new surgical practices were geared more toward the preservation of teeth, limbs, and life. The operation was no longer a solution to an emergency, but rather an everyday way of attending to the business of the body, whether this was the opening of abscesses, draining of fluids, inserting of setons, cauterization, or examining trauma. One of the most striking cases in this respect was the use of chloroform in women affected by what was known then as *morbid sensitivity*: a special sense of modesty which meant that the surgeons could not have adequate contact with their bodies. Doctor Miller explained the case of a female patient who suffered, at the same time, from an extraordinary sensitivity of the soul and a not less infrequent disease of the rectum. Although the psychic condition had left the physical one unattended to, when it reached a point that did not permit further delay, the woman agreed to let a doctor visit her. The story should not be missed:

> The patient I found in bed; curtains closely drawn; blinds down, everything as dark and close as possible. She would scarcely allow me to speak to her, or feel her pulse. However, with a little persuasion, chloroform-inhalation was begun; and very soon she was snoring. I had the curtains drawn; the blinds raised; the patient's position suitably shifted; and while the sick nurse kept up the needful amount of unconsciousness, I examined the fundament, found a fistula, probed it, cut it, dressed it; had the blind down, the curtains closed, the patients re-arranged, all as before the commencement of this rapidly shifting drama; and when the patient awoke, it was to find the nurse, the bed, the room, and herself, all unchanged, the only difference being that the fistula was somehow cut, instead of being whole.[41]

The fact that Miller referred to this operation as a "little comedy" leaves no doubt as to its dramatic nature. Even under the spell of chloroform, pain appears in the ritualized form of the theater. As the protagonist of the story, the patient disappears with the first inhalation, leaving her body at the disposal of others. For an indefinite time, her pain, but also her will, her preferences, and her consciousness, evaporate. Her opinions, fears, words, fears, gestures, and cries all disappear. The comedy is marked by a silence broken only by attentive gestures and measured voices. Unlike the prior proliferation of hands holding down arms or immobilizing torsos, the manipulation of the body no longer required the use or the abuse of force. On the contrary, chemical anesthesia was seen as yet another easily available technique for producing a state of insensitivity, semi-consciousness, unconsciousness, or trance, similar to those reached using other substances or practices. Taken as a whole, all these means of inducing sleep not only modified the economy of pain, but also its cultural and cognitive representation. The distance that had separated the anatomical lesion from the facial expression or bodily gesture grew excessively. A new route opened between emotion and experience: consciousness, which intervened to hide pain, to express it without feeling it, or, in an even less intuitive sense, to feel it without remembering it.

The disavowal of the main witness of pain, the person directly affected by it, did not depend merely on the generalized use of anesthesia. On the contrary, the history of the experience of suffering abounds in cases where direct testimony questions the most logical relationship between the lesion and the expression of pain. Neither the late medieval martyrs nor the ascetics of the early modern period felt pain from the burning torches or the punishment and maceration of their bodies. Likewise, during the Enlightenment, the feelings and emotions of those principally affected did not depend exclusively on the direct relationship between their bodies and the source of their suffering. Quite the reverse, their experience should be fair and proportioned so as to correspond not only to its cause but also to the idea each person has of himself or herself. The development of experimental physiology, which established a natural and direct correspondence between emotions and expressive signs, also faced time and again the spurious ways in which susceptibility, education, and sexual condition introduced strange elements into the system. The arrival of anesthesia emphasizes this fracture. The fight for professional legitimization and the more extreme debates related to the arrival of this technological innovation were produced under the cover of denouncing the other, or the other's body, as the depository for deliberate lies. Chemical anesthesia, which competes with other much less universal forms of treatment, also concerns the cultural history of deception. Personal testimony is not only questioned, but also inscribed in a system that makes it possible to denounce deliberate errors or conscious lies.

The oath that Eben Frost signed on 30 September 1846 legitimized Morton's etherization techniques. Gilbert Abbot's silence, as well as his involuntary grimaces, during the historical operation of October of that year also played their part. The first witness had to swear, the second to remain motionless. The triumph of anesthesia should not make us forget that in these negotiation processes the moral qualities of the witnesses acquired a new prominence. The history of pain cannot be written without taking into account the historical value given to direct testimony, and the cultural variations that governed its acceptance or rejection. In the previous chapter, we saw how the contemplation of the pain of others generates enigmas as complex as those of our own sensations. The possibility of being mistaken when weighing up the most evident signs of another's suffering, or when considering the other's groans in the framework of deliberate exaggeration or conscious lies, pushes us, more than toward skepticism, toward the metaphysics of suspicion. After all, what if they are tricking us? Aren't they perhaps pretending to be in pain or exaggerating their suffering? Is it not possible to think that women, for example, don't suffer in the same way as men, or that members of another race or culture do not feel pain in the same intensity or are unable to bear it as well as we can? Won't men never understand, for example, the pain of childbirth? Guided by certainty and supported by the distinction and clarity of their own states of mind, some philosophers asked us more than 300 years ago to call into question, at the same time, the existence of an external world and the honesty of others. Contrary to what we might think, we have had less difficulty living with the former than with the latter. The world of shadows in which we live has been no more than the ontological counterpart of the triumph of imposture. We live in a post-modern world where nothing is entirely true because no one is completely honest. The correspondence between words and things has vanished simultaneously with the moral integrity of the witnesses to knowledge. That is the reason why the social history of evidence has been studied through the social construction of testimony; and, consequently, in relation to the honesty of the person who upholds what he or she says above the questioned dignity of his or her own experience.[42]

Induced mental hallucination

Robert Hanham Collyer was born in 1814 in St Helier, the only city on the island of Jersey. Located off the north coast of Normandy, this small island had a sudden population increase in the eighteenth century as a result of wealthy families fleeing the French Revolution. Later, in 1852, the French writer Victor Hugo also went into exile there. The mixture of Norman, English, and French cultures situated Collyer on a sort of frontier.[43] A student of phrenology in Paris and of mesmerism in London, an indefatigable traveler, man of letters, entrepreneur, and keen experimenter, this dilettante could be just as easily found in Europe as in Mexico or Philadelphia. A friend of Whitman, Dickens, Poe, and other men of letters and artists, Collyer hardly ever appears in the history of anesthetics and his name would have sunk without trace had it not been for the fact that in 1877 he presented himself as the authentic and original discoverer of induced mental hallucination.[44] His pretension was backed up by the medical journal *The Lancet*, which had named him, seven years previously in 1870, as the first person to show the way for using anesthetic substances for surgical purposes.[45]

The argument as to who deserved this distinction, which we saw at the beginning of this chapter, and which Collyer joined surprisingly late, obscured some significant aspects related to the introduction and use of narcotic substances and gases. While historians of anesthesia, most of them anesthetists, tend to judge the past merits of this art according to the benefits they have given to the present, social and cultural historians of science tend to see, in the arrival of chemical anesthetics, a central element in the struggle for professional legitimization of surgical practices.[46] Whereas some historians place the emphasis on what was achieved with the discovery, others turn their attention to the efforts made to legitimize the new professionals, on occasions even calling into question the very importance of pain in these disputes.[47] And they may well be right. The priority was not always to alleviate pain, but the events that surrounded the appearance of anesthesia also led to a new evaluation of surgical pain and of the emotions related to its prediction, suffering, and collective distribution. One of the most important manifestations of this new economy of pain was the rift between subjective experience and objective expression of corporal suffering. On the one hand, the same bodily gestures did not always correspond to the same experiences; on the other hand, the same physical causes did not always produce the same expressive signs.[48]

The story of this curious character, who claimed to have lost a fair amount of his genuine contributions to science when he was attacked by bandits in Mexico, places the problem of surgical suffering in the murky waters of the cultural history of fraud. It concerns the barrier between scientific knowledge and mere verbiage, but it also affects the cultural value of suffering, the corporal signs of pain, and, above all, the limits of conscious experience.[49] Collyer's work revolves around elusive categories and short-term notions that appear for a brief while and then disappear for good or become completely modified in their scope of application. Suspended animation, syncope, catalepsy, apparent death, induced hallucination, etherization, anesthetic amnesia, hypnotism, and mesmerization were terms used to describe new sensory experiences that occurred halfway between consciousness and unconsciousness, reality and fiction, sensitivity and automatism.[50] The living, yet inanimate, bodies resting in surgical chairs and anatomical theaters opened up new cultural and emotional spaces where the old prescriptions and social conventions no longer applied. The anaesthetized body, alive and dead at the same time, vulnerable to unpunished manipulation, first required new forms of reliance; for allowing the body to confess its secrets to the surgeon may have been as intricate as allowing the soul to confess the body's secrets to the priest.

Like many of his contemporaries, Collyer inherited from the Enlightenment the fears, anxieties, and debates related to the uncertainties regarding the signs of death. His research stood at a diffuse cultural and cognitive border where social prescriptions, regulations, and conventions were held in suspension. His complex history consisted of a succession of events that, retrospectively, should have placed mankind in a position to free itself from the tyranny of surgical pain. To begin with, Collyer also looked with horror on any unnecessary manifestation of physical suffering.[51] Unless there was a purpose that justified it, pain always seemed abhorrent to him; it could not be justified either in the sphere of knowledge, as the vivisectionists sought to do, or in educational practices, as the colleges proclaimed. His marked "super-sensitive" nature (this was the word he used to describe himself) guided his actions throughout his life, leading him to search for a way of causing a state of *unconscious insensitivity* that could put an end to the torments that had accompanied mankind throughout the entire history of surgical practices. In this he shared in the new philanthropy that was flowering in the Victorian world, fostered by capitalism.[52] One of the most acute elements of this new sensitivity was the capacity to feel and suffer from the pain of others or the ability to anticipate the suffering hidden away in the surgeon's room. "There are thousands," he wrote, "who are so imaginatively sensitive that the mere anticipation of the necessity of Surgical Operation having to be performed, experience the greatest mental torture, much more severe than the most intense physical suffering."[53]

The most important events in the biography of this man of impetuous perception, impulsive actions, open nature, and unstoppable speech – as he was described by his contemporaries – are so tied to the inhalation of gases that both made a mutual claim on one another.[54] Not unlike something from a Dickens novel, Collyer describes almost over-dramatically his *nervous shock* when he had to leave his mother. His profound sadness only found consolation in the kind company of Humphrey Davy [1778–1829], a British chemist who had achieved a notable reputation through his research on the effects of nitrous oxide on the human body, and who later on will be considered by many to have taken the first step on the path toward the discovery of the sedative properties of ether.[55] The *Lancet*, for example, dedicated the first published account of this discovery to him. Although "laughing gas" (as nitrous oxide was known due to the fits of euphoria it caused in those who inhaled it) had only been used as a recreational drug, Collyer was never able to hear again the name of his protector, Davy, without being carried away by the most pleasant emotions. His personal story was constructed on unconscious mental impressions – hidden in the brain and produced during states of extreme sensitivity– that, having lain dormant for years, finally showed themselves when a more favorable occasion arrived. Unbeknownst to him, his first nervous shock had established a connection between the inhalation of gases and the use of anesthetic substances that would only much later become apparent.

When he attended his first surgical operation at the Middlesex Hospital, London, he was only 16 years old. Present in the anatomical theater were Herbert Mayo and Sir Charles Bell – who at that time was only acting as an assistant. On the operating table was a young woman, of about 25 years of age, with refined facial features, eloquent blue eyes, and a beautifully proportioned body. The surgeons prepared for the removal of a cancer of the cervix. Collyer recalls how he felt her heartrending cries, her screams of agony, the grinding of her teeth, the spasmodic twitching of her muscles, the distortion of her countenance. He saw how every feature was writhing in terror and agony, how her large eyes were imploring for mercy. Every fresh cry seemed to pierce his too-sensitive heart. The poor creature's voice became more and more feeble, and after some 25 minutes of intense suffering, she gave a long stifled groan; her eyes were fixed on his. She gasped and died. He felt sick and fainted. Collyer stated that while the death of the young woman had been the result of a *nervous congestion*, his fainting had been caused by another shock, also nervous. Given that both situations have the same physiological origin, the young man concluded that the woman's death could have been avoided if fainting could be produced on demand. There were many precursors to this case. To begin with, those in which a state of shock had resulted from a great physical effort were neither unknown nor infrequent, as the growing interest in sports clearly showed. In the second place, Collyer was convinced that a catatonic state could also be a consequence of the transmission of nervous fluid from one person to another, or from concentrating the mind on an object – as had occurred to him and as he explained in the phenomena of hypnotism and mesmerization. Last, but not least, it seemed possible to reach unconsciousness by inhaling narcotic or stimulant vapors similar to his mentor's nitrous oxide.

The transition from theory to practice did not center on pain, but on insensibility, unconsciousness, induced sleep, or nerve congestion. For most of the people involved, the problem consisted of reaching what was known as "suspended animation," a way to allow the soul to leave the body, without there being any substantive difference between the production of this state of hibernation through the inhalation of gases or the laying on of hands.[56] It is not therefore surprising that when the dentist William Morton went to Washington so that Congress would approve the use of his new anesthetic agent in the medical departments of the Navy and the Infantry, his initiative was rejected. Mutter, a doctor from Philadelphia who wrote up the official report, trusted that the National Congress would not give in to this new form of quackery.[57] His position, similar to Collyer's, made no distinction between mesmerization, hypnotism, and the inhalation of narcotic vapors. However, while for Mutter this confluence was a proof of fraud, for Collyer, on the contrary, the research should continue both into hypnotic induction and the inhalation of gases. Despite Mutter's opinion, the American Army began to use ether in 1847 on the battlefields of Mexico, without acknowledging either Morton's patent or his rights. A very similar response also appeared in the *American Dental Science Review*. In the view of its editors, one of the most extraordinary qualities of sulfuric ether was its capacity to make those that handled it forget the rules of conduct that distinguish the scientist from the charlatan. The surgeons at Massachusetts General Hospital, the editors said, no longer remembered that they did not invent either the drug or its use.[58] The new product, which was provided to all those who had enough faith to breathe it in and sufficient money to pay for it, brought into question not only rights and patents, but also the credibility of a profession that was fighting to establish itself as a respectable professional activity, one that could be comparable in its standards, its scientific attitudes, and its ethical values to the rest of medicine as a whole.[59]

The capacity to generate a state of trance, present in both ancient cultures and practices related to religion, witchcraft, and shamanism, found its modern form in the works of the Swiss Franz Anton Mesmer [1734–1815] at the end of the eighteenth century. Although a commission from the Paris Academy of Sciences discredited it, the idea that states of stupefaction or insensibility could be reached through the modification of certain magnetic fluids supposedly present in the body neither decreased in intensity nor in practice in the first part of the nineteenth century.[60] Partly due to its revolutionary nature, and likewise to the need to find some relief from the certainty of surgical pain, mesmerization was one of the most requested methods for avoiding surgical pain.[61] The Scottish doctor James Braid [1795–1861] tried to free it from its irrational connotations, re-baptizing it with the name "hypnotism." During the first half of the nineteenth century, there were many testimonies given by people who had entered states of unconsciousness at the hands of these new practitioners. Along with many other remedies for alleviating pain and improving symptoms of a great number of illnesses – something that Mesmer had already attempted – Braid considered that this new technique would also permit many patients to undergo surgical operations in painless conditions. If nature itself could produce states of unconsciousness, there should be no difficulty in producing hypnotic sleep at will. His work, published in 1843, included several references to dental operations performed on patients in a hypnotic state, in which he had managed to carry out the operation "with greatly diminished pain, although not entirely without pain."[62] In 1870, *The Lancet* echoed Mesmer's disciples' claim that certain individuals, though not everyone, could be hypnotized.[63] Although the evidence of painless operations was not conclusive, the magazine considered that there were many and very well-confirmed cases. In the decade of the 1840s alone, dozens of these were described. One of them especially deserves our attention.

In 1843, John Elliotson, professor of practical medicine at the recently founded University College Hospital in London and Chairman of the Royal Society of Surgery, published a small pamphlet on surgical operations performed using mesmerization. In the most controversial of these cases, James Wombel's leg was amputated above the knee while, according to those present, the placid look of his countenance never changed for an instant. Despite much favorable testimony from witnesses, most of the members of the Medical and Surgical Society of London expressed nothing more than incredulity and distrust. For Doctor Coulson, for example, the absence of expression or visible signs only indicated that Wombel was able to stand the torment of the operation with stoicism, keeping the magnitude of his suffering to himself. The young Doctor Blake, a surgeon who said he had witnessed the extraction of a tooth in a supposed hypnotic state, held the same opinion: he concluded that he had actually attended a play. Doctor Alcock, who had seen many patients submit to operations without voicing any complaints, refused to believe that this was a result of the laying on of hands. Doctor Moore, an expert in childbirth, asked whether there were any notaries amongst the witnesses – an insinuation that Elliotson could only find extraordinarily indignant. It would be the first time, he said, that a notary's statement would be required in a meeting of gentlemen. Marshall Hall, then already a celebrity, and Benjamin Brodie, one of the first to study pain without symptoms, felt inclined to favor the opinion of the French Royal Commission, echoed by the Academy of Sciences of Paris, which considered mesmerism a fraud.[64]

Despite all this, mesmerization had many faithful followers. In Calcutta, the Scot James Esdaile had witnessed more than 70 operations, carried out under the inspiration of Elliotson's writings, including all kinds of amputations, where he had noticed neither grimaces nor signs of pain.[65] Much of this material was published again in 1852, vindicating the favorable attitude of the Indian authorities toward mesmerization and contrasting it with the British stubbornness that was unable to recognize the truth despite having it in front of its eyes. Even after 1848, when mesmerism had already lost many of its followers, Daniel Tuke [1827–1895] in 1872 still lamented the fact that nobody had taken "psychic anesthesia" into consideration: "No one who has studied the history of anesthetics in all forms, doubts that, whether by inducing a profound and peculiar kind of sleep, or by merely rendering the patient insensible to a certain idea or train of ideas, severe as well as trivial operations may be performed without any pain."[66]

However, Elliotson's paper was already discredited. The members of the Society refused to attend the sessions at University College and did not want to take part in anything that might compromise their reputation. Brodie, for example, saw no patients at the University and went so far as never driving his horses through Russell Square. He preferred to think that just as there could be pain with no lesion, there could also be lesions whose natural expression might be hidden by the will. Marshall Hall used the same argument. Wombel, he argued, had taken his farce as far as he could; but as he lacked any physiological knowledge, his ignorance had led him to avoid movements that did not depend on the perception of pain, but on the spontaneous and involuntary contractibility of the muscles. His lack of argumentative coherence called the authenticity of his account into question, revealing the fraud. Physiology made confession unnecessary for discovering the lie: the body spoke the truth that the tongue sought to hide.

Doctor John Barnes, who had served in the Macquarie Harbor (Tasmania) prison between 1826 and 1827, knew firsthand the virtues of stoicism. Of the approximately 17,000 (yes, 17,000!) lashes that he witnessed during the 19 months he spent in that prison, what caught his attention were those received by a certain Thomas Hampden. He was whipped in June 1827 and tried to endure his 100 lashes without making a sound or moving a muscle. He didn't let out a single sigh or wail. The punishment was interrupted twice to check his pulse, but once it was over, he draped his shirt over one of his shoulders and, paying no attention whatsoever to the welts on his back, walked back to his cell with indifference. Although he wanted to return to work, he ended up in the infirmary. There, he confessed that the lashes felt like boiling water being poured on his back.[67] Some 80 years later, the Austrian philosopher Ludwig Wittgenstein used a similar example to deny the existence of private languages and solipsistic states of consciousness.[68] Unlike the entire philosophical tradition, which considered that the meaning of words (or gestures) regarding sensorial experiences referred to a private idea that consequently could not be known secondhand, and also unlike all those who thought that the meaning of words (or gestures) of these same sensorial experiences depended on how they were independently verified (through taking the pulse, for example), this philosopher held that if pain is learned, like language itself, the former could not be more private than the latter. Given that learning to feel and learning to speak were part of the same grammatical process, it was impossible to refer to sensations or to use words outside of the intersubjective rules that made the use of language and knowledge of the world viable. His position, later accepted by some historians of pain, was unthinkable in the mid-nineteenth century.[69] On the contrary, the members of the college of Surgery defended a form of functionalism based on physiological considerations. Given that the anatomical mechanisms responsible for movement were different from those that registered sensorial experiences, sensation and movement could remain objects for separate research.[70] In other words, the patient's movements were not what confirmed the presence or absence of sensorial pain.

The cases of Thomas Hampden and of Wombel are similar. Both had learned to control their expressions and contain their gestures. Their pain could have been *only theirs* if physiology had not been able to establish the presence of corporeal suffering and reveal what happened, so to speak, beneath the skin. But when obliged to choose between confession and proof, the new science found the latter far superior to the former. Physiology trusted external signs, like the pulse or reflexes, which could indicate the presence of sensations, making it impossible to hide or modulate them at will. Thus, along with the patient who complains too much or for no reason, the credibility of the person who does not complain when they ought to could also be challenged. As in the case of judicial torture, the witness's narrative has less value than the body's testimony. The latter is not governed by the logic of interest, but rather by the unbreakable laws of animal physiology.

The matter would have remained resolved had it not been for the proliferation of cases in which the patient's impassivity did not seem to be connected with any corporate interest or material gain whatsoever. The phenomenon was not new. At the beginning of the century, William Griffin [1794–1848] had already explained how the (subjective) perception of pain depended not only on physiological characteristics, but also on seasonal, cultural, or sexual ones. He based his arguments on the testimony of many military surgeons who had observed troops' very different ways of facing the scalpel depending on their nationality or state. Whereas Dupuytren, for example, considered that many human beings suffered from "hemorrhages of sensitivity," Brown-Séquard noted that the inhabitants of the New World were better equipped to put up with trauma and surgery.[71] Once it was accepted that human beings differ both in their susceptibility to pain and their capacity for withstanding it, there was not, nor could there be, a constant and necessary connection between stimulus and response. Even without taking into account the flagrant cases of deliberate lies or conscious concealments, there abounded stories of men, women, and children who withstood surgical operations with remarkable impassivity. Baron Percy, for example, witnessed an extraction of a stone from an elderly man who, although repeatedly impelled to scream, always swore that he felt no pain at all.[72] Some years later, the Scottish surgeon Brown described the case of a patient called Alie, who was subjected to a mastectomy while she remained immobile and silent. When the operation was over, she got dressed slowly, got down from the table and, speaking to the surgeons and the students in a clear, calm voice, she apologized in case her behavior had not been totally correct. Apparently, all the students began to cry like children.[73]

Susceptibility seemed to depend on the sensitivity level of groups of humans distributed around factors like sex, age, social extraction, and geographical provenance.[74] The capacity for suffering seemed to diversify in history, social geography, ages, sexes, and temperaments. Hence, it was reasoned, men and women did not feel pain in the same way, and neither did children or the elderly. The climate, habit, and individual states of mind could modify sensations of harm to the extent that the same stimulus would not always produce the same effect.[75] Even in the case of animal experimentation, Richet recognized that whereas many animals remained immobile when under surgery – their eyes staring fixedly and not moaning, as though immobilized by fear – on other occasions each incision, each tear, each strain was followed by a fight, and an attempt to flee.[76] In the face of their many differences, the experimenter Claude Bernard preferred certain breeds of dogs to others for his anatomical demonstrations. Even an animal like the frog showed, in specimens having the same weight, diet, and age, different reactions to the same stimuli. Given that this difference could not be attributed to the courage of each frog considered individually, it had to be concluded that pain was a purely central phenomenon that consisted of a "perception" (his word) that could exist even at a high intensity without manifesting itself in any external signs. In the case of vivisection, as well as surgical operations and childbirth, variations in the signs did not lead to a linear correspondence between visible signs, the expression of the emotions, and the intensity of the pain: "We would be making a serious mistake if we considered that a nerve had the same excitability when subject to laws of physics as a metal wire for conducting electricity," wrote Richet.[77]

The arrival of anesthetics only served to increase this debate. In accordance with different sensibilities and organic constitutions, the use of chloroform was not appreciated in the same way in all geographic contexts and social classes.[78] The calculation of the risks and benefits included factors such as sex, nationality, economic class, and temperament. Given that people have different personalities, it was widely accepted that they should also have different reactions and levels of tolerance. The different susceptibility to pain reached dramatic heights in relation to "race" or social extraction. Severe poverty, for example, supposedly had an enormous advantage in producing a state of lethargy, often connected with alcohol abuse, which served as a natural protection against sensations that would be unbearable for more refined social classes.

Unconscious suffering

As of 1846, patients no longer had to choose between the pain of an operation and the suffering of the ailment. Prior to the progressive introduction of surgical anesthesia, operations, extractions, and births were frequently described in terms of martyrdom. Fear led patients to doubt between the present awareness of their illnesses and the anticipation of the pains to come. Faced with the prospect of undergoing an operation, many suffered from nervous attacks, fainting, and convulsions. Toward the end of the eighteenth century, the young Doctor Bonnefoy from Lyon recommended that an operation be canceled when "patients went pale, their body suffered from shivering and their limbs began to tremble; when their teeth were chattering, when they had palpitations in their hearts and their stomachs and when their pulse was rapid, strong, and concentrated."[79]

The arrival of anesthesia did not assuage all these fears or put an end to all these uncertainties. The same technological developments that seemed to reaffirm hope in progress also brought with them new dangers and frustrations. On the operating table, in the surgical chair, at the moment of birth, a new calm took over a space that had until then been governed by violence and haste. On the one hand, anesthesia allowed people to contemplate an operation "with apparent tranquility which could not have occurred in the past by even the most courageous or stoic."[80] On the other hand, however, its appearance fostered a new climate of anxiety. After 1846, there were communications, discussions, tests, comparisons, more or less systematic experiments, and debates on the use of anesthesia and doubts regarding its dangers. A compilation of these testimonies shows disbelief, satisfaction, and surprise. The first woman who was given chloroform in childbirth, following 15 days of pain and one or two sleepless nights, had to be convinced that the baby before her was really hers. The fact that anesthesia avoided, at the same time, pain and consciousness, did not help to encourage its administration. The patient's whole life, including his or her physical and moral integrity, was at the mercy of the surgeon who might betray the patient's trust, either by error or incompetence.

Here we are not concerned with supposed abuse or fears related to bad conduct or intentions. The use of anesthesia brought with it other uncertainties and doubts. One of these consisted in determining whether the state of intoxication avoided sensitivity at all times or whether, on the other hand, it only affected the memory. The anesthetized patient could no longer confuse the physiological locus of the pain (in the brain) with the seat of the sensation (which could be any part of the body); but he or she could mistake the memory and the sensation. In other words, patients could suffer pains that they would not be able to remember later; or they even could have pain that, without being perceived, might leave a trace of corporeal suffering. In the first case, the pain is felt and not remembered. In the second, the body remembers a pain that passed unnoticed. The idea that Freud "discovered" the unconscious has made us lose sight of exactly to what extent the presence of sensations that were not part of consciousness was a problem treated and investigated in many other areas of scientific research. For Gustav Fechner, for example, "unfelt sensations" were a logical consequence of his empirical process for establishing perceptual thresholds. Given that the scale of sensation was continuous, there were certainly stimuli capable of producing physical reactions that did not reach the conscious mind. In the case of surgery, the difficulty consisted in knowing whether anesthetized patients would feel pain that they would not be able to remember later; or whether, even more dramatically, they could feel a pain that they were unable to express and that, like in the worst nightmare, they would forget upon waking. If everything went well, the journey would begin with the body leaning back in a chair or lying on a bed. Patients would inhale the gas, sleep, and remember nothing. If things went badly, they might never wake up. The hand of the surgeon putting a rag or mask on their face would be the last thing they ever saw. In the meantime, the body could be abused, sexually violated, or operated on by an incompetent or careless hand. Even more dramatic, the genuine and true effect of the anesthesia perhaps would not produce loss of sensitivity, but of movement and memory. In this case, there would be no difference between the effects of inhaling gas and the dreadful torment of being buried alive. Under the effects of ether or chloroform, patients would feel the same agonizing pain as without them, although they were of course unable to complain and, still worse, unable to resist.

Etherization was added to the long list of stories of confinement that inundated the Victorian imaginary. Journalism and literature of the time abound in young women locked away in dark convents, children in orphanages, passengers in tunnels, miners in claustrophobic passageways, prisoners in flooded cells, and sailors in ships lost in the immensity of the ocean. The tunnel, linked to the atavistic fear of entering darkness with the hope of seeing a light at the end of the passage, was the great metaphor for being buried alive. In 1844, two years prior to the appearance of chemical anesthesia, the American author Edgar Allan Poe described what it would be like to awake to find oneself inside a coffin.[81] Some 50 years later, the London Association for the Prevention of Premature Burial was founded.[82] As late as 1912, the engraver Richard T. Cooper echoed the anxieties associated with the inhalation of gases in a watercolor illustrating the effects of chloroform on the human body (see Figure 19). Like the caricatures that throughout the nineteenth century had shown pain personified in malicious beings, Cooper depicts a group of small demons who, armed with surgical instruments, torment the inert and unprotected body. Along with the dangers of exposure and vulnerability at the hands of a careless surgeon, the inhalation of chloroform could produce or even increase the effect it was supposed to avoid.

These fears shared many similarities with those that appeared at the end of the eighteenth century regarding another equally philanthropic invention: the guillotine. Following the numerous public executions in the years of Terror, the debate erupted in medical literature as to whether death occurred simultaneously with decapitation, whether the beheaded person lost all sensitivity following the swipe of the blade, or whether, in a slightly more technical way, the falling of the head coincided with the annihilation of consciousness.[83] In 1794, the anatomist Samuel Thomas von Soemmering, in his *Essay on the Torture of the Guillotine,* tried to demonstrate that, given that sensitivity remained following the passing of the blade, the guillotine could not be considered to be either a painless or humanitarian instrument. On the contrary, this form of capital punishment, which replaced the skill of the executioner with the efficiency of a mere mechanism, was no more than another torment, possibly the cruelest form man had ever imagined. Before falling into the basket, the head, separated from the body, still had time to feel its last and most dramatic pain.

Soemmering, who was by no means a dilettante, maintained a position that was supported by other surgeons who considered that there always remained a certain level of sensitivity and thought in the nerves and head of the beheaded criminal: "What a horrible situation, to contemplate one's own execution!" exclaimed the surgeon Sue.[84]

These experiences began with the reanimation of superior mammals and the application of electricity and galvanic currents to amputated legs and arms. Some of these experiments, like those that were later dreamed up by Mary Shelley for Frankenstein's creature, were carried out on human corpses in the military hospital at Courbevoie. Sue, who gave public courses on irritability and sensitivity, had reached the conclusion that there were various types of sensitivity: the first indicated sensation in the place of suffering itself; the second consisted of the consciousness of that sensation. He maintained that the nerves did not transmit the pain, but only the awareness of pain, to the brain, to the *sensorium*. The center of activity in the brain does not therefore suffer, but is responsible for knowing that the body is suffering, which means that a foot suffering from gout suddenly separated from the body will continue to suffer while it maintains its vital activities, and that the head will be aware of the pain until its vitality is likewise extinguished. Although most of the argument rests on the daily experience of mutilated people who said that they felt pain in their amputated limbs, the definitive proof in favor of this dual character of sensibility and, in consequence, in favor of the idea that the severed head maintained the consciousness of a pain that it was, however, unable to express, was provided by the execution of Charlotte Corday, the young woman from Normandy who assassinated Marat in the bath. An anonymous text explained how the executioner grabbed hold of the decapitated head, showed it to the crowd and slapped one of its cheeks. In the face of such offense, Charlotte Corday's face showed the unequivocal signs of indignation: "But let us return to the facts. The executioner held the head in one hand. The face of the young woman, which had been pale at the start, blushed on both cheeks as soon as she received the blows that the wretch gave her. Everyone was shocked by the change in color and called out angrily against this cowardly and barbarous act. And the color did not come from the blows, because everyone knows that hitting a corpse would never make its cheeks blush. Furthermore, only one of her cheeks was hit, yet both of them changed color in the same way."[85]

In the opinion of the new physiologists, these facts came to prove that nerves could be born, grow, and develop separately from the brain, that life and sensation were distributed throughout the nervous system and not only in the privileged parts, and, finally, that sensation was different from consciousness. It was not only that there could exist "unfelt" sensations, but also that these unconscious sensations showed the signs of pain through feverish movement or changes in color, as the case of Charlotte Corday demonstrated.[86] During the fourth and fifth years of the Republic, the Institute of France's Verbal Trials included a considerable number of investigations related to the distribution of sensitivity in the nerves and muscle fibers.[87] The majority of these experiments measured the time that sensitivity and movement lasted following the decapitation of different animals. A chicken whose head has been cut off, for example, could continue to move for one minute. Its heart continued to beat for four minutes. In all the experiences described, whether it was with a rabbit, a pigeon, a frog, or a calf, the movements of the head lasted less than those of the rest of the body. The heart continued to beat even when the first signs of death were already present. In some cases, the movements reflected apparent signs of pain. A pig continued to move for 1 hour and 43 minutes after it had been decapitated. In others, surgeons employed artificial electrical or magnetic means of reanimation. Pregnant females were also beheaded. In some cases, the mother's head was cut off first, before the fetus was decapitated.[88]

Just as the decapitated body felt pain that it could no longer complain about, the arrival of anesthesia suggested that the anesthetized body could be subjected to extreme suffering even if the patient were unable to protest or move. In both cases, the presence of unfelt pains should have been visible through the reading of other indicators, such as a fever, blushing, an increase in the pulse, or inflammation. Unlike decapitation, the inhalation of stupefying substances did not cause absolute states of insensitivity or unconsciousness. On the contrary, the effects of chloroform were expressed in degrees and not in absolute categories; they did not depend on a yes or no, but on a more or less: a very small dose did not provide the desired effect, whereas an overdose would cause certain death. In 1847, Simpson, one of the great defenders of anesthesia, identified five levels of unconsciousness. The first only brought about modifications in sensitivity, similar to those caused by a moderate intake of alcohol; the second affected motor activity and intellectual capacity; in the third, consciousness disappeared completely, and although involuntary reflexes remained, voluntary movements were no longer possible; in the fourth level, the only movements that could be observed were those of breathing and the heartbeat. In the fifth and final level, which Simpson had never observed with human beings, the respiratory movements became paralyzed. Under normal conditions, the patient, who could begin to speak on the second level, especially when returning from the third, often mentioned that he or she had been dreaming. Many patients said these dreams referred to early periods of their life. Others stated that they had dreamed about traveling.[89]

Since chemical anesthetics produced an altered form of consciousness similar to that observed in many other trances, be they religious, spiritual, natural, or supernatural, Simpson proposed a psychological investigation of some of the mental states induced by etherization.[90] The gauntlet was taken up by, among others, the psychology of William James: "Nitrous oxide and ether, especially nitrous oxide, when sufficiently diluted with air, stimulate the mystical consciousness in an extraordinary degree."[91] Or even in a more global way: "The sway of alcohol over mankind is unquestionably due to its power to stimulate the mystical faculties of human nature, usually crushed to earth by the cold facts and dry criticisms of the sober hour."[92] In the worst scenario, the question of whether the anesthetized body suffered without knowing appeared in many articles and texts on anatomy and physiology during the second half of the nineteenth century. Richet, for example, wondered to what extent the muscles, and especially the innervated muscles of the face, contract as reflex action without the will's involvement, or if on the contrary the same gestures could be interpreted as the expression of deep suffering. Although, even in 1877, the problem seemed unsolvable, the circumstance that some muscles contract during surgical operations with anesthesia – as had occurred in the first operation in 1846 – would suggest that the body continued to suffer without being conscious of its pain.[93] The matter was explored by Doctor Vigoroux; in 1861, he presented a memorandum to the Academy of Sciences in which he defended the idea that sensitivity was conserved during anesthesia. In his view, the heart continued to feel pain, even with greater intensity, which could be seen from the increase in the number of heartbeats.[94] Again, the difficulty consisted of determining whether the pain, being concurrent with some reflex actions, was always present in these movements or whether the movements could exist without it.

The evidence that corporal suffering could exist without consciousness came from a wide variety of sources. Simpson, for example, described the movements, the gestures of pain, and even the moans normally produced by uterine contractions in anesthetized women.[95] In his opinion, however, those patients did not suffer at all, despite the expressive evidence to the contrary. In favor of this stance, he argued that their gestures did not increase in proportion to the stimuli. And, given that the body could not contradict itself, the absence of a constant relation between the gravity of the lesion and the facial expressions suggested an absence of the perception of harm. The definitive argument, however, depended on the patient having no memory of what had happened when he or she woke up. The pain could have existed, without question; but since the patient couldn't remember it, the conclusion seemed obvious: "this pain, that is so fast that it doesn't leave a memory, is nothing, no more than an almost mathematical moment that should scarcely be taken into account," he wrote.[96] The implication was that the pain that lasts for a second, and the next second no longer exists, is not worth being calling pain. In other words: "provided that the memory disappears, the pain is practically unnoticeable."[97]

6
Narrativity

"The chief spring or active principle of the human mind is pleasure in pain."
David Hume

From the idea to the body

Objects do not lie, but appearances can be deceiving. The iconographic collection in the Wellcome Trust's Library holds a strange pasteboard measuring 40×25 cm. The front shows five scenes, some of which are very well known in the cultural history of torture. Although the images are numbered, it is difficult to imagine what we could learn from this sequence, which seems only to refer to the depiction of pain and humiliation in the body's geography. The pasteboard's owner has arranged the vignettes like hunting trophies, going so far as to encircle them with an elaborate border of maces and chains. There is a certain air of obscenity in this reiteration of images. Taken individually, each one has very little impact, but the set has far greater value than the sum of its parts. The group stands out for its diversity and suggests that pain, like Aristotle's being, can be expressed in many different categories (see Figure 20). If the front of the pasteboard is surprising, the reverse side is no less extraordinary. On the back there are no torture scenes, but rather three photographs of nude females in positions and attitudes characteristic of late nineteenth-century erotic illustrations. In two of them, which bear a slight resemblance to one another and might even have been taken by the same photographer, two women show their bodies with an air of submission, without the least feature of disapproval or defiance. The right hand hidden behind the back, the eyes lowered, the head leaning slightly forward or lightly lifted, the eyes looking out into space are some of the rhetorical strategies that allow the objectification of these bodies and their disposition as instruments of lasciviousness.

The first lesson to be learned from this pasteboard, collected by the anthropologist Edwin Nichol Fallaize [1877–1957], is that, here at least, suffering and

excitement are mutually implicated, whether because the representation of violence leads to pleasure or because beauty is experienced as a form of hurt. The
relationship between these images, the way in which they were put together,
and the fact that someone at some point decided that they should form the
front and back of the same material object, implies a deliberate transgression
of cultural and social conventions. Working at the Royal Anthropological Institute, Fallaize had a separate building where he received photographs like these
from all over the world. There, he classified them under the heading of "physical anthropology," at that time less of an academic subject than an excuse for
eroticism. Little is known of Fallaize. When his archives were opened in 1991
it was discovered that most of his 200 photographs were of naked women.
Perhaps there is no need to learn more. It is difficult to imagine what part
of his biography would shed light on this strange form of collecting. On the
other hand, however, perhaps we can make these objects confess; perhaps we
will be able to force them to explain the linguistic relationships and social
conventions imbedded in their production and in their use. If we were only
allowed to look at the reiterative scenes of torture, the cardboard would merely
be as obscure as its owner's life. But in looking at both sides of the pasteboard, its character becomes less cryptic, indicating how at least for Fallaize,
although perhaps for others as well, the obverse and reverse, pain and pleasure,
disfiguration and beauty, submission and violence formed some kind of spiritual unit that, eventually, could be turned into a real object. Our pasteboard,
almost forgotten by history, is a good example of what anthropologists call a
"solid metaphor:" a form of transferring emotional states into the opacity of
objects.[1]

The coexistence of pleasure and pain in a single material medium calls into
question the more conventional forms of ordering the world. The history of art
has also left us many examples of this confluence, although, unlike Fallaize's
pasteboard, the enigma of the canvases is not resolved on the other side of
the paintings. Even though the key to the mystery or the Rosetta stone of
the passions does not hide on the backs of the artworks, the representation
in European Academic art of implausible women in exotic or imaginary places
testifies to the unbearable persistence of an unsatisfied desire. In some cases,
like Bouguereau's *Nymphaeum*, the same body, seen from different angles and
points of view, suggests a vehement wish to show, in a single scene, all the different possible ways of looking at and emotionally possessing the same woman;
in other cases, like Wilhelm Trübner's *Caesar before the Rubicon*, the figurative
elements cannot hide the terrible pain of desire (see Figure 21). Some of the
paintings of Jean-Léon Gérôme [1824–1904] also share this characteristic. This
French painter, a member of the French school of the so-called *Orientalism*,
had already acquired a certain reputation for eroticism with his painting *Phryne*

before the Areopagus. This work from 1861 shows the trial of Phryne, a courtesan from Athens, at the moment when she was being defended by one of Plato's followers. Hypereides, for such was his name, disrobed his client and asked the judges if they would be capable of executing such a beautiful woman. When asked about the painting, Degas said that he considered it a pornographic scene; he based this opinion on the way that the painter had shown the prostitute hiding what must have been the cause of her glory and the origin of her fortune (see Figure 22).[2] Twenty-three years later, in 1884, Gérôme painted another woman in the same modest pose, covering her face with her right forearm, ashamed by her nudity and not daring to look forward. He did not paint her once, but twice. Previously, he had sculpted her in marble. In the first version of the painting, currently in the Hermitage Museum in Saint Petersburg, he painted the woman from the front (see Figure 23). In the second canvas, now in the Walters Art Museum in Baltimore, he painted her from behind (see Figure 24). Although the anatomical model is the same – a body modeled very similarly to that of Phryne – here we are not looking at a Greek courtesan but rather a vulgar slave from Roman times. In this new version, the Roman patricians are not debating the woman's life, but merely her price; they are bidding for the body that had been the model for Praxiteles' Aphrodite, the first watery birth of Venus as painted by Apelles. Between 1857 and 1884, Gérôme produced at least four paintings on the subject of slavery. In two of these he recreated the cruelty of the examination of a female slave's teeth. Using the same protagonists, Gérôme only changed the landscape of the scene, without varying any other element of the composition. The same fingers enter the same woman's mouth. It would be redundant to say that the slave woman is naked in both paintings. The unquestionable erotic overtones of these paintings only appear acceptable through the orientalism of ethnographic painting – an excuse that resembles Fallaize's human anthropology. It is inconsequential whether the fingers in the woman's mouth are Roman or Egyptian; all that matters is that they are not French.

Feminist historiography has tended to judge this type of painting as just another example of a pattern of sexual domination; an instance of how the female body has historically been abused.[3] Gérôme's images indeed have a strong emotive charge, linked to the representation of subjection and violence, that can also be found in many other similar artists – from *Brenin and his Share of the Plunder* by Paul-Joseph Jamin (see Figure 25) to *The Torment of a Martyr* by the Portuguese artist José de Brito or the *Christians before the Lions* by Herbert Schmalz. However, in reducing pain and beauty to a mere relation of gender domination, a great deal of the canvases' emotional significance is lost, almost as though it had never existed. Both the front and the back of Fallaize's pasteboard and the two perspectives of Gérôme's slave market embody a pictorial tradition and a set of social conventions that hide the tension between subjection and beauty. Violence against women is yet another form of excitation, but it is not the only one. The paintings of Judith, of Delilah, of Circe, or of Danaë, whose crimes against men were represented frequently in both paintings and novels, also followed the same pattern. Whether at the hands of Salammbô, of Medusa, of Salomé, or the daughters of Dracula, many men lost the signs of their virility, sometimes their heads, and in extreme cases, their lives. We see them poisoned, beheaded, shaved, humiliated, subjected, and turned into pigs. One of the most striking cases is that of Campaspe, also known as Phyllis, Alexander the Great's concubine. According to the medieval legend, she decided to seduce Aristotle to the point that he ended up as her beast of burden. The image of this woman riding on the back of the author of the ancient world's Logic, pulling on his bridle and beating him with a riding crop, was ever-present in the early modern Period and reached the height of its fame in the collection published in 1913 by Eduard Fuchs, including comments by the sexologist Alfred Kind (see Figure 26). In a very eloquent manner, this work was entitled *Die Weiberherrschafft*, matriarchy or female domination. In a similar way, Gérôme also painted truth coming to light from the depths of a well in the form of a violent, naked woman, armed with a hammer "to punish mankind." The painter was, in fact, was so fond of this work that he kept it hanging in his bedroom until he died (see Figure 27).[4]

In Gérôme's paintings as well as in the engravings of Aristotle and Phyllis, the visual representation rests on regulated and socially acceptable criteria, including the convention of setting the scene either in the Ancient World or the Far East. Exoticism provides the cover, placing the subjects behind the mask of anthropology or under the umbrella of fine arts. In either case, the real issue is not whether Gérôme himself, or any of the Europeans who praised and purchased these images, identified with Aristotle or with the Roman patricians, but rather the transformation of the voluptuousness of pain into a consumer product. The alternative images from Baltimore and Saint Petersburg open up a small window onto the cultural history of lasciviousness. The change in perspective lets us see the faces of the Roman patricians and, by extension, the lustful gaze of the European bourgeoisie, the lascivious gestures of the middle classes bogged down in pleasure and tarnished by the vices of misery, as the writer Émile Zola so graphically described them. Some years after Gérôme's paintings had been shown in the Paris galleries, Zola began what would become one of his most popular novels, *Nana*, with the description of the French bourgeoisie lewdly watching a courtesan stripping in a theater; a new kind of brothel that brought together "the Paris of letters, of finance and of pleasure, many journalists, some few authors, and several speculators, more kept girls than respectable women [...] a singular mixture composed with every kind of genius, tainted with every description of vice."[5] Like Gérôme's, Zola's realism sought to record facts and feelings; to show us the naked truth before an audience subjected, dominated, and captivated by the omnipotence of Venus, the tyranny of Nana or the nudity of Phryne.

Of all the possible responses to the inexplicable suffering of another – such as compassion, indignation, or shame – the bourgeoisie opted to turn the suffering of the other into an endless source for its own consumption. At the same time, it began to develop a tendency for obsessive identification with the victims. Severely punished in childhood, educated in the subjection to the new constrictions of the market – from the regulation of the workday to the economic forms of exchange – these witnesses to the exploitation and trafficking of slaves knew about submission, more than anything else, through their own experience. Given that pain guaranteed a form of life, and took part in education, the national economy, the colonial system, and everyday work, it was possible to subvert its cultural meaning and, more extremely, its physiological tyranny. Masochism, in a much broader sense of the word than mere sexual excitement, became a cultural icon. It was concerned with far more than obtaining pleasure in amorous encounters. Fully aware of this, Freud was forced to recognize the existence of both erotic masochism – which consisted of a veiled primary desire for destruction, opposed to the pleasure principle – and what he called "moral masochism:" an unconscious desire for punishment, the result of a feeling of guilt.[6] Far from being a phenomenon exclusively tied to the libido, this dark and uncontrollable desire for suffering was a social characteristic that sexologists and psychiatrists alike considered to be both geographically and historically universal. Its appearance depended on the constitution of a collective experience where pain and pleasure were no longer opposing terms or realities; where, as with Fallaize's pasteboard or Gérôme's paintings, punishment, humiliation, and defeat came accompanied by the proportion of forms, the sensuality of figures, and a longing for beauty.[7]

The philosopher Gilles Deleuze was right when he considered the idea, art, and the body as the three fundamental elements of masochism: "The ascent from the human body to the work of art and from the work of art to the Idea must take place under the shadow of the whip," he wrote.[8] He was mistaken, however, about the direction of this psychological trajectory. The whiplashes of voluptuousness do not move from the body to the idea, but from the idea to the body. And this idea, the idea that the masochist wishes to carve into his flesh, is not exclusive to his sexual condition. This global transformation of the experience to which the masochist aspires depends on a greater modification of the rules governing collective feelings and affections. Aspects as important as the development of sporting practices, which brought with it an essential dimension of controlled suffering, or the proliferation of shows and entertainment like the *Riesenrad* – the giant Ferris wheel built in Vienna in 1897 – formed part of a cultural climate in which masochism could flourish.

The history of the relationship between pain and pleasure cannot be undertaken without considering the material forms of emotional passions and obsessions, whether in Gérôme's paintings or Fallaize's photographs. The neoclassical taste for the connection between submission and pleasure took place within a cultural space that exalted sensitivity and the eccentric behavior of those same social classes that came together in the Paris Salons, the Universal Expositions, sporting events including the new Olympic Games, or Art Fairs. One of the great discoveries of the nineteenth century was accepting that objects had their own cultural story: a material biography in which their uses were inscribed and their meanings could evolve. Nineteenth-century social sciences could not have been developed without the premise that things, like words, share symbolic properties, cognitive and economic values, and emotional features. Neither political economy nor anthropology could have taken a single step without this reflection on the material conditions of exchange.[9] The works of art mentioned by Deleuze, halfway between the body and the idea, are just another way – though not the only one – of showing how emotions leave their traces on the surfaces of objects.

Fetishism

The entrance into circulation of the terms "masochism" and "sadism" – in the 1890 edition of Austrian psychiatrist Richard von Krafft-Ebing's [1840–1902] *Psychopathia Sexualis* – coincided with the invention of sexual perversion as a medical, legal, psychological, and psychiatric category.[10] Never before had there been so much literature about normal behavior and the pathological types of sexual exchange. To begin with, procreative sex was set in strict opposition to the variety of infertile pleasures. Whereas the former was "normal" and sanctioned by both the Church and Science, the latter was marked by the most conspicuous signs of perversion: the stains left by the human seed spilled in inappropriate, dirty, or illicit places. The study of so-called "peripheral sexualities" – deviations from what was considered normal sexuality – did not stop at behavior, but also included the conscious or unconscious personality of those who practiced non-procreative sexuality and, more extremely, of those who enjoyed sexuality without sex. "The sodomite had been a temporary aberration; the homosexual was now a species," wrote the historian Michel Foucault.[11] Psychiatry gave rise to human groups, dissimilar not for their morphological appearance, but because of their functional attitudes. After its first appearance in 1886, subsequent editions of *Psychopathia Sexualis* began to attribute psychiatric concepts to new collectives. Instead of serving people, words were now used to subject them. Some found themselves trapped forever in the new taxonomies: sodomites, sadists, masochists, fetishists, necrophiles, and pedophiles. All of them were marked by a deviation of their instinct and by an anti-natural preference for non-procreative pleasures.

It was not complicated to differentiate between the normal and the pathological; it was sufficient to equate the normal with the procreative. What was more difficult was to institute some form of order in the garden of heterodox passion. Krafft-Ebing distinguished four main groups of sexual deviations. With the exception of the first, the so-called "paradoxia," which consisted of sexual excitation without the use of the reproductive organs – such as sexuality in infancy or old age – the three remaining groups were defined using a criterion based on the modification of their threshold of desire. Like the monsters of the Renaissance, human beings sinned through excess, defect, or transposition. Here there was nothing new under the sun. Deviation could be the result of an absence of sexual instinct ("anesthesia"); an excess of desire ("hyperesthesia"); or be provoked by inadequate stimuli. In this last condition, which the Austrian sexologist called "paresthesia," patients found pleasure in contact with persons of the same sex, with animals, with corpses, or through the contemplation or possession of objects or artifacts.[12] In the most extreme cases, lubricity was the result of a transformation in the emotional meaning and the sensorial qualities of the more or less everyday objects that, in their new psychological perception, became protagonists of the libido.

This emotional transformation in the social meaning of objects worked as a spell that was not exclusively cast on the objects of sexual behavior. Some 40 years before Fallaize collected his images of nudes under the pretense of physical anthropology, and 60 years before Krafft-Ebing defined sexual paresthesia, Karl Marx [1818–1883] explained that commerce of goods depended on the social relations inscribed on the objects of exchange, like a second nature: an emotional assessment he didn't hesitate to describe as *fetishism*.[13] The term had previously been used to describe a passion for collecting or adoring relics and holy objects, saints' and martyrs' bones and entrails, which were supposed to have healing or supernatural powers. In the case of goods as well as relics, these objects became "sensitively suprasensitive" things. It didn't matter that they were "suprasensitive" – Marx's own expression – because they reflected social relationships or because they were enchanted with supernatural powers. Fetishes possessed an added value, a metaphysical secret, which went beyond their material composition and, as a result, beyond their directly perceived properties: "So far no chemist has ever discovered exchange value either in a pearl or a diamond," Marx wrote, not without irony.[14] Suffice it to say that no one has ever discovered it because this value is not a visible, but an invisible property; it is not material, but social; because it is not public, but secret. And yet, although it is invisible, social and secret, it is an essential property in the process of exchange.

The title of the chapter in *Das Kapital* that describes this phenomenon is "The Fetishism of Commodities and the Secret Thereof." At the beginning of the twentieth century, Sigmund Freud [1856–1939] offered an interpretation of this suprasensitive "secret" in psychoanalytic terms, relating it to his theory of sexuality and childhood traumas.[15] In 1905, he had already dealt with this subject in his *Three Essays on the Theory of Sexuality,* discussing the aberrant impulse toward objects, which he himself considered to be "perverse to the normal sexual aim."[16] In this respect, nothing had changed in a hundred years. The Austrian doctor had in mind the cases reported by Alfred Binet, Charcot, and other French psychiatrists who had used the concept of the fetish to describe the devotion for a loved one's possessions: their shoes, their feet, their handkerchiefs, their underwear, a lock of hair, or, as was the case with Emma Bovary, her landlord's cigarette case. Although, in principle, anything could acquire the category of sexual object, the first clinical proceedings described men masturbating at the windows of shoe shops in Vienna or renting prostitutes' boots without requiring any of their other services.[17] The records depict the case of a salesman who had his first sexual experience with a woman who neither undressed nor removed her shoes. From that moment on, the gentleman was impotent unless a woman presented herself to him dressed in exactly the same way and under the same circumstances. In all cases, although in some more than others, certain objects took on a symbolic and emotional charge that changed their uses and modified their forms. They not only exhibited *improper* properties, they were also related to their owners by means of rituals that had nothing to do with their production, consumption, or exchange.[18]

The first scene in Sacher-Masoch's novel, the literary text that would become the model for sexual masochism, also shares in this new form of enchantment. The novel opens by describing the apparition to an anonymous narrator of a statue wrapped in furs, much like the young woman painted by Titian. The action, which takes place as if in a dream, includes all the elements of sexual paresthesia. As in the myth of Pygmalion – where the sculptor achieved a world in which he felt both loved and excluded – this novel also produces a gap between an alienated man on one side and the humanized stone on the other. Even before the rock comes alive, the sculptor succumbs to the attributes of his own creation.[19] Gérôme himself, who in the words of Flaubert showed "a total absence of what could be called moral atmosphere," also found some delectation in the myth.[20] True to form, he produced at least two oil paintings and one sculpture on the theme. Unlike the Pygmalion of the Enlightenment, the narrator of Sacher-Masoch's novel does not want to educate the statue, but rather to be educated by her; he does not want to discipline her, but be disciplined; he does not want her to serve him, but to serve and adore her; he does not want a slave, but a cold-hearted and brutal woman who will humiliate and despise him. He does not want a Venus; but a Phyllis. As in "The Eternal Idol," Rodin's sculpture from 1889, the statue does not kneel at the feet of its creator; it is the creator who, holding his hands behind his back in a recognizable gesture of submission, like the highly erotized women in Fallaze's photographs, begs at the feet of his work. Some years later, Théodore Rivière represented the same scene, but changed the characters. Instead of Pygmalion and Galatea – a story known in Europe through Ovid's *Metamorphoses* – he depicted Matho kneeling before the priestess Salammbô. In this case, the young soldier is not concerned with the indifference or derision of the daughter of the Carthaginian Hamilcar Barca. Unarmed and humiliated, the mercenary can do no more than cry out "*I love you! I love you!*" (see Figure 28).

This obsessive repetition of man's submission before woman was inscribed in a variety of materials, such as paintings, sculptures, or literature – as in the case of Flaubert's novel, which popularized the story of Salammbô. But this was not the first time that men fell to their knees before a statue. For Alfred Binet, the new passion for the Pygmalion myth came to replace the worship and adoration of Virgins in Catholic Europe.[21] Devotion remained intact, although no longer as a supernatural passion, but as a perversion of the instinct. Perhaps it was not a coincidence after all that one of Gérôme's companions in his travels to the East had the idea of producing a work that could be a massive object of adoration. On his return to Paris from Egypt, Frederic Bartholdi made some small-scale models before creating the definitive work, a 46-meter-high sculpture (not counting the pedestal) that was erected in the New York Bay in 1886. Probably no statue in the world has been brought to life as often as the so-called "Statue of Liberty," one of the great fetishes of the American nation.

With regard to the uses of pain, fetishism concerns us for various reasons. In the first place, the psychic association between suffering and pleasure exceeds the narrow boundaries of sexual pathology. The arousal of the libido using inanimate objects takes place mainly within the limited category of sexual perversion, but the connection extends much further. When the French psychiatrist Alfred Binet [1857–1911] recognized the voluptuousness of pain as a form of fetishism, he did not mean that the latter was foreign to sexual behavior as a whole, or that it was only present in pathological conditions. Whereas in normal sexuality fetishism was, so to speak, polytheistic in its choice of objects of worship – not becoming obsessed with a single thing or quality – in pathological behavior, the obsession turned into a compulsive adoration of a single part of the body or some other object or artifact, whether it be velvet, furs, feet, ears, fists, or high heels.[22] In the correct proportion and in the precise context, these forms of objectifying psychic obsessions – the way in which objects acquire meanings – were never pathological. On the contrary, they could open the doors of literary criticism, artistic judgment, or the new markets.

Secondly, the masochist's reification only comes about as the counterpoint to the personification of his objects, as the way in which they acquire social properties and animate features. Making the distinction between persons and things was never an easy task – still less if we look simultaneously at the history of slavery and the trafficking of goods – but the border becomes even more diffuse when looking at a deviation of the instinct that fantasizes about animated objects and reified persons. Here the nineteenth-century version of the Pygmalion myth takes on a new hue. Whereas for Enlightenment thinkers what was difficult was to animate the statue, such that it would be able to reach ethical and aesthetic ideas based solely on sensations, for the followers of Sacher-Masoch, on the contrary, the greatest difficulty was to reify the sculptor.[23] Behind the new reading of this myth pulses the vehement desire to transform ideas into matter – a psychological fixation with certain objects or some of their properties, which leads almost inevitably to the need to accumulate them. Whether we are speaking of a photograph collection, as in Fallaize's case; a collection of perspectives, like Gérôme's; of commodities, as described in *Das Kapital*; clinical histories, as collected in the *Psychopathia Sexualis* by Krafft-Ebing; or erotic images, like those Eduard Fuchs amassed, fetishism is always a collector's affair; it accumulates objects and, more specifically, objects of *the same kind*. Therein resides the quintessence of compulsive consumerism. The treasures collected must resemble one another; they should have some common characteristic that makes them belong to the same group. They are not, and cannot be, the same object; but neither can they be a collection of heterogeneous things. Emotional properties, financial and aesthetic values, and in some cases, sexual desires are hidden in their size, their design, and the material properties of which they are made.

In the museums of Europe, it is not difficult to find objects related to the material history of suffering that simultaneously contain some element of voluptuousness. Let us take, for example, the carved marble figure shown in Figure 29. This piece, which measures about 18 centimeters in height, looks like a decorative object or an ornamental representation of an instrument of execution. Nothing is known of its author or provenance. It could well have been made at any time between the sixteenth and nineteenth centuries. The sharp points on the inside of the sarcophagus, whose articulated blades can be closed at will, menace the nakedness of the young woman who, in a gesture of modesty similar to the protagonist of Botticelli's "Birth of Venus," seems not to have quite managed to cover herself. Her right hand rests on her thigh while the other falls beneath her ribs. As with many other similar objects, this figure forms part of a history of compulsive reiteration, of the need to accumulate the same psychic object.[24] In Sir Henry Wellcome's collections in London we can still find many similar items. In their day, some of them were instruments of torture, but their use value was pushed into the background as they acquired a new life that did not depend on use or exchange. As with many other fetishes, they became luxury items, and for that very reason: they were exclusive, authentic, and useless.[25] On the one hand, the masochist's testimony positions itself as the greatest denunciation of social convention, a vindication of a private sphere that does not depend on social rules or regulations. On the other hand, the objects exhibit the tastes and preferences of those who collect them, placing us in relation to those human beings with whom they maintain isomorphic similarities. This is so because people construct objects as much as objects construct people. Therefore, for every suprasensitive object, in Marx's terminology, there will be a suprasensual person, using Sacher-Masoch's terms. And on the contrary, for each of Fallaize's pasteboards, there exist people with a public and a private side. There is nothing strange in masochism becoming a cultural industry related to the production of fetishes.[26] These same mixed objects, which now form part of the market, in their affected ideas of what was correct and organized. At the same time, we should not be surprised that they were amassed: repetition was always the best way of expressing difference.[27]

The normal and the pathological

In 1904, the same year that Charles Féré [1852–1907] introduced the term *algophilia*, the English sexologist Havelock Ellis [1859–1939] published his *Love and Pain* as part of his *Studies in the Psychology of Sex*.[28] For Ellis, as for other authors, deviation was not a quality but an excess. Behavior became pathological only in the intensity, not the nature of the desire.[29] There was not a leap between genuine perversion and normal sexuality, but rather a scale, a succession of degrees, the intensity of which determined the presence or the absence of deviation. Paraphilia conformed to a universal pattern of conduct that human beings shared not only throughout geography and history but also with the animal kingdom as a whole. There was an imaginary curve between healthy sexuality and morbid desire, wherein human drives progressed from the normal to the pathological. In the best tradition of the so-called "Broussais principle" – which considered illnesses to be the result of an excess in the normal functions of different organs – sexual deviation occurred as a result of gradual modifications which, in appropriate doses, were not in the least bit pathological. On the contrary, Ellis, like many of his colleagues, always began by showing the natural, geographical, and historical universality of the relationship between suffering and pleasure. This universality of behavior revealed judgments and values relating to the boundary between reality and fiction, the feminine and the masculine, and, more generally, between the East and the West. The new medicine of sex did indeed construct perversion; but it did so by delving into an intermediate space where the relationship between normal behavior and pathological deviation did not correspond to a boundary that was put up once and for all, but rather to a liminal space where advances were made by imperceptible gradations and steps from desire to reality, from dreams to facts, or from normal sexuality to pathological behavior. Like many other paraphilias, sexual masochism arose as an excess in the intensity of desires and drives present in normal sexuality.

On the one hand, ethnological proofs and biological studies found the connection between sexuality and pain well rooted in scientific evidence. The aggressive behavior observed in animals in heat seemed to suggest that suffering and violence were part of their mechanisms of excitation. On the other hand, ethnographic observations permitted defending the universality of this impulse. It didn't matter that these observations included reports on mentalities considered "primitive" or of marginal or poorly educated social classes: the introduction of harmful elements in amorous encounters responded to a natural impulse that, in more mitigated forms, lived on even among the most civilized human beings.[30] Whether through the study of literary sources or legal texts, the connection between pain and pleasure seemed to be a cultural universal, an indelible part of amorous relations, distributed across a strict sexual division. For many experts, male brutality toward women, along with women's acquiescence and desire to be brutalized, constituted a well-established fact of society and history. Ellis, for example, wrote that among Slavic peoples, women "feel hurt if they are not beaten," while among the Italians of the Camorra, they only feel loved when they are treated badly.[31] "Women love to be conquered [...] and the less refined ones love not only to be mastered, but even to be beaten," wrote Charles Féré.[32] The male propensity for violence naturally met with the females' delight in punishment and their natural disposition toward obedience: "the tendency to find pleasure in subjection and pain is often faintly traceable even in normal civilized women," Ellis concluded.[33] So long as it was in the proper amount and in the right proportion, there was nothing either pathological or reproachable about it. On the one hand, he wrote, "When the normal man inflicts, or feels the impulse to inflict, *some degree* of pain on the women he loves he can scarcely be said to be moved by cruelty."[34] On the other hand, a woman who enjoys some degree of violence cannot be thought of as a masochist. The interesting expression in both cases is "some degree;" for those passions that remained within these limits could not lead to denunciation or commiseration. Given that there was a fine line between the right amount of pain and excessive violence, abuse was not uncommon; as a magistrate wrote: "If anyone has doubts as to the brutalities practiced on women by men, let him visit the London Hospital on a Saturday night."[35]

The first implication of this gradual understanding of sexual paresthesia at the turn of the nineteenth century was that masochism was regarded, at least initially, as an almost exclusively male condition. Scarcely one in ten of the cases quoted by Krafft-Ebing had a woman as the protagonist.[36] The desire to suffer, which constituted a universal characteristic among females, was, however, a voluntary perversion in men. What for some implied a deviation, for others was purely natural. The difficulty masochists found in fulfilling their desires was something women were born with. The former wished to be dominated; the latter had to be dominated even if they did not want to be. Given that, secretly at least, females found pleasure in submission, to speak of masochism in women would simply be redundant. When Freud introduced the expression "feminine masochism" in 1924, it was obvious that he was speaking principally about a masculine condition. The behavior, in which males adopted the role that, in his opinion, came naturally to women, was more accessible to observation and less problematic. This point of view was later shared by Freud's disciple Theodor Reik, in the first book comprehensively dedicated to masochism.

In the second place, the idea that masochism operated in a continuum, as an excess of normal sexuality, also implied that it was difficult to place it within a determined referential sphere. The expression "sexual instinct," in referring to both the field of conduct and the realm of desire, confused again and again what fell within the context of observed behavior and what formed part of the internal psychic profile. Dreams of servitude and humiliation, for example, could by themselves constitute a deviation of instinct, but they did not seem to be material for clinical study. The implications of this diffuse border between what is only desired and what is also performed affected the whole economy of pain in the nineteenth century. At the same time, it made the relationship between women and suffering problematic. Whereas, according to Ellis, most women deemed any kind of physical suffering to be abhorrent, even the most civilized among them could have dreams that included elements of violence. Likewise, in order to account for the sensorial delight in the pictorial or literary representation of suffering, it seemed necessary to coin a conceptual term to describe the enjoyment of the spectacle of violence – algolagnia – an emotional reaction that was not linked to the sensation of protection or the desire for safety, but rather to the transformation of experience through the contemplation of suffering.

Charles Féré – famous for having written a study on hypnosis, with Alfred Binet, in 1877 – reported the case of a 23-year-old woman who attended a bullfight while visiting Spain.[37] At that time, there was already a lengthy list of foreign writers who had taken on the Spanish "fiesta," whether to praise or to revile it. In the case described, at a moment when the bull seemed to have killed the bullfighter, the young woman became sexually excited, and reached orgasm in a matter of seconds. Although she considered the spectacle barbaric, she could not resist returning to the bullring on other occasions, which almost always ended in the same result. When she left Spain, she incorporated the scenes into her dreams. In his *Evolution and the Dissolution of the*

Sexual Instinct, Féré deemed that the young woman's behavior responded to an instinct for cruelty present in society as a whole.[38] There were many, he argued, who enjoyed observing someone else's pain, took pleasure in reading stories of the most abominable cruelty, and had a particular predilection for the images they represented. In his view, mere exposure to bloody scenes was enough sometimes to reach orgasm. Even though this pleasure in contemplating pain was nearly always manifested in infancy, as in the case of Sacher-Masoch, it was not unusual to come across the same passion in older people. Damiens' dismemberment in 1757, for example, was described with enjoyment and delight in the *Memoirs* of the Italian Giacomo Casanova, who was present on the day of the execution.[39] The Marquis de Rays, famous for his successive and failed colonial expeditions, was overcome by a fondness for cruelty while reading Suetonius' lives of the Caesars. Caligula's savagery, Nero's bloodletting, and Tiberius' orgies, far from horrifying him, gave him delight. No doubt they also comforted him during the long periods he spent in prison toward the end of his life. The subject of Krafft-Ebing's case number 41, which we will examine later, began to have fantasies about domination while reading *Uncle Tom's Cabin*.[40] Some of the passages, and, who knows, maybe some of the illustrations too, gave him erections.[41] And this is not a unique case. For Sacher-Masoch, the construction of desire depended on the emotional values attributed to objects from the pro-slavery and repressive world of Eastern Europe.[42] The whips, animal skins, and, generally, everything that was considered in Vienna to be part of the culture of cruelty of Tsarist Russia made him sigh. In its mitigated forms, a single drop of blood was enough to unleash the most sophisticated forms of pleasure. In more exaggerated cases, arousal took place through the contemplation or mutilation of corpses, human beings, and animals. Without entering the area of criminal conduct, Doctor Lacassagne described the story of a man who could only be sexually stimulated at funerals.[43] Ellis, for his part, mentions a woman whose greatest satisfaction came from tearing off her lover's clothes and biting him until he cried out for mercy.[44] Between these two extremes, there abound in society, culture, and the arts many other forms and manifestations of natural violence. On many occasions, deviation was hidden beneath the guises of popular traditions or sports. On others, it was disguised under the shadow of anthropology, where the recreation of imaginary places in Africa and Asia had a privileged position, both for the exhibition of exotic beauties and for the most sophisticated forms of punishment and execution.[45]

One of the images of the peoples of the Congo River shows a strange form of capital punishment, apparently practiced by the Ba-Yanzi (see Figure 30). The condemned man is seated, tied, and anchored to the floor by six stakes. Each pair of them guarantees the immobilization of his body through cords tightly bound to his ankles, knees, and arms. His body is pulled upright by the force of a net placed over his head and around his neck. The rope attached to the net has been tied to a thin, flexible trunk buried in the ground and pulled so taut that it looks like it is on the verge of breaking. The executioner is about to cut his neck with a large machete. The scene implies that once the tension of the rope is broken, the trunk will pull on the rope so strongly that the decapitated head will be flung into the air. The image is not dated, but the North American anthropologist Walter Hough described a similar execution process in a short article published in *Science* in 1887.[46] The reasons behind the image's production cannot be told as we have very little information on the authors of the picture, the explorers Edward James Glave and H. Ward.[47] Neither do we know whether the drawing is of a real execution or, on the contrary, if we are witnesses to an imaginary scene. Perhaps this figure can tell us something of the European view of the African colonies, but its private use is what makes it worth studying here. In the field of ethnography, it resembles other similar scenes showing the European culture of colonial violence, and, even further back in time, the tradition that, framed by the dark legend of the conquest and colonization of America, represented indigenous torture and sacrifices as a way of legitimizing the Spanish Crown.

The same applies to the European fascination with Chinese tortures (see Figures 31 and 32). It was probably through the Universal Exhibitions that small groups of wooden sculptures were commissioned, depicting scenes of public life and domestic customs, along with different forms of execution and punishment.[48] These small models could well have been merely informative, like the images of Eastern punishment so popular in Europe dating from the times of the Portuguese martyrs in the seventeenth century, which became especially popular at the beginning of the nineteenth century. One of the most detailed of them appears in a volume entitled *Punishment in China*; this book, which contains a bilingual text accompanying a set of images, was published anonymously in 1801 and attributed to George Henry Mason.[49] Its 22 engravings generally lack ornamental elements and are more concerned with the proper proportionality of crime and punishment than with the Early Modern period's spectacle of cruelty. Although the author claims to be aware of far more severe punishments in China – related to such grave crimes as regicide, treason, rebellion, parricide, and sedition – he claims that depicting them would be an unseemly affront to his readers' sensibilities. Instead, the selected images are related to minor crimes like theft, mistakes in interpreting and translation, or the absence of modesty (see Figure 33).

Nothing in all this imaginary recreation of physical suffering had anything to do with cruelty or was ethically reproachable. Mason's pictures and the Ba-Yanzi execution were publicized in the context of anthropology or of a legitimate curiosity about the cultural customs of distant places. On the one hand, there was nothing pathological about the mere contemplation of these exotic punishments. On the other hand, the possible condition did not have to lead necessarily to the criminalization of behavior.[50] On the border between reality and desire, pathologies depended on gradual intensifications of a normal sexuality that, having a pathogenic rather than ethical origin, did not constitute a crime, but rather an illness. On many occasions, those who were sick did know of their condition or were aware of it. Ideas and acts of cruelty produced sexual arousal, and vice versa: arousal was accompanied by a propensity for violence. But cruelty was never the objective. On the contrary, as Havelock Ellis wrote somewhat grandiloquently, the aim was always "the joy of being plunged among the waves of the great primitive ocean of emotions which underlies the variegated world of our every day lives."[51]

Masochism and asceticism

The social universality of the connection between pleasure and pain discussed above is merely the counterpart to its historical universality. Sexologists approached these new pathologies as categories of behavior that, far from being isolated cases, had well-established precedents. Prior to the publication of Krafft-Ebing's work, medicine had at its disposal a historical repertoire of sensory enjoyment of harmful practices going back at least 300 years. The relationship between pain and knowledge, pain and salvation, and pain and truth constituted three ways in which physical suffering was used as a sign and a medium. Although each one of these relations had its historical particularities and specific spheres of application, their areas of overlap mostly depended on a positive assessment of human suffering. The German poet known as Novalis [1772–1801], for example, found it surprising that humanity had not paid more attention to the intimate connection between lust, religion, and cruelty, and the similarity of their ends or objectives.[52] Some of these points of contact helped psychologists of the early twentieth century to trace connections between sexual deviation and religious behavior through a retrospective medicalization of ascetic experience. In *The Varieties of Religious Experience*, for example, the psychologist William James [1842–1920] mentions with disdain, or even disgust, the lacerations and punishment of the flesh endured by some of the most important mystics of the medieval and early modern periods.[53] Although the desire for mortification was clearly pathological, James sought to make a distinction between those who, like the fourteenth-century mystic Henry Suso, had not managed to transform their torment into a kind of perverse pleasure through an alteration of sensibility, and those who, like Marguerite Marie Alacoque in the eighteenth century, appeared to find an extreme bond between pain and pleasure. While the former withstood pain as a kind of penitence, the latter considered that the greatest penitence was to spend a day without agony. For one, physical suffering was yet another rung on the ladder of asceticism; the other transformed her afflictions into the only way to live: "Her love of pain and suffering was insatiable. She said that she could cheerfully live till the Day of Judgment, provided she might always have matter for suffering for God; but that to live a single day without suffering would be intolerable."[54]

The connection between masochism and religious asceticism had already been discussed in many places and by many authors prior to James' work. The American psychiatrist James Kiernan, for example, linked the flagellating practices of monastic life with passive algophilia, and many other colleagues saw the mystics' stigmata and insensitivity to pain as being not unlike the most frequent symptoms of hysteria.[55] In 1866, Georges Gilles de la Tourette published the autobiography of Sor Jeanne des Anges, Mother Superior of the Ursulines in Loudon, with a preface by the illustrious Dr Charcot. The book's title left no doubt as to the nun's psychological state: *Sor Jeanne des Anges, Autobiography of a Possessed Hysteric.*[56] For the psychiatrists at the Salpetriêre Hospital in Paris, the pains in her side about which the Spanish mystic Teresa of Avila had written so profusely, seemed to be none other than hysterical cardiopathy.[57] Far from being a physical manifestation of the transverberation – the curious way in which the arrows of God's love pierced the saint's heart – her cardiac pain corresponded to the pattern of chronic and unspecific suffering frequently observed in nervous disorders: "the pain from this wound was so keen that it tore sighs from me [. . .]; but this incredible martyrdom made me, at the same time, enjoy the softest delights so that I could not find the moment to wish it were over," wrote the Spanish saint.[58]

Even when psychiatrists made retrospective diagnoses emphasizing the moral and emotional enjoyment of pain, there was no shortage of opinions suspecting more graphically that, as in Fallaize's pasteboard, veiled desires for sexual satisfaction hid behind the enjoyment of mortification. When, already in the twentieth century, the philosopher Lacan pointed out the eroticism of Bernini's statues of Saint Teresa and Saint Ludovica, he was not discovering anything new: "You only have to go and look at Bernini's statue in Rome to understand that she's coming, there is no doubt about it," he wrote.[59] Once accepted that the libido could also be induced by stimulation of the buttocks, many authors rushed to trace a line of continuity between ascetic flagellation and sexual arousal. In Krafft-Ebing's opinion, for example, the desire for purity was so entwined with sensual fantasies that even Maria Maddalena de Pazzi, the Florentine nun whose pious life had been the model to imitate during the seventeenth century, came close to losing her virginity on many occasions.[60] For many other psychiatrists, a positive assessment of mortification was linked, consciously or unconsciously, to sensorial delight.

The anonymous author of the *History of Flagellation*, for example, considered that many confessors who had initially used flagellation as a religious act ended up using it to gratify their promiscuity. On various occasions, along with the lack of modesty and morality in practices where abuse was not infrequent, the libidinous nature of ascetic behavior became clear. The Franciscan Cornelius Adriassen, for example, managed to convince several women, single and married alike, to submit to being rubbed with a rod on their thighs and buttocks.[61] And this was not an isolated case. In the history of depravity and the loss of values connected to chastity, the story of the Jesuit Girard stands out. His relationship with Mademoiselle Cadière was well known during the Enlightenment. His name was used sarcastically in one of the most widely read libertine novels of the time: *Thérèse Philosophe*, whose title was a mocking reference to the biography of Teresa of Avila. The rituals of degradation imposed by the confessor in Leopoldo Alas *Clarín's* nineteenth-century novel *La Regenta* obeyed the same principle. Only through shamelessness and lewdness can the spiritual adviser of Ana Ozores – the novel's protagonist, subjected to the moral authority of her confessor – convert her suffering and humiliation into a source of sensorial delight and personal reaffirmation.

This comparison between sexual masochism and modern asceticism was largely based on retrospective diagnosis. The immediate intention was never to shed light on the past but to use the past to understand the present. Appropriately or not, asceticism and masochism shared sufficient elements to make it plausible to place one as the precedent of the other. To start with, both practices rest, at least in principle, on the desire for submission, the apparent indifference to and even voluptuous enjoyment of harmful practices. They are both also concerned with the invention and manufacture of objects related to the exercise of punitive practice. Their designs range from the simple use of tree branches from nearby forests to more sophisticated tools. One of the most renowned modern Italian saints, Luigi Gonzaga [1568–1591], for example, acquired a notable reputation as a seasoned manufacturer of instruments of punishment. Soon thereafter, Father Paolo Segneri [1624–1694] designed a device that he used to carry out his spiritual exercises. He called it the *"excoriater,"* the liberator of filth. It consisted of a tin box in which a round cork was embedded, with at least 50 pins and needles protruding from it.[62] Artisanal models included a wide variety of objects, from chickpeas fixed in sandals to pins and hair shirts of varying shapes and sizes.

Of all these tools, the one with the greatest popularity and symbolic value was, of course, the whip or scourge. The history of this object, or rather group of instruments, concerns religion, justice, education, and sexuality, among other practices.[63] From the *Lupercalia* of ancient Rome to the appearance of algolagnia, human beings appear to have repeated the same gesture over and over again, leaving identical marks from different whips across their backs. It is not surprising that psychiatrists found the need to explain the physiological and psychological mechanisms underlying a thousand-year-old activity that, despite counting Church Fathers among its practitioners, had also become one of the most requested services in European brothels. In some of them, a curious instrument was used, a kind of stocks or flagellation pillar.[64] Even toward the end of the nineteenth century, there were still people who considered that moderate beating could have a tonic or stimulating effect.[65] The scenes of flagellation in *Fanny Hill*, published in 1748 and considered by many the masterpiece of English erotic literature, described behavioral habits regarding the secret history of impotence. For Mr Barville – one of the characters in the novel – flagellation was not a punishment, but rather a therapeutic procedure capable of mechanically producing an erection through the over-excitement of the buttocks; the only way the young man knew to make what the female protagonist initially took for "an impalpable or at least minute object" into something as large as her surprise.[66] In this scene Cleland echoes the works of Bartholine, or Heinrich Meibom, whose essay *A Treatise of the Use of Flogging in Venereal Affairs*, published in repeated editions following its first appearance in 1669, had defended *ad nauseam* the use of flagellation as a sexual stimulant.[67] Other works in this mold included Paullini's *Flagellum salutis*, and the French doctor Amédée Doppet's *Aphrodisiaque externe*, published anonymously in 1788.[68] In 1818, the Italian Benedetto Mojon in his *Treatise on the Usefulness of Pain* asked himself how many 60-year-olds did not owe the honor of fatherhood to this clandestine practice.[69] Although it was not the case with Mr Barville, whom Cleland depicted at a little over 20 years old, at the beginning of the nineteenth century the considerations of Salgues and other French doctors, who had described in all detail how men had made recourse to similar procedures in order to obtain "joys that outraged nature did not allow them without the intervention of pain."[70]

Along with this therapeutic use of flagellation, other authors pointed out that its popularity was rather due to psychological factors. For Havelock Ellis, for example, the spectacle of suffering was a stimulant for sexual feelings even when the whip did not come into contact with the flesh.[71] The mere imaginary recreation sufficed to provide arousal. This change in perspective had its importance, not only due to the abundance of scenes of flagellation in erotic literature, in the lives of the saints, and in paintings – beginning, of course, with the flagellation of Christ – but also because those who felt the blows and those who watched them shared in the same emotional benefits. Unlike the cases of Meibom and Doppet, for whom flagellation was a direct physiological stimulus provided it was administered in "moderate quantities," for Ellis, the mere contemplation of this ritualized form of suffering could produce, against all physiological logic, a significant increase in sexual arousal. While the connection between pain and pleasure was explained through an elaborate Hippocratic theory, echoed by some paramedical essays in the early modern period, the relationship between vicarious pain, which was felt indirectly, and sexual emotion constituted a privileged example of sexual paresthesia.

Flagellation was, however, a significant social peril, both in its physiological and psychological uses. To its function as an amorous tool, one had to add its use in the educational system. The word "discipline," which had already been amply accounted for in modern asceticism, was also central to teaching. The centrality of corporal punishment to education, the correspondence between pain and gain, was of medieval origin, but it would live on until the late twentieth century. On contemplating Mr Barville's practices, Fanny Hill felt that the young man was condemned to "have his pleasure lashed into him, as boys have their learning."[72] Away from its religious or penal implications, physical punishment regulated education.[73] Although it affected all social strata, the most ritualized forms of discipline had the elite as their protagonists, as only the most sensitive or *suprasensitive* people could transform physical suffering into an educational benefit. The English parliamentarian Sir Charles Adderley, for example, wrote in his *A Few Thoughts on National Education and Punishment* of 1874 that pain was essential in the healing function of punishment. Following the maxim "spare the rod and spoil the child," the high bourgeoisie and the aristocracy found ample reasons to be satisfied with their childhood beatings. For some American students there was no greater point of pride than having the colors of their flag, red stripes and blue bruises, across their buttocks. For others, the use and abuse of the cane depended on the possible implications it had on future sexual behavior, and on its ability to awaken libidinous passions in both the punisher and the punished. The English doctor William Acton [1813–1875], an expert in venereal diseases – including spermatorrhea or the involuntary emission of semen – echoed some of these fears in *The Functions and Disorders of the Reproductive Organs*. Originally published in 1857, the book was employed in the educational system after its third edition. According to Acton, caning boys on the buttocks excited their sexual feelings and led to masturbation.[74] For someone like him, who had made the custody of seminal fluid a respectable and remunerated activity, most of the students' physical activities, such as jumping or climbing, also led one way or another to *chiromania* or "hand mania." The difference now stemmed from the fact that the temptation of the teachers was added to the danger to the pupils. The experience of English schools is especially relevant here. Havelock Ellis, for example, cited the case of one Udall, headmaster of Eton, whose name appears in the *Dictionary of National Biography*. Famous for frequently beating his pupils for no apparent reason, he eventually confessed to engaging in sexual practices with the boys under his charge.[75] To judge by the comments of other psychiatrists, this was not an isolated case. On the contrary, there seem to be many older schoolteachers who had abused flagellation as a way of unleashing their own instincts.[76]

While this form of punishment could foster active algolagnia in those carrying out the beatings, it could also provoke passivism in those who felt the burning of the leather, the sting of the cane, or even the warmth of a bare hand on their own flesh. Sometimes the first hint of sexual excitement comes from receiving a beating, wrote Krafft-Ebing. So, in the face of the dangers this punishment poses, it would be preferable if parents, teachers, and nurses avoided it altogether.[77] When the *History of Flagellation* was published anonymously in 1888 – really no more than a copy of Boileau's treatise – the author recognized that the main motivation for writing and publishing his work was to get rid of these practices, whether employed for punishment or penitence: "A period will, sooner or later, arrive, at which the disciplining and flagellating practices even now in use, and which have been so for so many centuries, will have been laid aside, and succeeded by others equally whimsical."[78] Despite his intention, this text, as many other similar pamphlets, seethes with an undercurrent of eroticism. Its detailed descriptions of the beating of children often cross the line from denunciation to obscenity. Readers' continuous demands for the most intimate details did not go unnoticed by either the editors or the authorities. This was one of the reasons given by the English psychologist Alexander Bain to promote the modification of punishment procedures and the elimination of whips and canes from schools, the army, and the navy. He also promoted the use of electrical charges for executions. Given that the tool of punishment was invisible and left no traces on the body, it could not cause any kind of delight.[79]

But let us return to asceticism. The aforementioned similarities between penitent practices and sexual masochism cannot hide their many differences. The same mortification gestures join together very different realities. To begin with, masochism is always a gregarious activity that requires the participation of another playmate. The pleasure of this other is never irrelevant. On the contrary, it constitutes an essential part of the ritual forms of suffering proper to sexual paresthesia. The masochist may beat himself alone, but his vice is not solitary. On the other hand, although the ascetic penitent can always find a way for his suffering to reach those outside his cell, his punishment is mainly self-inflicted. In the second place, masochists never seek any kind of pain through deprivation, whether through fasting, not speaking, or any other physiological limitation. For the same reason, they never take an illness or natural pain as part of their agonic search for pleasure. In the third place, and more important still, masochists, unlike ascetics, never aspire to be unique; they never wanted to serve as an example or follow a model of behavior. Far from trying to distinguish themselves through their deeds, masochists are tormented by the loneliness of their conditions. There is no historical evidence of the connection between ascetic practices and sensual pleasures. To suggest that the European mystics felt any kind of sexual arousal could have had a certain psychiatric interest at a given moment in time – undoubtedly aided by a notorious anti-clerical feeling – but it lacks relevance or historical basis. Imputations such as these can tell us nothing about God's servants in the early modern period, but they do reveal a few things about the way in which nineteenth-century psychiatrists put some order into the garden of sexual heterodoxy. Last but not least, even when the relationship between both practices was governed by theatrical criteria and a set of rituals that limited the amount of pain or prevented physical suffering from being produced outside of a socially meaningful context, the will of the ascetic was shown to be always unbreakable, whereas the will of the masochist had to be continually broken. For Magdalena Pazzi, for Teresa de Avila, for the *Mujer Fuerte*, writing was a form of obedience. Suprasensualists' confessions, however, never intended to become an example. On the contrary, the masochist wrote to leave evidence of his desire for submission and obedience.

The power of the idea

Before being subjugated by another human being, the masochist is dominated by an idea – an idea much more powerful than any person. Unlike asceticism, where salvation and mortification go hand in hand, masochism is not interested in pain, but in the global transformation of experience. In the context of its sexual practices, it aspires to such a radical modification of the sensorial universe that even physical suffering can be modulated, transformed, and, in the extreme, converted into pleasure. Though suffering conditions the arousal, it is not the final purpose of the desire. The masochist uses it as an instrument, but does not take it as the central part of his experience. The harmful feeling, the hurt, is maintained as long as it can be counteracted by a psychological re-evaluation that distributes it as a global emotion or experience. In the context of sexual arousal, suffering is not a sensation, but rather a fetish. In the same way that any other object can be transformed before our eyes into something different or acquire an unexpected value, such as an amulet, a talisman, or an idol, pain can lose its tautological character. Pain is not just pain. Ideally, at least, the torment becomes a sensorial illusion that is not bound by the principles of identity. "The relation [between pleasure and pain] is not of such a nature that what causes physical pain is simply perceived as pleasure, for the person in a state of masochistic ecstasy feels no pain," wrote Krafft-Ebing.[80] There is, therefore, no direct and essential relationship between masochism and suffering, but rather between masochism and a psychic or emotional state of voluntary renunciation and humiliation. It is not pain that is the cause of pleasure. The masochist does not describe his fantasy in these terms. Neither are we dealing here with a mere positive evaluation of physical pain. Rather, it is a much more generalized process of re-elaboration of a sensorial perception, through which physical suffering, against all physiological logic, is not felt as pain. This is the description we can find in *Venus in Furs* and other similar works. Severin, the main character in Sacher-Masoch's novel, serves as a perfect example of this curious sensorial re-composition. When Wanda beats him and asks him if it hurts, he replies with conviction: "No! [...] Pain that you inflict on me is pleasure!"[81] Even when the lashes of the whip cut into his flesh and keep burning, the only thing they cause is delight.

The idea that the masochist wants to inscribe on his or her body – that pain feels like pleasure, not like pain – is not achieved without effort. On the contrary, realizing this dream requires a monumental endeavor. Here again masochism takes a different route from the mortification of ascetic practices. For while in the latter, the way to salvation begins with the body, and moreover the body is always present – even if only to deny it, torment it, and destroy it on the road to divinity – the masochist's body does not stand as the beginning of anything. On the contrary, it is rather the inevitable end of everything. The masochist's flesh, far from being a reality to be denied or rejected, is the place where desire crystallizes. The body is not the means; it is the end. The way in which the masochist wants to modulate his experience has nothing to do with Platonism. His path is not an ascending path – one that would take us from bodies to ideas – but rather a descending one, from ideas to bodies. Light, truth, and beauty are not beyond the cavern. The paradise of pleasure does not lie outside the world of shadows, but deep inside the cave, in that intermediate place where the masochist, no longer himself, behaves as a being without will, without identity, almost as an object.

The "Detailed biography of a masochist," the case study number 41 that opens the 11th edition of Krafft-Ebing's work, is particularly exemplary.[82] Although some authors have pointed out that "sexual masochism first began to appear in isolated cases around 1500, [that] it began to spread during 1600s and [that] it became a widespread and a familiar feature of the sexual landscape during the 1700s,"[83] in the narrative of this correspondent from Berlin there is nothing to support such an affirmation. Not only does our author not know what "sexual masochism" is, his account also helps to elaborate on it. His very well-structured text begins by relating his familiar psychiatric background and profusely describing his sexual desires in childhood and prepubescent masturbation. As though he wanted not only to write, but also to interpret, he hesitates between advancing a theory of hereditary predispositions or infantile drives. He does not know whether to blame nature, culture, or both. Not even his descriptions of the facts are free of evaluations. He constantly makes value judgments on his fantasies, practices, and wishes. He is especially concerned that his desire for subjection is made manifest as a kind of unstoppable fantasy or fancy. He has waking dreams. He imagines he is a prisoner, at the disposal of a woman who uses her all-encompassing power to wound and subject him. The beatings are mixed with even more severe punishment, designed to test his obedience.[84] And he loves it. In this he resembles his literary counterpart, Severin. Far from identifying with the bloody tyrants and inquisitors who tortured heretics, they both liked to imagine themselves in the role of the victim, especially if violence was dealt by the hand of women historically considered lascivious, beautiful, or cruel. They wanted to turn into the slaves of the beautiful women they loved and adored; they wanted a kind of slavery in which pain and physical abuse would form an integral part of their fantasies.

Underneath this kind of narrative unburdening there is something unique, authentic, and unmediated.[85] As in other conditions, the illness acquires a historical form. The masochist's drama does not belong to the field of experimental physiology or psychology, but rather to those other kinds of knowledge that, like psychiatry, sexology, or dynamic psychology, depend on the narrative drawing up of testimonies.[86] This is what that the psychologist and the criminologist have in common with psychoanalysis: case studies built upon the history of experience. Any cure must pass through the biography of the emotions, either through literary works or through clinical records. In this respect, there is no substantial difference between literature and life. Each one is a recreation that, in its paroxysm, imitates the other. On the one hand, paresthesia, like the Romantic novel, lets itself be seduced by the temptation of the impossible. On the other hand, literary sources, in addition to their reflection of practices and behavioral models, also contribute to the construction of collective identities. In both cases, confession presupposes concealment, a deliberate lie, a dysfunction between the social sphere (with its regulated conventions, rules, and forms of conduct) and the interior life (with its dreams, desires, and illegitimate behavior).

In the case of masochism, the literary model par excellence was Sacher-Masoch's *Venus in Furs* – a novella published in 1870 that told the story of Severin and his desire to be subjugated by Wanda von Dunajew. Our Berlin correspondent had also read Rousseau's *Confessions* with pleasure. He did not judge either its literary merit or its philosophical pretensions. His reading of this French author meant that he could find another person, a famous writer in this case, with emotions and desires similar to his own. The sensation of loneliness was mitigated by the presence of another human being who, by having the same tastes, could be considered to be the same kind of person, or as he himself describes it, to be suffering from *the same condition*. The passages that Rousseau included in the first book of Part I of his *Confessions* – where he explains that the beatings he received from Mademoiselle Lambercier at the age of eight determined the desires he would feel for the rest of his life – helped to encourage the feeling of belonging to a group connected by the same fears and subjected to the same frustrations. In other personal experiences our correspondent finds emotions he can access and to which he can relate.[87] In this respect, if Rousseau was a discovery, Sacher-Masoch reached the level of a revelation. It was especially in Severin's *Confessions* that he saw his own weaknesses, fantasies, and fetishes reflected.

Against all odds, the Berliner found his equals in the pages of novels and in other clinical records.[88] He felt like a member of a group, not in real life, but in the printed word. A small glimpse of happiness can be observed in the melancholy of his prose. After all, the primary experience of masochism is not pain, but loneliness. Unlike other paraphiliacs, the masochist cannot act alone. Like the onanist, he lives in isolation, but his vice is not solitary. The fulfillment of his fantasies requires the intervention of another who knows how to interpret his silences. This turns the masochist into a genuinely heteronomous being. In his search for a playmate, he behaves more like a lamb than a wolf. He does not want to impose his will, but to lose it. He is not governed by the logic of violence. On the contrary, he needs a pact, an imaginary commitment with another who will take on the role of his master. Within the limits of this alliance, which is binding on both parties, a global re-evaluation of experience will take place, a new way of perceiving the world, in such a way that the most primitive and universal of all sensations, pain, will no longer feel like pain. That is the idea – the idea that the masochist wants to inscribe upon his body. We should not find it strange to read that the narrator of *Venus in Furs* falls asleep reading *The Phenomenology of Spirit*. Simplicity is not exactly one of the characteristics of Hegel's book, so there is a certain maliciousness in Sacher-Masoch's giving us a reader who is unable to cope with the text. However, Hegel's work also touches on the drama of the story that would follow in the novella. The experiences of consciousness – the subject of Hegel's book – require an analysis of the dependent relationship between master and slave, which is the subject of Sacher-Masoch's story. Hegel suggests that neither of these two characters could be what they are, nor know what they are, without the active intervention and recognition of the other. Not even the master has sufficient power to escape from this phenomenon of mutual dependence. Identity and conscience are marked by the presence of a reciprocal agreement, by a ritualized and dramatized form of conduct.

Within this contractual form of desire, the will finds limits. To begin with, the realization of desire is at the mercy of a well-defined set of rhetorical and ritual elements. Success or failure depends on the rigor and care with which the representation is performed, the way in which the suffering is meted out, and the procedure designed for exerting pain. There is an air of comedy in sexual masochism because, in its primitive form, it cannot reject its theatrical qualities. For physical suffering to be experienced as psychic pleasure, the amount of pain, its economy, and the means of submission to its dominion must be regulated. There can only be enjoyment if the brutality is kept within certain limits and if it is meted out in accordance with regulated schemas. What is still more difficult is that the actions, even if implicitly measured, should appear to have an air of improvization. In this sexual ritual, we witness a triple deception. In the first place, the master must behave in accordance with the expectations, limits, and desires of the slave. In the second place, this must be done as though the slave's pleasure had no relevance whatsoever and was, in fact, dispensable. Finally, both the master and the slave must forget the constitution of their pact or the provisions of their agreement. Any prior alliance must be ignored. Arousal depends on the scene developing as though the theatre itself had no rules, and as though the comedy did not exist. The masochist not only questions the laws of physiology, but rather, in salacious bewilderment, also wants to willingly forget the same norms that have just been agreed upon.

It is, however, obligatory to comply with the rules. There are no exceptions. When the deception becomes visible and the plot is uncovered, suffering appears in all its crudest intensity. This pain that flourishes in the midst of the simulacrum cannot be diminished. The blows hurt as all blows do. Once the deception has been exposed, submission only causes shame and beatings only produce harm. Like a bad actor unable to hide his reliance on the prompter, the scene takes on a both tragic and ridiculous tone. All we can do is to cover our face so as not to see, and above all, not to be seen. The breaking down of its theatrical elements gives masochism the air of an *opera buffa*, in which the beatings cause only pain. In the case history of Krafft-Ebing's Berlin correspondent, there was no place for any kind of hope. There was no future to his life other than desolation and defeat. Unlike Severin, Krafft-Ebing's case 41 could not awaken to his pain for the simple reason that he had never stopped feeling it. His careful, elegant prose is full of intrigue. It is not just any story, it is a suspense novel that begins, as do all novels of this kind, with an introduction of the characters. The world, he tells us, was divided into two: on one side his imagination and on the other his fancy. The first was sensual, noble, intellectual; the second aesthetic, ignoble, sensitive. Both led him, alternately, to the arms of a virgin or to the feet of a Venus. Sad reality and vain hope look askance at one other. He knows that there is no pleasure in a world governed by social conventions. There is only pleasure in the imaginary and furtive underworld of his secret dreams and his lonely vices.

The dissonance and separation between case 41's inner world and his noble aspirations marked his adolescence and his youth. Absorbed in daydreams, he often walked alone in forests where he could beat himself with fallen branches. In these escapades, he was not looking for pain, but seeking to delight in his own imagination. Incapable of finding women who would behave in accordance with his expectations and desires, he found only desperation and frustration. In brothels he met with only repugnance and aversion. "All these comedies with prostitutes, which to the normal man appear as simple madness, are to the masochist only meager substitutes,"[89] he wrote. When he finally managed to get over his shyness and prepared himself to be beaten, kicked, and humiliated, the result was no more than a deception: "the blows caused me nothing but pain. The situation repugnance and shame."[90] Desperate, he sought out more experienced women and gave them more precise instructions.

He noticed that they did not lack experience and that predecessors with similar tastes had paved the way. But the value of these "comedies" – our Berliner himself uses this word – continued to be problematic: the scenery interfered with the satisfying of his desire. This led to an even more extreme form of self-deception, so that the beating could be enjoyed spontaneously and not as the result of a studied staging. Sexual satisfaction depended on this premise: "The more perfect the self-deception, the more perfectly the pain was felt as pleasure."[91] The perception of pain could only be overcome once the punishment had acquired symbolic value. This was not his case. His visits to prostitutes always ended up with the same result: he did not feel the least arousal and he could not get an erection. The impossibility of finding satisfaction with what he called a "real woman," together with his inability to carry out the sexual act – what our author calls in Latin *imissio penis* – was compensated by the ever more violent presence of his fantasies. Whereas his attempts to sleep with a woman seemed to him senseless and unclean, his secret activities gave him almost daily ejaculations. In his case, as in many other similar narratives, the distance between desire and reality was insurmountable, with no glimpse of a connection between the vehemence of his desires and the loneliness of his existence.[92]

This story gives us a characterization of the conditions that would become, in the hands of Krafft-Ebing and others, a dysfunction of the sexual instinct; at the same time, it also provides a glimpse of the genuine suffering that plagued the Berliner throughout his life. "[...] I was convinced that my ideal would not allow me to come close to its realization," he wrote. "As for the essential element of masochism, I am of the opinion that the ideas (i.e. the mental element) are the end and aim."[93] His conclusion is full of desperation: "Whether there is such a thing as a possible transformation of these masochist's dreams into a romantic relationship, I do not know."[94] His text teems with descriptions of his dissatisfaction, his impotence, the difficulty of making his fantasies come true, and, at the same time, his need to live under imposed rules, the internal and external struggles to make his conduct seem normal, which always ended in feelings of frustration and shame. Expressions like: "I began to suffer;" "it caused me nothing but pain;" "what was done to me was brutal, repugnant, and silly" appear frequently. The description becomes even more vivid when its author considers there is nothing anti-natural in his ideas. In no way do his sexual preferences offend his sensitive taste. Quite the reverse, he considers himself to be a person with noble sentiments and refined aesthetics. In this he has much in common with his colleagues from this section. Many had lost any hope for the future, whereas others considered their lives to be hell and their existence to be a misery. In some cases, frustration came from their inability to cross the line and ask for a decent woman who would "perform flagellation."[95] However, even when all the standards of decorum have been broken, on the other side there is nothing but pain and shame.

Imprisoned in his unhappy consciousness, the masochist vacillates between his obligations and his desires. He wants to be real and normal at the same time, but he cannot become either one or the other. On the contrary, his condition worsens the more effort he makes to fulfill his fantasy. And vice versa, the possibility of realizing his dreams decreases the more he settles into a familiar environment. This unsolved duality explains why, in these paraphilias, there is finally no substantive distinction between real and purely imaginary pain. The latter has the same cognitive and clinical relevance as the former. The drama of the masochist consists of the terrible, and usually failed, attempt to find a solid base on which to transfer the idea to his body. His continuous failure – his inability to stop feeling pain as pain – is expressed as a troubled confession or a clinical history.

This entrance into the universe of private experience had very clear implications. Although the stories were individual and unique, psychiatry would turn them into a universal pathology, a deviation of the instinct that affects the entire history of mankind. The compilation of desires, frustrations, and attitudes, for the most part away from the public eye and limited to private life, sometimes helped to establish a diagnosis and (almost never) a treatment, but it allowed for the construction of a paramedical category that permitted the cataloging of subjects and the objective study of their public behavior and their private experience.[96] This medical category could only be achieved by means of reiterating testimonies, so that the repetition of stories would give way to an exemplar, or an ideal model, into which the rest of the cases could be subsumed.[97] There is something particularly sinister in the collection of clinical records related to a kind of pathology itself governed by a desire of collecting objects and fetishes, but this was precisely what the successive editions of Krafft-Ebing's book entailed. His *Psychopathia Sexualis* contained hundreds of confessions collected in a single volume. As a whole it offered an unadorned vision of the ostracism, the incomprehension, and loneliness of its protagonists. The informants, like insects pinned beneath the glass case of this new repository, had reflected a great deal on their condition and had consumed large periods of their lives in trying to understand their sexual impulses. Furthermore, they had formed part of the book of their own free will. In the best confessional tradition, they were willing to reveal the most intimate part of their lives, to sell the same secrets that made them feel observed and judged. Outside the glass case they were lost. In the pages of this new treatise, they could finally meet one another, all together for the first time – subjected, humiliated, perhaps finally pleased.

7
Coherence

Pain, by its very intensity, may end up altering reason.[1]
There is nothing, including hate, that cannot adopt the form of a word.[2]

Elusive entities

Almost 300 years ago, the Irish philosopher George Berkeley [1685–1753] called into question whether anything could exist independently of the psychological processes necessary to perceive it. In his *Three Dialogues between Hylas and Philonous*, he defended the impossibility of conceiving of a world outside of our own sensorial capacities. In his opinion, all the properties of objects, both the *secondary qualities* – such as color, smell, flavor, or taste – and the so-called *primary qualities* – like shape, movement, or solidity – only existed in the mind: they were no more than perceptions. Among the arguments he used to convince the reader that the exterior and interior worlds were inextricably linked to our perceptual capacities, one stands out in particular: "Because intense heat is nothing else than a particular kind of painful sensation; and pain cannot exist but in a perceiving being, it follows that no intense heat can exist in an unperceiving corporeal substance."[3] Like many other philosophers before and since, Berkeley used harmful experiences as probative examples. Given that pain does not exist separately from consciousness, he maintained, heat does not exist independently of its perception, and so on. This departing premise for his reasoning, however, is more than questionable. By affirming a connection between pain and consciousness, Berkeley denies the possibility of pain that cannot be perceived, which makes it impossible to speak of unconscious pain. Equally problematic is the fact that the argument does not allow clarification as to whether the mere awareness of pain, independent of any other objective manifestation, in and of itself constitutes a guarantee of pain's existence.[4] Although the supposed impossibility of *unconscious pain*, and the supposed existence of *only conscious pain*, led to profound philosophical queries, it is not philosophy we need to look at to resolve them, but history. Chronologically, Berkeley's reasoning has been challenged by at least two counter-examples. In the first place, there are pains that do not correspond to any anatomical location. In the second place, there is also suffering that does not manifest itself consciously. In both cases, there is a disagreement between structure and function or, more generally, between geography and history. The patient's anatomy does not coincide with his or her narrative. Or vice versa, the patient's story does not correspond to any place in which one could visualize his or her experience. In one situation as much as the other, the credibility of the experience depends on a form of argumentative coherence – the patient's, doctor's, or both. If the pain is only conscious, the doctor may not believe the patient. If the pain is unconscious, on the other hand, it might happen that the patient does not believe the doctor.

Let us start with the first option. The presence of symptoms that are not related to a visible injury or morphological alteration has historically caused a great deal of distrust. In these cases, patients do not have only one problem, but at least two. The possibility that *their illness* will never be given the status of a disease where the cause and the treatment are already known adds to their physical complaints. The absence of an explanation for the abnormal bodily behavior, an explanation that could refer to a visible morphological injury, causes a great deal of tension between the person suffering from the ailment and the person trying to cure it. Pain – much like fevers, dizziness, and other unspecific symptoms – increases not only the patient's anxiety, but also the anxiety of all those involved in his or her diagnosis, treatment, or care. The shadow of fabrication that floats over the way in which patients describe their ailments is offset by the suspicion of professional incompetence with which their eyes incredulously interrogate the doctor. Whereas the physician may suspect that the patient is exaggerating or lying, the patient may doubt the doctor's professional capacity and competence in making a correct diagnosis. Without the determination to recognize that instead of saying "you do not have" the doctor should be saying "I am unable to see," the clinical gaze can turn anxiety into a matter of personal responsibility. In the most extreme cases, that which patients perceive as science's inability to define the cause of their ailments, the doctor converts pain into an ontological problem. If he or she can't see it, it's because it isn't there. Furthermore, if he or she can't see it, the explanation must not be in the patients' bodies, but rather in their psychological makeup, or more extremely, in their moral attitude. The tension between the *supposed* symptom and the *supposed* absence of injury, between subjective experience and the objective knowledge of the illness, turns pain into a problem that is at the same time cognitive and moral. As long as the ailment lasts, objectivity is questioned and, so to speak, suspended. While the patient continues to complain, the symptom itself may become the illness, or in other words, a *syndrome*.

The distinction made by medical anthropology between *illness* and *disease* is particularly relevant here.[5] The first, *illness*, includes all symptoms as the patient perceives them, lives them, and especially the way he or she talks about them. Pain is not only one of the most frequent elements in the subjective experience of an illness, but it is also one that has historically held the highest diagnostic value. On the other hand, disease refers to the way in which different symptoms are grouped together into theoretical frameworks that allow for identification and treatment. These theoretical frameworks, ordered into families and genres, allow for general knowledge about them as well as for the study of their specific variations. The birth of clinical medicine at the end of the eighteenth and the beginning of the nineteenth centuries was broadly based on this dichotomy between the patient's account of discomfort and the objective knowledge of the disease provided by science. Between the story of symptoms as narrated by the patient, and the objective inscription of the ailment on the bodily geography, clinical medicine prioritized the latter, giving a greater importance to the disease over the patient. Just as our bodies are a more or less gross alteration or modification of an anatomical-ideal model, private experience introduces spurious elements into a pathology that the patient could only speak about approximately. Rather than *listening* to the patient, the doctor should *see* the disease.[6]

The narration of symptoms and its inclusion in a taxonomic system produces tension between two social and cultural forms of understanding illness. One is geographical, the other historical. Whereas the doctor learns to read the body like a map and recognizes its pathological signs, patients take notice of their symptoms within the confines and subservience of a narrative. While one establishes a system of signs, indices, and correspondences, the others understand their illnesses within the rhetorical form of discourse. This narration, no matter how sophisticated, is based on the comparison of two minimum elements: *before* and *now*. That is the reason why the discourse of pain is never presented in an isolated form, such as "this hurts" or "that bothers me," but is rather constructed in comparison to past experience: "I was fine *before*, but *now* I'm not"; "*Before* I felt this way, *now* I feel a different way." The definition of pain given in the first writings on the matter, such as those by Petit, Griffin, and Bilon, were not established on the basis of any other consideration and employed no other guiding principle. This temporal delimiting of harm, expressed in a discursive form, led to the inevitable consequence that *to feel* was also *to judge*.

For so-called psychogenic pains to make their appearance in the history of medicine – at the hand of Otto Binswanger, a professor of psychiatry at the

University of Jena – diseases no longer needed to be defined only using morphological lesions or damage, but also through functional accidents and forms of somatization or guidelines of behavior of a psychological origin. That is, it was necessary for clinical medicine, linked to the search for morphological correspondences between symptoms and bodily ailments, to allow the appearance of symptoms without visible ailments – symptoms whose only source of credibility depended on the patient's discursive coherence. Although the cultural space that allowed the framing or naming of these pains only arose in the second half of the nineteenth century, research into the corporeal effects of emotions had a long historical and iconographic tradition (see Figure 34).[7]

As early as the eighteenth century, various physicians and surgeons, in reflecting on the influence the mind exerted over the body, had concluded that both on a sensorial level and in the context of mobility, the ways in which emotions could produce physical reactions were extraordinarily varied. In 1787, the Medical Society of London awarded William Falconer for providing a list of diseases that could be cured or mitigated by exciting the affects or passions. The list included nervous diseases such as mania, melancholy, and epilepsy, but also many others that today we would judge unrelated to the mental faculties, for example scurvy. Investigation into the possible psychogenic nature of pain also gave rise to strange experiments. Some members of the Society for Psychical Research, for example, investigated the possibility of inducing pain through suggestion, going so far as supposedly managing to transfer the sensation from one subject to another.[8] For Desault, the increase in aneurisms and heart ailments was always related to the evils of the Revolution.[9] In his opinion, whereas anger accelerates the circulation of the blood, multiplying the efforts of the heart, terror, conversely, debilitates the vascular system and by preventing the blood flow from reaching the capillary vessels causes the pallor that so explicitly captured some years later the French painter Géricault. The pallid faces and rouged cheeks that proliferated during the reign of Louis XV grew pale as a result of anxiety, resentment, fear, and revenge.

Along with "only conscious" pain, first neurology and later psychiatry postulated the existence of cognitive activities and psychological traumas of an unconscious nature. In part connected with studies on suffering without visible morphological injuries and in part as a result of research into certain psychiatric conditions – especially in the case of different kinds of hysteria or other neuroses – the history of unconscious or subconscious pain and the history of nervous pain ran along parallel courses.[10] On some occasions, pains with no known disease diversified into a broad spectrum. This is the case of neuralgia, or a painful tic, but also that of causalgia or rheumatism, acute as well as chronic. Likewise, many discussions were centered on frenalgias, hysterical, hypochondriac, or melancholic pain, or the abnormal modification of sensorial thresholds. Many of these illnesses appeared in the twentieth century with other names and under different cultural categories.[11] Hysteria and hypochondria, for example, became considered dissociative syndromes. Neurasthenia, which was formulated by the North American electrotherapist and doctor George Beard [1839–1883] at the end of the nineteenth century, shares notable diagnostic similarities with chronic fatigue syndrome and even with fibromyalgia, whereas many cases treated in relation to nervous disorders in conditions of shock would be defined as post-traumatic stress, with retrospective diagnoses, for example, in situations of paralysis caused by soldiers' fear in the First World War.[12]

The historian Andrew Hodgkiss called these pains: "pains with no *bichatian* lesion," that is, with no *morphological* lesion. After all, these pains did have a lesion, whether it was of a functional nature, the result of a nervous irritation, or the product of a psychological trauma.[13] In the last of these, the difficulty would consist of determining how we can account for physical or psychological traumas that have been memorized or inscribed in emotional states.[14] In the first, the problem lies rather in how to establish the way in which emotional states can, without the use of the will, produce symptoms that do not correspond to any morphological lesion. In both cases, the automatic relation between the mind and the body, which operates without the intervention of consciousness or the will, inverts medical practice, which becomes obliged to focus on the patients' narratives instead of looking at the physical signs inscribed on their bodies.

Identity

For the first time in this book, although not for the first time in history, the harmful experience is, at the same time, certainty and truth: the truth of a certainty and the certainty of a truth.[15] Representation, mimesis, sympathy, correspondence, trust, and narrativity are tied to the subjective expression of the person who, at the same time, feels, judges, and suffers. This historical tour through the *topics* of harmful experience will have caused the reader no shortage of frustration and unease. Whoever has read this far will have found *something else*, but not the subjective sensation and emotion linked to the person who suffers. Throughout the previous pages, the reason that perhaps prompted you to read in the first place has been missing. In the first chapter, pain was absent from the representation of violence and from those saints that smilingly accepted the ritual destruction of their bodies. In the second chapter, suffering disappeared beneath the will for servitude and the desire for obedience. The impartial spectator in Chapter 3, who constructed his or her scale based on distance and impartiality, looked on but did not suffer. Neither the women in labor nor the anaesthetized bodies of the nineteenth century complained in adequate proportion. The women, as a result of the supposed exaggeration of their gestures, and the anaesthetized bodies, due to their suspended animation and catatonic state. Although the masochists' suffering took the form of a story, their autobiographical narration did not look for pain, but rather subjection. These *topics* of experience allow us to understand the conditions under which suffering becomes significant, but they do not refer to the very awareness that, here and now, there is someone who suffers.

The relationship between pain and consciousness depends on the most sophisticated form of conviction – certainty – that vindicates the most ancient form of correspondence – truth. In a similar way, it is also necessary that the realm of scientific knowledge, which pretends to have the monopoly of truth, claim for itself the universe of certainties, not through mechanisms of objectification, but through the appropriation of the patient's testimony. Illness should become a disease, just as the subjectivity of experience should become an objective fact of knowledge. Although in the best possible world every well-defined set of symptoms would correspond to another set of probable diagnoses, the history of medical practice is full of cases where a symptom refuses to be classified under the rubric of a well-defined entity that is treated with standardized therapeutic procedures. This lack of concordance between the experience of the illness and its objective classification and treatment – which is part of the history of anxiety itself (both the patient's and the doctor's) and appears in varying degrees throughout the history of medicine – is especially relevant in cases of mental illness. In *The Death of Ivan Ilyich*, probably the most explicit novel ever written on this dissonance, the Russian writer Leo Nikolayevich Tolstoy [1828–1910] established the definitive incommensurability between pain as illness and as disease, as certainty and as truth. The equation between both terms – the presence of pain and the absence of an explanation – is completed in this short novel by another equation: the inversely proportional relationship between the intensity of the pain and the amplitude of consciousness.

For those who have not read Tolstoy's 1886 novel, it is perhaps worth giving a brief description of its content. Ivan Ilyich is a normal, middle-class civil servant who, following a professional promotion, calmly decides to do some work on his new house. His days of poverty when his salary seemed insufficient to satisfy the demands of his children or the requirements of a nonconformist wife, are over. Now, though, everything has changed. His work situation has positive repercussions in his private life, and pride victoriously takes over from humiliation and bitterness. Ilyich is so filled with a sense of well-being that he even takes the time to do things that he would previously have rejected as trivial, not to mention impossible, like hanging curtains. *Previously* there was no money for curtains, nor anywhere to hang them. Above all, there had been no need for adornment. Life was lived from day to day out of necessity. *Now*, however, internal and external decoration form part of his reformed moral scenery. His wife, his children, his superiors, and his new subordinates are all witnesses to the transformation of a man who, until recently, had been just another example from darkest, deepest Russia: the "life of Ivan Ilyich was most simple, most ordinary and, therefore, most terrible."[16] The main character represents above all the triumph of objectivity. "Ivan Ilyich very soon acquired the art of eliminating all considerations irrelevant to the legal aspect, and reducing even the most complicated case to a form in which the bare essentials could be presented on paper, with his own personal opinion completely excluded and, what was of paramount importance, observing all the prescribed formalities."[17] His lack of subjectivity extends into his family life and serves as the epicenter for an inanimate life that Tolstoy describes as though it were a still life painting.

When Ilyich is hanging his curtains, he has a small accident, an event without importance, a light bump. He feels a little pain, a minor nuisance, and then nothing. The feeling seems to mislead his memory. After all, what is a small knock? Who hasn't banged themselves slightly from time to time? It hurts a little, it passes, and that is that. As anyone else in his position would do, Ilyich wants to get on with other things. But the pain returns. First, it comes back infrequently, but then, little by little, it grows more intense. What had been nothing, because it couldn't have been anything, turns into something to worry about, and then becomes a matter for clinical investigation. After a few days he goes to the doctor. The civil servant wants more than a diagnosis; he demands an explanation. He has a right to one. After all, it is incomprehensible that something that is nothing could cause increasingly more frequent and intense pain. Unfortunately, everything seems to indicate that it is too early for a diagnosis. At most, a few incomprehensible medical words blend together with his despair. Ilyich dares not ask the ultimate question and when he finally does it in private – with *"Will I be cured?"* – he rejects the answer. Maybe the problem isn't the illness, or whatever it is. It must be the doctor. His wife knows a different one. They decide to call him. They think that he'll know what to do. His reputation precedes him. They hope that if they contact him he will turn up, and everything will be solved in a matter of days, weeks at most. One diagnosis follows another in a gibberish of technical terms, but Ilyich is no longer interested in them. They seem incomprehensible to him. His point of view disappears in the academic jargon. What is more, he no longer wants to know what is wrong with him, but wants it to stop. Something that wasn't in his body before has gotten there and somehow someone must find a way to get rid of it. If he can't get it out of his body, then there must at least be a way of hiding the symptoms. Or at least stopping the pain! Being able to live with the illness has now become a priority over finding a cure for the disease. Let's forget the cause, the origin, and let's go to the symptoms; let's only be concerned with the consequences. What Ilyich wants, initially, is to live *like he did before*. But as the illness increases, he would be happy just being able to live. A decrease in his personal identity goes along with an increase in pain's means of expression. In this inversely proportional relationship between pain and consciousness, the one-time civil servant will be turned into a scream without a cause: the greatest sign of the disproportion between suffering and decorum, between nature and culture.

Tolstoy's novel is disturbing because suffering is its only protagonist. It is not just, as Berkeley claimed, that pain can only exist in consciousness, but rather that, in being only consciousness, pain surpasses it, and finally annihilates it. We know of the destruction through a narrative that, against all logic, does not take place in a precise anatomical place. Far from being perceived, the pain uses perception to manifest itself. The different stages that Ilyich passes through do not imply that his ailment might not come from some internal injury that could perhaps be observed in a post-mortem dissection. The narrative tension in Tolstoy's tale, however, increases with this absence, and reaches its climax in the extreme sounds of laments and cries. The illness can't be seen, but it can be heard. For medicine at the end of the nineteenth century, this trauma could be related to an imperceptible functional lesion of the nervous system or to a prior psychological event, also of a traumatic nature. In both cases, the pain was only a phenomenon of a previous, invisible, and unconscious injury, for which there existed no cure. What would Berkeley make of all this?

Nervous pain

The presence of a pain or, more generally, a set of symptoms that cannot be related to any kind of structural lesion, appears in a good number of books and literature on nervous disorders in the nineteenth century.[18] One of the first doctors to study these disorders systematically was Benjamin C. Brodie [1783–1862]. This professor of Surgery at St. George Hospital, London, UK, began his *Lectures on Nervous Affections* of 1837 by explaining the case of a middle-aged woman who complained of a constant and severe pain, which she traced to a spot about three or four inches in diameter beneath her last left rib. For Brodie, who had already worked on the diagnostic value of pain, especially with regard to diseases of the joints, the area where the woman felt the sensation had no reason to correspond to the place where the symptoms originated. The discomfort could be due to a peripheral trauma of the affected nerves, a functional lesion in the brain or the spinal cord, or, in the strangest cases in which it was not even possible to establish a direct communication between the nerves and the affected parts, the pain, known as sympathetic, could derive from the brain and be transmitted through the secondary nerves.[19] The ailment could be as far away from the sensation as the patient was from knowledge. The distance between the experience and its nervous origin opened a cognitive and emotional barrier between the physician and the patient. The latter's incorrect testimony regarding the localization of his or her own symptoms constituted no more than a confirmation of the former's prerogatives. The physician knows but doesn't feel; the patient feels but doesn't know.

The study of these *local hysterical affections*, as Brodie called them, was based on a different principle from the one that had guided clinical medicine until that point. Rather than looking for the illness in the features left by morbidity processes in the organs and tissues, anatomical examination served only to confirm the absence of lesions and morphological damage. The doctor looked for a sign, an indication, a trace, but given the impossibility to find any of these, the invisible and, finally, the non-existent, acquired a cognitive value. Even when pathological anatomy and the anatomical–clinical method – which sought a lesion for every kind of ailment – could maintain their explanatory capacity, diagnosis was supported by the confirmation of an absence. There was nothing on the other side of the patient: no rash, no lesion, no fever, no inflammation. Nothing. This "nothing," as in "nothing is wrong with you" – or at least, nothing is wrong with you in the place you're complaining about – questions the patients' groans and the subjective narrative of their illnesses. In those cases where it was possible to identify a lesion that explained the symptoms, the body would have very little story to tell. In hysterical affections, on the other hand, where pain was not accompanied by any other manifest sign, such as inflammation or fever, the lack of corporal coherence constituted a proof in favor of the existence of a functional lesion. The patient told a story that had, we could say, very little body.

The clinical gaze, forced to choose between what patients describe and what their bodies report, continues to take the side of the latter, although the correspondence (between words and things) has given way to (functional) coherence as a form of clinical investigation. The reasonability of the choice is beyond any doubt, for on what morphological structure could the diagnosis be confirmed? To what organs or tissues could the symptoms refer? In ruling out morphological injury, the medical inquiry must modify the patient's narrative. In the clinical histories compiled by Brodie, those who arrived at London Hospital suffering from one pain very often left the premises suffering from another. Following a careful examination, the surgeon concluded, for example, that the young lady who arrived at his surgery complaining of a hip injury was suffering from nothing other than a hysterical condition. The woman thought, mistakenly, that the pain was located in her joints when it came, in fact, from the nervous system as a whole.[20] Her sufferings, which to a large extent appeared to be rheumatic in origin, did not worsen with movement or pressure. She complained and, on occasions, cried out when the doctor's hand exerted pressure on the affected area, but she also did so when he examined another part of her anatomy. Even if the pain was being felt in the hip, she also protested when her ribs were examined. The complaints were the same when he scrutinized her thighs or studied her ankles. Although she had constant and, at times, unbearable pain, which appeared to suggest a serious lesion in the bones or the joints, her laments frequently disappeared when she conversed about topics other than those that caused her ailment.

This does not mean that the symptoms were not significant or that the ailment was imaginary. Far from it, the pain was real, almost no one doubted that. Despite patients' not knowing the source of their ailments and attributing them to the wrong place, Brodie did not question the presence of the pain, nor did he put aside symptomatic remedies, such as the application of belladonna or friction with camphor, sometimes used jointly with a tincture of opium. As the origin of the disease was unknown, the treatment was palliative. In any case, Brodie considered that the best remedy was prevention and the most essential thing for recovery was that the patient's mind not be constantly occupied with the subject of his or her ailments. Alexander Turnbull [1794/1795–1881] was of the same opinion. This physician tackled extensively the symptomatic treatment of nervous pain through the application of veratria, a remedy obtained from the roots of *Aconitum napellus*, whose active component is aconite, a neurotoxin. Its use was recommended whenever colchicums, quinine, iron carbonate, moxa, the cutting out of the nerve, and even amputation had failed.[21] The prescription of these treatments demonstrates the degree to which Brodie's position, among others, constantly distinguished between the correct form of understanding illness and the clinical response that should be provided to the patient. Given that the certainty (of the illness) does not coincide with the truth (of science), surgeons should work with the same intensity in both directions, seeking to solve the first while attempting to understand the second. This duality between the diagnosis, which limits the patients' testimony, and the treatment, which after all bestows them with some prerogatives, is also demonstrated in other forms of linking the virtues of the narrative to the properties of the body. Apart from the immediate correspondence between the (subjective) discomfort and the (objective) lesion, the search for the locus of the pain could proceed in three different directions. To start with, the interrogation of the dead could replace the questioning of the living. Secondly, one had to consider that the seat of pain might not coincide with the place of sensation, but it might rather be invisible and remote. Finally, both surgeons and physicians had to find forms of managing the patient's body that, calling its argumentative coherence into question, could still postulate the existence of some functional illness.

The advantage of examining a dead body is clear, given that the cadaver, unlike the patient, neither talks nor lies. Although many of the patients examined by Brodie were subjected to the scrutiny of an autopsy, the post-mortem examination confirmed the absence of any morphological lesion. On their inside, there was nothing. It is a far cry from the story of the surgeon John Hunter who, convinced that he was suffering from a cardiac malfunction, asked his disciples to take out his heart once he had died to confirm what he had already postulated as the true cause of his death. In one of the strangest obituaries ever written, one of his assistants dedicated a few paragraphs to Hunter's life, while most of the text concentrated on details of the anatomical dissection of his heart. As might have been predicted, his body proved Hunter right, even after his death. Brodie's cadavers, however, betrayed his patients. The carefully dissected bodies showed not even the slightest trace of any morphological lesion; there was no anatomical indication to relate their pain with an illness of the organs. The same body that had tormented them in life betrayed them in death. For Brodie, at least three-quarters of the cases of female patients who came to his office complaining of their joints were suffering from nothing more than hysterical pain.[22] Their dissection opened a space of refutation where geography could rebel against history. The border separating the interior from the exterior operated as a dividing line between absence and presence, between the certainty (of pain) and the truth (of knowledge).

For John Hilton [1804–1878], author of a work on physiological rest, when the pain was not accompanied by an increase in temperature – the local symptom of inflammation – it had to be referred to a remote cause located far from where the discomfort was felt, and therefore far from the patient's subjective evaluation of his or her pain.[23] The perceived hurt could be the external sign of some distant disorder capable of producing an effect through the sinuous distribution of the nervous channels. In this vein, while the patient identified the place where pain was felt with the source of the ailment, the doctor, on the other hand, should distinguish between the ailment's subjective and objective localization. Given that any pain has a different meaning, from that caused by a speck of dust in the eye to sympathetic pain, the surgeon's first task was to carefully point out this new place and this new residence. Knowledge of the disease thus began with an evaluation and normalization of the symptoms, with their inclusion in a code that would allow distinguishing the nature and location of the affected nerves, and finally, with the attribution of a diagnostic value to the results obtained, for, unlike patients,

> who judge of the position of their own disease, most frequently, by the situation of the most prominent painful symptoms, or those most palpable to their senses; we surgeons, relying upon our knowledge of the true cause of the symptoms, judge of the seat of the disease by a just interpretation of the symptoms through the medium of normal anatomy.[24]

For François Louis Isidore Valleix [1807–1855], famous for having written a monumental treatise on neuralgias, it was also essential to distinguish between those spontaneous pains always present (although in varying degrees of intensity) and those pains that were provoked, either by the patient's movements or the surgeon's manipulation of the body. The former, the spontaneous, could fluctuate between a dull, continuous pain to a sharp, intermittent pain. The latter, the provoked pains, could be precisely located or, on the contrary, could be distributed or extended through numerous nerve endings. With this kind of pain, one also had to observe the direction, frequency, violence, and extension of the pain, for even when the pain could be considered the principal and nearly most important of all the symptoms of neuralgia, the diagnosis rested on the doctor's correct interpretation of the patient's subjective testimony.[25] While there is no doubt that the truth hides in the body, it has no relation to the words, cries, or lamentations of its most relevant witness. On the contrary, Valleix argued, the gestures and signs of suffering can easily be contaminated by preconceived ideas, by the way in which the patient believes his ailment should manifest itself, or by other interests that, working either together or in isolation, suppose some form of material or emotional gain. Even when patients do not deliberately lie, they are always trapped in an ocean of ingenuity. Their body, so to speak, does not belong to them. Their expressive signs do not refer to a place, but rather express an insurmountable contradiction between what they feel and what they do not know.

Based on a classification previously established by Brodie concerning lesions of the spinal cord, Herbert Page also showed a special interest in those pathologies that, even when they produced severe symptoms, could not be attributed to any morphological lesion either before or after a post-mortem evaluation.[26] Page, a surgeon who worked for the London and North Western Railway Company, took into account the studies previously undertaken by John E. Erichsen [1818–1896], a Briton of Danish origin who had in 1866 published a study on lesions to the nervous system caused by a shock from a railway collision.[27] The term "shock" had a deliberately ambiguous meaning, and could refer to either a psychological blow or a physical shaking. The shock could be the result of a panic attack, but also of a concussion or brain damage. Here we are particularly interested in those accidents in which, along with the dead and injured, there were other passengers who suffered from long-term unspecific symptoms, despite their not having any structural damage or lesion. Without being able to relate the symptoms to any kind of anatomical lesion, these patients' ailment went on to become a condition known as "railway spine." Although Page did not agree with Erichsen regarding the ultimate cause of these disorders, the work of both doctors led to the establishment of a legitimate diagnosis for certain symptoms that, in Page's words, condemned the patient to a "life of pain, misery and uselessness."[28]

Both Erichsen's and Page's work had an added value, given that the majority of their patients not only sought to recover their health, but also wanted economic compensation. Both surgeons had to relate an experience of a subjective nature, such as the presence of symptoms with no lesion, to an invisible lesion in the spinal cord or a psychological trauma that could give the patients the right to an indemnity. The objectivity of the symptoms thus took on the form of financial profit. Or in other words, the unit of analysis to measure pain was no longer the nervous impulse measured with sophisticated technological instruments, but rather the distribution of indemnities according to the independent judgment of the company's experts. For even if their patients want, in principle, to be freed of pain, they also want to be believed. Once all doubts have been dispelled, the expert judgment will establish a directly proportional relation between pain and payment. For the patient and for the lawyers, the subjective experience of the illness is transformed into an economic appraisal, so that the intensity of the pain is no longer measured in *daps*, as Fechner intended, but in bank notes.

Let us look at the case of S.W., a tall man with a strong constitution, who was the victim of a severe collision. As with many other similar clinical or medico-legal records, we do not even know the date or the place of the accident. Prior to the publication of his book in 1898, Page had worked for nine years for the London and North Western Railway Company. The accident must have happened at some point between 1879 and 1896, but it is really impossible to know. In those years alone, British railways counted their accidents by the dozen, and there were more than a few deaths and injuries in cases of derailment or collision.[29] From the standpoint of the logic of financial gain, these accidents did not prevent the railroads from continuing to be profitable. At the same time, many voices protested against their unlimited power of destruction and their numerous signs of violence.[30] The image of a machine expelling smoke could not better express this ambivalent character of progress as linked to servitude to the machine, its limitations, its schedules, and its constrictions. On the one hand, mass transport had the disadvantage of placing the passengers in large agglomerations where it was necessary to learn how to behave collectively, in accordance with regulated systems of social action. On the other hand, the railways cut through the landscape, not finding a place within it, but forcing nature to change. Of all the most evocative figurations and symbolisms of the new fears produced by the railway, the tunnel occupied a privileged position. With its entrance into darkness and the uncertain expectation of a victorious departure, with its libidinous image of anti-natural penetration, the greatest anxieties of railway transit built up inside it (see Figure 35).[31]

Following his accident, S.W. ended up with bruises all over his body and received a heavy blow that tore the skin of his face and fractured his nasal bones. After the event, he entered a state of nervous depression, with a feeble and rapid pulse and an inability to eat or sleep. He was greatly disturbed by the death of a friend who was sitting beside him at the moment of the fatal mishap. His anguish was so great that the scene came back to his mind over and over again.[32] Curiously, some of these symptoms had already been published in the medical magazines of the day. There were often articles in the press regarding railway safety.[33] In a climate of growing concern regarding this uncontrolled mode of transport, some publications paid special attention to the trains' excessive vibration, the carriages' heat and the locomotives' smoke. It was not only that the movements of the train seemed to be involved in the production of nervous disorders, the changing distance of the objects observed during the journey also allegedly caused excessive activity that led inexorably and unconsciously to the destruction of the organs. In 1862, the prestigious medical journal *The Lancet* argued that the trains' continuous oscillations and vibrations could have serious consequences for the passengers' health. In extreme conditions, cerebral or spinal concussions annihilated organ functions. In their more moderate forms, the same blows could lead to a disease that, much later, could manifest itself in the form of paralysis.[34]

Although the corporal injuries healed quickly, nine weeks after the accident S.W.'s mental condition showed clear signs of instability. He complained about depression and sadness, as though some great concern prevented him from recovering. He felt uncomfortable with doctors and burst into tears frequently. His voice had become very weak, almost inaudible. He said he slept badly and continually awoke from nightmares. The narrative of a man that had once been healthy, lively, and robust became more and more moribund. Fifteen months after the accident, he was still unable to work and four years later, his doctor recognized that he would never be the same again. His appearance had also changed. His healthy looks and strong hair had given way to a much older, more haggard face. His symptoms had worsened over time. He now had palpitations, lack of sleep, and continual fatigue to add to his general lack of vitality. No one, however, had been able to identify any lesion whatsoever, either in the brain or in the spinal cord. Page affirmed that he had little doubt that this prolonged illness was not due to any bodily injury, but rather a mental shock, perhaps brought on as a consequence of fear.[35] Unlike Erichsen, Page maintained that fear itself could cause somatic effects such as those described above, and that there was nothing to suggest that this shock was related to any morphological injury that might be discovered during a post-mortem evaluation.

The history of *railway spine* has been described in the context of the so-called psychodynamic revolution that took place in psychological practice during the second half of the nineteenth century. Both Page and Erichsen were aware that concussions in the spinal cord, brain, or backbone were frequent in other accidents of everyday life – such as falls, blows, and carriage or horse accidents; they were also aware that the alarming situation created by railway accidents had increased the frequency of these injuries, which had become proportionally more numerous and more severe. The polemic faced by both specialists was based not so much on the fact that one (Erichsen) proposed an organic explanation while the other (Page) opted for a psychological justification, but rather on the order of causation. For Erichsen, physical shock caused psychic disorders, while for Page, fear and anxiety caused organic trauma. Regardless as to whether the trauma was physical or psychic, both surgeons bolstered a new form of testimonial trust: a relationship between the doctor and the patient which was no longer mediated by mechanical forms of objectification, but by the veracity of the patients' account, by their visual gestures and signs, by the conviction with which they expressed their symptoms, their family background, the opinion of those who know them, their position in the working world, or the criterion of other colleagues who had examined the case. Without this relationship of trust there is no clinical case, and far from finding ourselves faced with one of the chapters in the cultural history of nervous pain, we would be looking at a section of the difficult and problematic cultural history of deceit. Page understood that without this initial axiom that judges and considers the accounts given by his patients as genuine cases, there is no discussion or development possible: "we premise that we are dealing with perfectly genuine cases, where none of the circumstances, as far as we were able to learn, threw doubt on the bona fides of the patients," he wrote.[36] However, how could the expert have the conviction that the case presented to him was real and not feigned? How could he establish the true nature of the patient's account?[37] For both Page and Wilks, the author of a treatise on illnesses of the nervous system, there was no general rule. The daily task of the doctor consisted of deciphering the meaning of pain and establishing its real or subjective nature: "no rules for diagnosis can be laid down; every case must stand on its merits."[38]

Page dedicates the whole of his book's seventh chapter to the evaluation of symptoms as the patient describes them, and the suspicion as to whether the illness might be an exaggerated or feigned one.[39] Following the customary literature on imagined illnesses, he argues that the majority of cases related to the fabrication of symptoms are discovered because the patients either have insufficient anatomical knowledge or fail to know some of the symptoms that accompany their supposed ailments. That is, in the absence of sufficient correspondence between the verbal account and the examination of the body, coherence alone should allow the doctor to distinguish between real and faked pain. The impossibility of finding a morphological reference that could explain the symptoms requires the defense of a truth that is not constructed through correspondence with the world (or better put, with the body) but rather through the internal coherence of the patient's words. What use is a dynamometer or a sphygmomanometer, Page asks himself, if the patient's account is no more than the result of interest and imposture? On the contrary, "the reality of many of the symptoms, lacking all vestige of objective sign, depends upon the veracity and good faith of the patients."[40] Furthermore, we must remember that "to the patients themselves [the condition] is very real: the pain, the stiffness, the palsy, are to them as great as they are described [...] and though we may regard these symptoms as of little moment in themselves, we must not look upon them as altogether feigned."[41]

Not even improvement following the awarding of financial compensation can necessarily be considered to be a sign of falsifying illness. For isn't the compensation an explicit acceptance of the reality of the patient's subjective symptoms? Is this public recognition not perhaps a way of eliminating incredulity and suspicion? Might not this social acceptance of the illness lead to a general improvement in the patient's condition? For Page, the improvement of the patients, much more willing to deceive themselves than to deceive others, takes place in a "completely unconscious" manner.[42] Here too, the narration of these symptoms, and the way in which they are felt, is mediated by the patients' capacity for imitation, by the process of sympathy described by the philosopher Adam Smith in his *Theory of Moral Sentiments*. This is part of the nature of the "stigma," the word Pierre Janet used to describe the symptoms of hysteria. Nervous illnesses imitate symptoms, especially from the publicity of similar cases frequently mentioned in the press. Even in the worst of cases, patients do not invent their ailments, but copy them from the cultural matrix in which both they and their symptoms relate to one another. Rather than being a fabrication, the symptom is experienced more as an always-imperfect copy of a cultural model that it ought to resemble.

Pierre Janet was also fully aware of this process of mimicry when he discussed hysterical patients' supposed fabrication of one of their most characteristic symptoms: anesthesia. Janet reasoned that in the absence of structural lesions, one would be inclined to think that these patients did in fact feel what they claimed not to, or see what they said they did not. Undoubtedly, one might think that the insensitivity was simulated, as were perhaps the rest of their claims. However, he asked: how is it possible that in all civilized countries of our milieu, hysterical patients decided to imitate the same symptoms from the Middle Ages to the present day? What's more, he concluded, if we are dealing with a fabrication, it should be the doctors and not the hysterics who are held primarily responsible for such a deception. For it is the doctor who, through his questions, suggests the "correct" responses to the patient; it is the doctor who prompts a particular experience of symptoms that are always inextricably linked to subjective evaluations and cultural conventions. The problem does not consist of distinguishing between genuine and false symptoms, but rather of clarifying which of these are faithful copies and which are not. In cases involving subjective (unobservable) symptoms, this tends to happen *a posteriori*, prompting us to ask ourselves whether bedridden patients' rapid recovery, once they have obtained financial compensation, might not serve as an objective proof of a moral rather than a nervous disorder. But neither in these cases nor in those of a supposedly voluntary exaggeration of symptoms was Page able to establish a clear dividing line between the real and the faked. After all, "we must remember," he wrote, "that the exaggeration may be, and in fact it is, neither desired nor assumed. Exaggeration is the very essence of these emotional or hysterical disorders which are so common in both sexes after the shock of a collision."[43]

Unconscious pain

The history of unconscious pain begins with two words: trauma and stigma. Prior to the nineteenth century, a trauma was an anatomical lesion and, more specifically, a fracture of the bones or joints. Stigmata, on the other hand, made their appearance in the world of mysticism, as signs of the passion that divine action inscribed on the bodies of the devout. In both cases, natural actions and supernatural passions left visible marks on the corporeal geography. From 1224, when Francis of Assisi received stigmata from a six-winged cherubim, there was no shortage in Catholic Europe of cases of mystics whose bodies acquired the wounds of Christ's Passion. Catherine of Siena, the Spaniard John of God, or the German Katharina Emmerick were just some of the precursors mentioned in the Salpêtrière Mental Hospital. In the nineteenth century, Marie-Julie Jahenny and, above all, the Belgian girl Louise Lateau joined the ranks of their fellow hysterics. One of the followers of the neurologist Charcot, Désiré Bourneville [1840–1909] studied some of these supernatural phenomena in depth, reinterpreting them in the light of mental illness. Under the general title *Diabolic Library*, he published and evaluated ancient documents related to religious phenomena. Little by little, the supernatural signs were transformed into diagnostic elements. At the same time, a word that had been employed in physiology and surgery – "trauma" – was displaced toward a psychological use.[44] A first phase of this transposition began with studies on somnambulism at the end of the eighteenth century. Later, considerations on psychogenic amnesia were added to the list. Physical blows began to cohabitate with psychological dramas linked to the tendency to hide memories from consciousness.[45] Trauma expressed itself as a kind of amnesia similar to a paralysis, just as partial paralysis, so frequent in some mentally ill patients, began to be understood as a different kind of amnesia. There were not, then, two sets of phenomena, mental and physical, but rather two manifestations of the same phenomenon related to the connection between states of consciousness and the construction of personality (see Figure 36).[46]

The notion of "hysterical trauma" was popularized by Charcot, and around 1893 Sigmund Freud and Joseph Breuer extended the concept of "traumatic neurosis" to hysteria in general. Pierre Janet, for his part, used the term "stigmata" for all of the essential symptoms of hysteria: the result of ideas that had become disassociated from the consciousness but remained there, like parasites feeding on subconscious experience. When Freud met Charcot on his first visit to Paris in 1885, the ideas of this "young and poor human being, tormented by ardent desires and dark sadness" (as he described himself) were determined by the diversification and study of mental illnesses, as well as by his doubts with regard to what was then called the "neurological approach."[47] Already by that time, he was increasingly convinced that some so-called nervous illnesses had their origin in a psychological pathology. The same symptoms seemed to lead to very different diagnoses when observed from the point of view of neurology or from the standpoint of psychiatry: "More important Viennese Authorities than I used to diagnose neurasthenia as a brain tumor," he wrote. Not long before, he could have done the same.[48]

Much has been written about Freud. Curiously, the Freud prior to the formulation of psychoanalytic theory paid much more attention to pain, both in its symptomatic and psychological aspects. Although the strict formulation of "unconscious pain" came later – in a theoretical work of 1923, *The Ego and the Id*, which to a certain extent came to rephrase some of the ideas contained in his *Beyond the Pleasure Principle* of 1920 – Freud reflected upon suffering in his earliest writings: in *The Psychic Mechanism of Hysterical Phenomena* and in his *Studies on Hysteria* from 1895.[49] Five years previously, in the "Psychic Treatment (Treatment of the Soul)," he drew a clear dividing line between the failure of neurology and medicine's unilateral emphasis on the corporeal, which was unable to account for the proliferation of the symptoms observed in medical practice. His reasoning was based on two well-corroborated facts. Firstly, it seemed impossible to deny the existence of a significant number of patients whose symptoms could not be traced to any morphological lesion. Secondly, the existence of these symptoms could not be questioned. On the contrary, the clinical histories of these patients showed an overabundance of ailments:

> These patients cannot do any intellectual work due to their headaches or lack of attention; their eyes hurt when they read, their legs get tired when they walk, they feel dead pain and they sleep; they have digestive ailments, they vomit and have gastric spasms; they cannot defecate without laxatives, they have become insomniacs, etc. They may simultaneously or successively suffer from all these ailments or from just some of them.[50]

From these two asseverations, Freud understood that these people were suffering from the same disease; they could not be treated as patients with illnesses of the stomach, the head, or vision. Likewise, their symptoms did not correspond to nervous or functional diseases; on the contrary, all the pathological, visible, and conscious signs came from the altered (and unconscious) influence of their state of mind.[51] Along with sensitive discomfort, Freud postulated another pain of a psychological (but unconscious) nature that would allow us to account for symptoms and behaviors of a neurotic nature.

Before Freud, the idea of this "unconscious pain" had already made an appearance, both in the field of experimental psychology and in physiology and psychiatric practice; it was also present, though in a mitigated form, in Nietzsche's genealogy and in the works of Schopenhauer, as well as in the works of many experimental psychologists and physiologists, who postulated the existence of sensations, including harmful sensations, beneath the threshold of perception. Subsequently, in addition to the pain of a conscious nature that accompanied any organic lesion, psychoanalysis distinguished between psychogenic pain, neurotic pain, and psychotic pain, all three of which had an unconscious origin.[52] Philosophers have reflected extensively on these matters, at least as much as psychoanalysts have.[53] This is not strange at all. The well-established early modern dichotomy that made any intellectual activity a conscious activity found two clear refutations in pain without lesions and unconscious pain. In the first case, the difficulty consists of knowing what might be causing the pain, given the apparent absence of a lesion. In the second case, the problem stems from how we can assume the existence of a lesion – or, more descriptively, a trauma – that is not accompanied by consciousness. Given that we tend to identify pain with consciousness, the idea of unconscious pain seems counter-intuitive, even absurd. Inasmuch as we consider that suffering has an etiology that always refers back to a morphological lesion, the possibility of a pain without a lesion appears to place the ailment against a metaphysical backdrop. In these cases, as we have seen, the looming doubt about the testimonies of others becomes even more pointed. The same formula that establishes the content of our consciousness with absolute certainty allows us to call into question any experience of suffering that is not accompanied by visible proof. In the case of unconscious pain, the line that leads from symptoms to treatment also changes. The patient keeps going to the hospital as a result of a proliferation of symptoms – including physical pain or other diffuse and unspecific forms of suffering – but the clinical practice is now based on recovering a memory that, like a trauma or a fixed idea, is preserved in the body but not in consciousness.

Pain relates to psychological illnesses in three different ways. In the first place, physical suffering also appears as a clear diagnostic sign. Because the doctor confronts the ailment through the patient's narration and historical description, the illness can be mental but the first manifestation is always physical. Paul Briquet [1796–1881], for example, who studied more than 400 patients at the Hospital de la Charité in Paris, considered that pains in the epigastrum (or upper part of the abdomen), on the left side of the thorax and along the left vertebral canal, were a constant manifestation of hysteria (see Figure 37). More than 60 pages of his treatise were dedicated to the identification and evaluation of these pains, whether they were cephalalgia, rheumatic pain, or pleuralgia. The anesthesia, spasms, convulsions, and hyperesthesia that characterized the nature of this illness could be present or not, but rachialgia or back pain appeared so often that Briquet considered these pains universal in all hysterics.[54]

For Étienne-Jean Georget [1795–1828] as well, the most extraordinary manifestations of hysteria always led to a continued experience of chronic pain.[55] A student of Pinel and Esquirol, Georget, who had proposed the study of neurosis based on features such as chronicity or low mortality, considered that while the convulsions or cries disappeared after each attack, the cephalalgia ran its course continuously.[56] Although hysterical behavior could include convulsive movements or nervous attacks, the most common of its symptoms manifested as a constant and untreatable pain. A similar occurrence marked hypochondria, one of whose expressions was *periodic migraine*. In the case of epilepsy and the so-called nervous, spasmodic, or convulsive asthma, some of his patients described a strong and permanent sensation of heat on the head. Some others made reference to a psychological suffering, to which there existed no clear empirical correlation. All of them recounted how their days revolved around a vortex of sad ideas. One of them had desires to shun everyone, felt like crying, and had strong contractions in the stomach area:

> above all my head aches; it takes a great effort to get my ideas together, they seem to pass by quickly; they cross one another. Some days I feel very depressed, horrible sometimes; days when I can see no way of getting out of the state I am in, in which I feel no will of any type; acting like a machine, with no pleasure at all, and only because I have to act.[57]

Madame D, a woman with a strong character, also felt incapable of attributing her sadness to any external circumstance:

> I am worn out, I do not have the least desire to eat although I feel the need; I am sad when I rest, I sob in my sleep without being able to remember when I wake what dream caused my tears. [...] I don't feel a pain that I can locate in any particular place. Sometimes, my vapors come upon me suddenly and manifest themselves through a sharp pain, sometimes piercing my chest or my side, sometimes in my stomach, rarely in my head unless I feel dizzy. When this invasion happens so suddenly, I think I am threatened by a serious illness; I feel distressed, worried and I set to medicating myself to combat the ailment I am afraid of having. Often all this dissipates after weeping for what I thought was a close and certain death.[58]

These patients' narratives show a symptomology that, more than anything, questions the logical order of causation. Given that the symptoms do not stem from any morphological lesion and do not fit into any physiological pattern, the patient tends to think – not without reason – that the proliferation of unconnected sensations, some of which are very painful, will end up driving him or her mad. The doctor, on the other hand, considers that a psychological disorder is the only thing that could account for the proliferation of symptoms. The patient understands that if the symptoms could be eliminated, his or her psychological discomfort would also disappear. For the doctor, on the other hand, if it were possible to resolve the psychic trauma, the physical symptoms would go away. The problem for both of them is that the experience does not refer to any other reality outside consciousness and that therefore the distinction between causes and effects cannot be made according to a chronological order. What the doctor perceives as a "somatization," the patients experience as a result of the proliferation of symptoms, a crazed way in which the patients' bodies, but not the patients themselves, spontaneously produce the most undesirable effects with no apparent motive. In both cases, the illness calls a patient's identity into question, as well as the dividing line that distinguishes fact from fiction. On the one hand, the patient's distrust of the doctor, who is unable to identify a lesion, ends up being applied to the patient him/herself, obliged to live with unspecific symptoms and private experiences. While in traditional clinical medicine, the doctor could observe the (always deficient) way in which the ailment manifests in the body, it is now the patient who cannot understand the circumstances that seem to make him or her responsible for his or her own ailments. The patient's experience refers back, over and over again, to something that is not outside but inside of him or her, something that does not seem to exist beyond the narrow limits of his or her consciousness.

In this progressive reduction of experience, Georget's patients, for example, end up heeding nothing but their own pain: "The patient normally understands everything that is going on around her; but with regard to the pain that is destroying her, she does not respond to any question; she has no idea that is not the pain itself."[59] The first implication of this curious narrowing of consciousness is that there is no significant difference, nor can there be, between real and imaginary pain; in the same way, there can be no significant difference between *being* sick and *believing* one is sick.[60] At the same time, like in the story of Ivan Ilyich, the continued presence of the symptoms establishes an inversely proportional relation between pain and personal identity, which manifests itself especially in the use of language: "The muscular system enters into convulsion, the use of the senses and the reason is interrupted. Some of the patients give out sharp cries, or a characteristic scream which is similar to the howling of wolves: most of them call out, screaming, for their mother."[61] Here also, the intensity of physical suffering decreases the sphere of consciousness and limits verbal expression. Between the articulate use of language and piercing screams, expression becomes metaphorical. In the case of the patients described by Georget, when the cephalgia becomes unbearable, when the brain no longer has intellectual and moral existence, suffering is communicated through complex expressions: some feel that they have an anvil crushing their heads, others feel they are being beaten by hammer blows, others that their brains are boiling, as if they were touching scalding oil. The sensations are not described with the proper terms of popular psychology, but rather through a twisted correspondence to imaginary worlds. Like the writer Marmontel, who complained that for seven years he had suffered from a pain that had pierced him to his soul *like a stiletto*, the patients describe their ailments in relation to realities they have not actually lived; their logic takes on dramatic shades of the "as if," a theatrical form of the projective imagination. At the end of the process, screams replace words. Whatever their age or condition, they all howl for their mothers. Like in the Greek tragedy *Philoctetes*, the presentation of the characters occurs in a diatopian, uninhabited space, with no easy landing.[62]

In the second place, if pain constitutes one of the most decisive diagnostic symptoms in hysteria, so too does the lack of response to harmful stimuli. The sense of touch remains, but the patient either does not recognize pain or experiences it disproportionately. During the last quarter of the nineteenth century, cases of this strange sensorial condition, which may be systematic, localized, or general, appeared more and more in specialist literature. Of the almost 600 patients examined by Doctor Auzouy – most of whom were demented, *imbéciles*, and melancholics – more than half showed different levels of cutaneous insensitivity.[63] Thus what during the Middle Ages or the early modern period might have been construed as proof of supernatural involvement – either related to witchcraft or to mysticism – now became a sign of hysterical behavior. In the case of the so-called *convulsionnaires* of Saint-Médard – famous in Paris at the beginning of the eighteenth century for remaining for two to three days with their eyes open and staring fixedly and their faces as pale as a corpse's – their bodies seemed totally insensitive to pain. Not even when they were subjected to the severest tortures did they complain or show any signs of suffering.[64] In the nineteenth century, the explanation for these phenomena came initially from Daniel Tuke and was later seconded by Pierre Janet himself.[65] Their contemporaries, however, had already described this behavior as hysterical vapors.[66] There had also been frequent cases of cutaneous insensitivity linked to the so-called test *de la piqûre*, a form of torture that consisted of piercing or puncturing supposed witches' or sorcerers' skin with sharp instruments. Even though the Parliament of Paris prohibited the practice in 1603, its use still appeared in the trials concerning the supposed possession of the Ursuline nuns of Aix in 1611. A stake pierced the flesh of Father Louis Gauffridi, the supposed guilty party, "without the wretch feeling anything."[67]

Pierre Janet, who had written his doctoral thesis on involuntary acts, began to use the term "automatism" to refer to physiological phenomena that were both independent of the will and the reflexive consciousness. In the same way that the body produces reflex movements, he argued, not all sensation must be accompanied by conscious perception.[68] Unlike Wundt, who considered sensations to be primitive states of consciousness, Janet thought them to be experiences that included the personality, the body, and the social position.[69] To feel was not only *to live*, as physiology had suggested since the Enlightenment, but *to know that one was alive*. Whatever the nature of sensorial processes, one could not disregard the conscious or unconscious personality responsible for combining stimuli and generating perceptions. On the contrary, one had to start by recognizing that the absence of sensations always occurred in relation to a group of objects or stimuli that formed a system. The patient may be conscious, for example, of the presence of an indeterminate number of persons in a room, but be unable to distinguish some of them. Similar to a state of somnambulism, he or she distributes sensitivity in accordance with a pattern that unconsciously determines the choice of impressions. From this standpoint, hysterical anesthesia, including its historical manifestations, consists of nothing more than a pathological form of absent-mindedness that prevents the sufferer from connecting certain sensations with his or her personality. In Janet's interpretation, far from being an organic lesion, anesthesia resulted from a contraction of (or a decrease in) consciousness.[70] In the face of certain stimuli, he argued, the patients see and feel things that they are not capable of perceiving, and therefore they do not react or complain when they are pricked, pinched, or burned. What he proposed about anesthesia also applies to most of the symptoms of the allegedly "nervous" illnesses, which can only be interpreted and understood in light of personal identity. When the patient has no interest in the pain, the sensation disappears, even from automatic mechanisms.[71] This occurs to such a degree that not even attempts to recover sensitivity through an increase in the stimulus's intensity – for example, through the application of electrical shocks – produces the desired result.

The absence or excess of sensitivity does not determine the nature of the illness, it merely constitutes the most visible expression of a psychological problem of which the patient is unaware. This becomes still clearer when instead of looking at anesthesia, we examine the opposite modifications of sensitivity such as hyperesthesias or hyperalgesias. In these cases, some parts of the body demonstrate such delicate sensitivity that the patients feel the most terrible pain from the slightest touch or lightest contact. Substances or objects that under normal circumstances cause a banal sensation, like for example a sheet of paper, now cause intense pain.[72] For Janet, if the symptoms are painful, so is the trauma that triggers them. The daily sensation that these patients experience as perpetual torture is, in his estimation, connected to a set of terrifying ideas and memories: "They are, as we said, hyperesthesias caused by fixed ideas."[73] Memories or remembrances, those parasites of consciousness, generate so much fear and pain that their presence culminates in a perpetual distraction, or more generally, in a narrowing of the field of consciousness. Since not all psychological phenomena are equally perceived, a good number of them will be never perceived at all. This implies that subconscious states are nothing more than the reflection of a dissociated personality:

> We have described acts and sensation that the subject seemed to ignore completely, being absolutely out of her personal perception. These totally subconscious phenomena formed, through their development and combinations, a second psychological existence, on occasions a second personality that was seen at the same time as the normal personality.[74]

While Pierre Janet focused his attention on secrets and anxious emotions fixed in the mind, Freud's first writings also related the symptoms of hysteria with previous emotional traumas. For both authors, there was a triggering element that, through a sort of imitative process, made chronic a pain that, under normal circumstances, would have been momentary.[75] As in the story of Ivan Ilyich, or S.W.'s agonizing tale, what was nothing, because it had been nothing and couldn't be anything, ends up absorbing the totality of consciousness, settling in the body as a syndrome: "the memory, the image of a past pain, seems to be associated with a particular sensation and it is reproduced automatically as soon as this signal appears," Briquet wrote.[76] The connection between this triggering element and the symptom may be real or symbolic, so that a moral pain may cause neuralgia just as a mere apprehension may also cause vomiting.[77] Thus, for example, a painful emotion that arises during a meal (but is repressed in that moment) causes nausea that lasts for months in the form of hysterical vomiting. The neuralgia may be the consequence of a mental pain, and the vomiting may be the result of a feeling of moral apprehension. In both cases, these psychological traumas do not act in isolation, but rather they join together to create a single history of suffering that is simultaneously conscious and unconscious: conscious in that we cannot deny the dramatic proliferation of symptoms, unconscious insofar as the symptoms can only be explained through the remote presence of a psychological trauma. The illness should be understood as an illness of the memory inasmuch as the memories that trigger the present suffering are not *at the patient's disposition*; on the contrary, they are memories that the patient *wants to forget* and that consequently are "deliberately repressed from conscious thought."[78] The symptoms of hysteria therefore constitute *mnemic symbols*, that is, indications of repressed memories.

Regardless of whether repression (in Freud's terminology) or dissociation (in Janet's) is responsible for the clinical symptoms, the recovery of traumatic memory also brings with it an enormous amount of suffering. Along with pain as a symptom and unconscious pain, this is the third sense, the third form in which pain and psychological illnesses are connected. In the case of

Madame D., the return of long-forgotten memories was accompanied by violent headaches: "We have seen Madame D. cry out in pain, suffer from vertigo during which she could not remain on her feet and we have seen her delirious when she recovered an important set of memories. These symptoms decreased and even disappeared when the memories became clearer."[79] In her case, as in many others, if suffering forms part of the illness's development, it also constitutes an inevitable element of the healing process. The recovery of the memory, of the perceptual space, as much as the re-unification of split personalities, is not achieved without an enormous amount of suffering that consists, precisely, of putting into words the affliction, making the psychological trauma at the same time clear and present. Given that hysterical patients principally suffer as a result of their reminiscences, the psychotherapeutic treatment would provide a way out for the strangled memory by means of a coherent verbalization of the past. In his *Psychotherapy of Hysteria*, Freud recognizes that all these repressed ideas or remembrances have in common "their distressing nature, calculated to arouse the affects of shame, of self-reproach and of physical pain, and the feeling of being harmed; they were all of a kind that one would have preferred not to have experienced, that one would rather forget."[80] The forgetting, however, has not been complete or sufficient; hence the proliferation of symptoms. We cannot get rid of the continued and constant physical pain, the sensorial anesthesia, or the hyperalgesia without verbalizing and recalling a past that continues to be present.

It never ceased to strike Freud (who was educated as a neuropathologist) as odd that his clinical histories read like novels.[81] Those that he included in his studies on hysteria – the cases of Elisabeth von R., Lucy, Katharina, and Emmy von N. – pointed toward the linkage between those histories and their symptoms. These latter always end up by slowly revealing a (metaphysical) secret or a strange body. The process of bringing these repressed or unconscious memories to light is itself wrapped up in an enormous amount of suffering. In order to exhume a buried city (as Freud called it), or archaeologically recover the remains of a distant past that lies buried and protected, we need new forms of physical and symbolic violence. On occasion, the assault should take place by provisionally eliminating consciousness. In almost all occasions, it should occur through the use of words. Given that the patient has "swallowed" her psychic trauma, which lives on in the form of anxiety, horror, or shame, she will have to be forced to "vomit it out" by means of a cathartic process that will free her from the poison responsible for her physical symptoms. This process, which Freud called "abreaction," consists of the linguistic and affective recreation of the traumatic memory. It is not enough to remember, it is necessary to remember so as to forget.

This relationship between memory and forgetting permeates not only the dynamic transformation of psychology, but also the philosophy of the second half of the nineteenth century. "It is possible to live almost without remembering, indeed, to live happily; however, it is generally completely impossible to live without forgetting," wrote Nietzsche in *On the Use and Abuse of History for Life*. During the previous century, philosophers had endlessly discussed the relationship between the involuntary nature of forgetting and the voluntary nature of memory. To think, for Nietzsche, and later for Foucault, was to think about history, not a history that turned the past into archaeological flotsam or an unchangeable monument, but rather a critical and essential history to feed the living. There are many similarities between Nietzsche's text and one of the most enigmatic phrases that closed the posthumous work of the philosopher Immanuel Kant. When this Prussian thinker dismissed his butler after 40 years of service he wrote in his diary: "Remember to forget Lampe." In the face of a loss that he seemed unable to understand – but about which he couldn't, it seems, stop thinking – the philosopher of the categorical imperative assigned himself the difficult task of forgetting Lampe.[82] For Freud, memory should not only reach conscious remembrances but also all those that were inaccessible to patients in their habitual psychic state. To bury the memory of the butler required a voluntary exercise, a cure that could only be achieved once the repressed and forgotten memories had been linguistically and emotionally recreated. We must remember so as to forget all that which, despite having been falsely erased from consciousness, still interferes with it like the walking dead in the world of the living.

8
Reiteration

Nothing is so soon forgot as pain.[1]

Hell

In an article published in December 1832, Professor Elliotson – the same man who defended the use of mesmerization in surgical operations – described a neuralgia resistant to all forms of treatment. This clinical history alternated between medical specifications and the inability to produce not only a cure, but also a temporary relief from the symptoms. "I am sorry to say I did no good whatever, or at least only produced a temporary alleviation from time to time," he wrote. The illness was present in the legs, arms, and wrists, as well as on the right side of the face, in the submandibular nerve. Though the patient had been in this predicament for some years, his ailment had its beginnings in the more distant past. At the outset, the pain – agonizing, lacerating – was concentrated in the index finger of the left hand. It was so acute that the slightest friction produced a very violent reaction, as though someone were running a penknife along the finger, like an electric shock. The agony was such that the patient, a journeyman printer aged 32, bit off the whole fingernails of his healthy hand, as if with this gesture he might free the other from its extreme suffering. The doctor, who did not know the immediate cause of the ailment, made no reference to hypnotism or mesmerization. On the contrary, he attempted to reach a diagnosis based on the negative elements that emerged in the examination: there was no inflammation, redness, or increase in temperature. "There is nothing whatever to be seen," he said, "but yet there was agonizing pain."[2]

Having dismissed the search for a cure, Elliotson attempted to alleviate the symptoms. He began by administering iron carbonate mixed with a fourth of morphine chloride. He also applied a solution of cyanuret of potassium to the finger. Faced with no noticeable improvement, he increased the dose to a grain of morphine, got rid of the iron and started with strychnine, first topically and then orally. Since the patient's general health began to deteriorate without any significant change in the neuralgia, he then began a treatment with arsenic. When the amount of morphine had reached eight grains a day, the agony was so great that the patient begged for the opiate in larger and larger doses. Otherwise, he said, he could scarcely exist. "He appeared to be an excellent man, a man of a strong mind, but in his agony the tears were seen running down his cheek." Extracts of jimson weed or belladonna also proved to be ineffective. Amputating the finger would not solve anything, as it was a matter, Elliotson wrote, of a "chronic disease, and the reason why you frequently cannot cure it is that it is often connected with some organic affection. I know that, after death, nothing has been found; just as after epilepsy and paralysis."[3]

In the same way that pain without a lesion suggests the presence of a psychological dysfunction that we could categorize as hallucinatory, chronic pain also breeds distrust. The presence of an ailment that begins but doesn't end calls into question the rational schema that has served for centuries as the framework for the subjective experience of falling ill. The ritualized form that the drama of suffering has always acquired finds here its most extreme refutation – at least after the moment in which reconciliation, relief, and the body's reintegration into the community is forever postponed. Unlike the dramatized form taken on by the experience of acute pain, Hell – for there is no other way to describe this place that can never be left – is not a border, but rather a state: an ultra-mundane residence wherein the body suffers mercilessly and eternally without the slightest glimpse of a solution or an escape. On the inside of this tunnel, suffering is simultaneously acute and chronic, human and superhuman, reiterative and perpetual. Faced with the everyday experience of illness, anesthetists, surgeons, psychiatrists, and social service professionals have always understood this particular kind of anguish as being an exception, an anomaly occurring within an already transitory state. Not only is it infrequent, but also clearly abnormal: a form of suffering that contradicts the protocols that, through the appropriate treatment, leads from the symptom to either cure or death.

For a long time, the only way definitively to avoid this interminable torture was suicide. Reconciliation, the phase always considered by anthropologists as the last stage in this rite of passage, did not appear in this kind of experience. Although Doctor Falret [1794–1870], who theorized on the matter at the beginning of the nineteenth century, held that physical pain was borne with more resignation than its moral counterpart, his book contained many examples of human beings who had taken their own lives as a result of prolonged suffering. A woman who felt as though her flesh was being bitten and devoured by packs of wild dogs hung herself with a rope tied to her bedroom ceiling. Another, who suffered from rheumatism and couldn't bring herself to commit suicide, never ceased to beg her friends to put her out of her agony. A third, who was suffering from uterine cancer, poisoned herself with grains of opium, and so on. In the dozens of cases of hypochondria studied by this expert, what drove the men and women to make attempts on their own lives was not indifference or weariness of existence, but "the real or imaginary pain that, having destroyed the harmony of their faculties and taken disorder to their will, led them to sacrifice the most precious of their gifts."[4] Together with the innumerable causes that trigger a suicide – among which our author cited temperament, age, sex, education, reading novels, masturbation, the passions, marital tensions, love, ambition, humiliation, anger, gambling, or religious beliefs – Falret also added prolonged and incurable physical pain. The concatenation of sufferings culminates in the same pathological conduct to which the sociologist Émile Durkheim would later dedicate one of his most famous books.[5] In the cases of both Falret and Durkheim, suicide was not evaluated from a moral standpoint, but it was studied as a behavioral form belonging to anomic and socially disintegrated beings. Like the monsters of the early modern period, who wore inscribed on their bodies the signs of the rupture in the natural order that had made them possible, the suicides' behavior was a mere reflection of their illegitimate origins. Their life conditions expelled them outside the community and placed them beyond history. This is how the suicide was frequently depicted: on the edge of a bridge, on the brink of a precipice, on the boundaries that separate the social from the asocial and life from death (see Figure 38).

The appearance of pain as an object of medical practice, the pharmaceutical industry, and the cultural market is a twentieth-century phenomenon. Only then did pain – the *faithful friend*, the *cry of life*, the *punishment of God*, the *weapon of Christ*, the *punitive instrument*, the *educating rule* – come to serve as the object of research programs and welfare institutions. In our time, although still to a limited degree, the experience of harm has found a corporate materialization and a space for scientific development. We need only look at the growth in recent years of units specializing in palliative care to confirm the extent to which pain now has its own instruments, societies, and institutions.[6] Clinical and academic interest in this new object of study brought about the 1967 founding of the *Intractable Pain Society*. The magazine *Pain*, an offshoot of the International Association for the Study of Pain, began to be published in 1974.[7] For its protagonists, the appearance of this new medicine seemed to be the culmination of a process, the last chapter of a narrative sequence that had led human beings from the logic of resignation to the technology of resistance. Following the abolishment of surgical suffering in the mid-nineteenth century and the widespread introduction of analgesics in the consumer culture of the twentieth, what remained to be found was an effective treatment to combat the suffering associated with incurable or terminal illnesses, as well as those that are now known as fibromyalgia, rheumatoid arthritis, facial neuralgia, or post-traumatic syndromes, that is, the different varieties of prolonged or untreatable physical agony. Surgeons and neurologists always interpreted their history thus: as a result of the proliferation of anomalous phenomena that their inherited theoretical framework seemed unable to explain, but also as the necessary culmination of a broader historical process that included the arrival of the humanitarian and enlightened gaze to the *lectus doloris*, to the bed of pain and death.

On many occasions, this "humanitarian perspective" was implemented by the use of opiates in terminal patients, in other words, by the (not always socially accepted) policy of providing the patient with the necessary instruments and substances to decrease suffering. In 1890, the doctor Herbert Snow was already arguing for the generalized use of opium in treating incurable cancer.[8] Three years earlier, William Munk [1816–1898] had also begun his pioneering treatise on euthanasia, vindicating the medical management of death; this included putting at the patient's disposal the necessary means to avoid agony. Unlike Snow, who based his recommendation on the quality of life of people affected by tumors, this English doctor and historian considered that opium should be used both to alleviate pain and to soothe the feelings of weariness and despondency, the exhaustion and anxiety that sometimes accompanied the final journey.[9] The art of dying, which had since antiquity been an occupation connected with religious orders and welfare laws, had to be secularized and make use of the knowledge medicine and science had to offer.

Almost 100 years later, in a 1982 publication, Patrick D. Wall and Ronald Melzack sought to account for the same pain that had tormented Elliotson's patient and hundreds of other human beings before and after him.[10] Their text used as its starting point the distinction between acute pain, which had been one of the visible signs of illness since antiquity, and chronic pain, which they described as an illness itself or, more precisely, as a set of symptoms. In the 1980s, many members of the scientific community – physiologists, neurologists, or anaesthetists – recognized that whereas acute pain could maintain some level of utility – at least as far as to allow anticipating the presence of some underlying condition – chronic pain could only be interpreted as a disorder which caused a great deal of suffering for the patient, his or her family, and society as a whole, without any clinical justification for its presence whatsoever.[11] Although the material space of this new illness began to fill rapidly with divisions and subdivisions of harmful syndromes, the first taxonomies had a dichotomous nature. Medicine began to distinguish between useful pain and useless suffering, between laboratory pain and clinical anguish, between peripheral and central pain, between pain in the limbs and pain of the internal organs. Certain other conditions, like the suffering associated with an incurable illness, took on a new visibility. The scholar Marcia Meldrum holds that from the mid-nineteenth century to the present day, pain has been the object of three related medical discourses: the symptomatic relief of acute pain, the treatment of severe pain in the terminally ill, and the management of chronic pain in cases of migraine, rheumatoid arthritis, trigeminal neuralgia, and other syndromes of an unspecific nature.[12] The key word here is "related," for although each of these lines of research had its own development, the medicine of pain has always been built upon their zones of confluence.

The history of untreatable chronic pain does not in all cases coincide with the history of terminal pain; likewise, the history of acute pain does not in itself lead to a new clinical conceptualization of chronic suffering. Each one of these realities has its own historical development, subject to national and local variations. However, the new conceptualization of pain and its progressive institutional materialization depends in part on these mutual relations. The acute, the chronic, the terminal, and the unspecific can only be understood from the conditions that allow the parceling out of experience, the subsequent multiplication of names and theories, the building of a new scientific community, the institutionalizing of treatment, and the appearance of a new group of people: sufferers of chronic pain. More important still, this entrance of science into Hell, the linguistic and institutional materialization of a medical practice linked to the study and treatment of chronic pain, presupposes, along with the creation and the manipulation of a family of harmful syndromes, the temporal annotation of a life experience that, instead of being interpreted from the point of view of the logic of defeat, aims at a new reconciliation.[13] Unlike acute pain, chronic pain does not cross over cultures or historical periods; it is not a universal phenomenon in either history or culture.[14] Of course, the existence of persistent suffering, manifested throughout continuous periods of time, is not exclusively connected to twentieth-century medical practices. Headaches, backaches, pain in amputated limbs, so-called causalgias, and neuralgias have always existed. But this does not mean that we may consider those people who suffered from such ailments in the past as "ill." Although we may be tempted to think that the chronic nature of pain has affected humanity as a whole throughout history, it is not necessarily true that those who suffered from chronic ailments were always considered *sick with them.*

The name

Although the distinction between acute and chronic pain was already present in Romantic physiology, it only emerged explicitly in the second half of the twentieth century. The International Association for the Study of Pain, founded in 1973, depended so much on this distinction between the transitory and the chronic that when pain achieved full visibility in the field of clinical research, it did not do so as a single object, but as many.[15] Its appearance coincided with the partial dissolution of what until that time had been called by the name of "pain." It was not the first time in history that the development of the sciences was linked to the speciation of its objects and the proliferation of words. At the beginning of the nineteenth century, the new science of anatomical malformations relegated the old monsters of the Middle Ages and the early modern period to the spaces of fiction and the culture of the spectacle, so that when physical deformations linked to embryonic development began to be systematically studied, the strange and infrequent beings that had populated Natural History books went on to join the ranks of freak shows and libraries of fantasy literature.[16] As the development of scientific teratology progressively eliminated the interest that these preternatural phenomena had aroused through the ages, it also generated a complementary effect, in the sense that those features that had previously been interpreted as signs of supernatural intervention or evidence demonstrating normal functioning of the organism now became a privileged object of scientific study. For this reason there was never really such a thing as a science of monsters, but rather of anatomical malformations. As concerns its clinical development, the history of pain also follows a similar path: from the (natural or supernatural) signs of injuries or morphological lesions to the constitution of an object of research proper, human suffering dissolved into a typology of intermediate beings or harmful syndromes.[17] Some of these, like causalgia, phantom limbs, or trigeminal neuralgia, were already long known by medicine, although not always under these names. Many others, however, appeared along with the new subdivisions and led to the multiplication of theoretical frameworks and explanatory hypotheses.[18] The so-called "theory of specificity," for example, allowed an accounting for the majority of types of acute pain – such as contusions, lacerations, or fractures – but was of almost no help in complex clinical cases. Partly as a reaction to this theory, from 1894 onward a new explanatory model understood pain as the joint result of specific harmful stimuli and of mechanisms related to the stimulus's intensity. This is the reason that some authors considered pain to be an affective quality that should be distinguished from tactile sensations. For the American Psychologist H. R. Marshall, for example, far from being a sensation, pain was an emotion that could be unleashed by an infinite combination of causes. For almost all clinicians, however, pain was a sensorial aberration that, because it manifested in a plurality of states, made treatment excessively difficult.[19]

The transformation of (natural) signs into (clinical) evidence was not difficult. The cultural materialization of the new object of study was much more complicated. In 1986, the Association for the Study of Pain offered the first large-scale classification of the so-called "chronic pain syndromes."[20] Fibrositis, burning mouth syndrome, and tendinitis were added to an ever-diversifying list of syndromes such as migraine or persistent backache. The world filled up with new inhabitants: allodynia, painful anesthesia, dysesthesia, hyperalgesia, hyperesthesia, paresthesia, neuritis, or peripheral pain all described realities that until then had only had a literary existence, hidden away in the incomplete, sometimes incredible, tales of the human beings affected by them.

Even when the diagnostic value of the pain was not questioned, (chronic or terminal) suffering dissolved into a family of experiences that far exceeded, when they did not contradict, the theoretical elements that formed the basis of the relationship between the (physical) lesion and the (psychological) experience. This was always the first problem:

> Doctors are willing to admit very quickly that pain is a defense mechanism, a fortunate warning that alerts us to the dangers of an illness. But what is it that we are calling a defense mechanism? Defense against whom? Against what? Against the cancer which so often produces symptoms when it is already too late? Against heart conditions that are always developed in silence?[21]

Thus the surgeon René Leriche [1879–1955] attempted to repudiate the false concept that associated the presence of pain with a necessary evil that, especially in France, had served as the basis of physiological research into pain since the beginning of the nineteenth century. The semiotics of groans, the translation of expressive gestures into clinical signs, had made it possible among other things to speak of animal suffering or of pain in infancy, but it was never capable of explaining what might be a warning sign for a trigeminal neuralgia or what the suffering accompanying a carcinoma might be protecting against. When pain was resistant to all categorization and treatment it lost its meaningful character, not only in the (obvious) sense that it could no longer be interpreted as the sign of a hidden lesion, but also to the extent that science did not have the necessary elements to visualize it.

This was also true as concerns cancer. Just as the illness multiplied into a plurality of varieties, medical discourse sought not only to identify the cause of the illness, but also to clarify its development and, in many cases, search for palliative treatments.[22] The same ailment was broken down into a multitude of names that, like epithelioma, blastoma, rodent ulcer, fibroma, or lymphosarcoma, coexisted with more primary classifications. In a very general sense, tumors seemed to be divided into benign and malignant, as well as painful and silent. This last distinction, although extraordinarily simple, had an enormous relevance given that while some tumors develop painlessly or with only a little discomfort, many others, even those of the same type, cause extreme and prolonged suffering.[23] The verification of long-term illnesses that could run their course without symptoms was merely the counterpart of the proliferation of (also long-term) symptoms to which no disease corresponded, or at least no "curable" disease.

Both the cases of lesions without symptoms and symptoms without illnesses demonstrate a triple process of concealment related to experimental perspective and clinical practice. The emergence of pain medicine inverted the historical process that had washed its hands of the patient's testimony, shown no interest in chronic internal pain and, most importantly, had also ignored the severe and incurable pain of entire population groups. The institutional materialization of chronic pain and its simultaneous medical, clinical, and cultural understanding depended upon the inversion of this triple process of concealment that limited the patient's testimony, paid no attention to terminal pain, and showed even less interest in resolving or palliating the suffering of marginalized groups and disenfranchised classes, including among them, no less, the class of terminally ill patients.

On the one hand, the physiology manuals published in the second half of the nineteenth century scarcely referred to visceral pain, that is, to any pain that did not easily fit in with laboratory practices and their attendant mechanical procedures of experimental objectivity and manipulation. Although this internal pain was much less exceptional than external pain, physiology preferred to concentrate on the study of the infrequent, while the everyday – those pains felt in an organ and that were the result of stimulating the central nervous system – took on overtones of exceptionality. On the other hand, the efforts to objectify illness had hijacked the patient's narrative qualities along with all his or her narrative resources. The testimony of the *sens intime*, scarcely verbalized and almost always dramatic, only became comprehensible through the logic of mental illness. Unlike today, a psychological dimension to physical suffering was not recognized, but rather those suffering from chronic pain frequently ended their days in oblivion or in the psychiatrist's notebook.[24] In 1919, James Mackenzie [1853–1925] distinguished two methods of understanding and treating illness: the laboratory approach, which sought to comprehend the signs of the disease by reproducing it experimentally, and the hospital medicine approach, which understood the symptom in relation to the patient's life.[25] For John Ryle [1889–1950], one of the exponents of the new social medicine, the physician should not *see* the disease in the patient's body, but rather *understand* each sick person in the context of their illness. His clinical approach did not depend on mechanical procedures, but rather on the education of the (doctor's) senses and the accumulation of (patients') testimonies. On the one hand, hospital medicine should rest upon meticulous examination, exhaustive interrogation, and detailed description of the experiments that nature spontaneously practiced on the human organism. On the other hand, the very resistance to a treatment that the patient experienced as hell ought to lead the physician to redefine his or her ends and goals.[26] The health care professionals' task consisted of curing when it was possible, and alleviating suffering when it was not. During the first years of the 1960s, Cicely Saunders's experience with hundreds of terminally ill patients led her to defend a similar vision of illness.[27] In her view, ignorance of the causes, along with the fact that the disease would inevitably lead to death, did not hinder the development of a program of palliative measures. On the contrary, to confront what Saunders called "total pain," medicine should begin by privileging the position of the patient and stop considering death as a failure that called for no intervention whatsoever. Her position marked the culmination of a stance already present in the hospital sphere: "Our inability to construct a perfect theory of pain cannot be an apology for ignorance of known methods of coping with it," Spender wrote in 1874.[28] René Leriche had also begun his *Surgery of Pain* by affirming that, although humanity had been subject to pain in all time periods, very few advances had been made in its treatment.[29] Twenty years later in 1957, Doctor K. D. Keele declared that pain had only recently begun to constitute a problem in and of itself.[30]

Last, but not least, the unequal distribution of harm across different sectors of the population also led large groups of people to become socially invisible and clinically forgotten. This latter form of concealment not only concerns the history of medicine, but reflects a much more wide-reaching phenomenon related to the cultural elaboration of chronic pain, which had a particular incidence in the bodies and ways of life of the most vulnerable sectors of the population.[31] Mid-nineteenth century working-class children in London, for example, appeared "pale, delicate, sick [...], many suffered from illnesses affecting their nutritive organs, curvature and distortion of the spinal column and deformity in their limbs."[32] Workers' bodies were also prematurely aged and stooped. At least starting in the second half of the nineteenth century, more and more testimonies appeared regarding the ways in which each profession seemed to bestow its workers' bodies with the signs of the mechanical and monotonous repetition of their working life. It was not only that each profession had a particular "physiology" – as some of the old authors of Romantic treatises had written and which certain modern chroniclers seemed willing to confirm – but also that the repeated movements of professional activity, combined with the use of chemical substances, deformed the worker's body to such a degree as to cause morphological lesions. Some of the anatomical casts kept in the Museum of Hygiene in Dresden compare the hand of an electrician, a mechanic, a milkman, and a housewife, with the ideal shape the hand would have had if the person had enjoyed a different life and, especially, a different working life. The result provides a disheartening portrait of the way in which time passed for these manual (an apropos name in this case) laborers. The wax models show the silent pain that devoured these bodies to such an extreme that they became an almost indistinguishable mass of defeated remains (see Figure 40).

Silenced in many other areas of medical and physiological research, chronic pain in industrial Europe fills many pages of political economy and journalism. Outside of medicine, the most incisive of all testimonies on the pariahs of the new urban centers was provided by Friedrich Engels in *The Condition of the Working Class in England*, first published in 1845.[33] His testimony was yet another naturalist literary description, in whose pages the physical and psychological despondency of the world's disinherited masses came together.

In Victorian society, the chronicler Henry Mayhew found a "painful unifor-mity" in the lives of the underprivileged classes. Whatever their profession, age, or the conditions of their existence, the accumulation of cases enabled the discovery of common features in the detailed description of underprivileged individuals' and groups' forms of survival that, on many occasions, narrate the conditions of their existence in the first person and in direct speech. This portrait of the landscape of everyday life resembles the strategies employed by painters of the quotidian. In his artwork of 1854, the Austrian F. G. Waldmüller, for example, depicted a woman lying on the floor near a cradle where her baby was sleeping. As in many other similar scenes, the observer enters into the inti-mate territory of a semi-conscious body that has no reason left but its hardship (see Figure 41).

The majority of people who have spent their lives gripped by pain find no place in the history of medicine. For the same reason, entire books and mono-graphs have been dedicated to many other human beings that today we would not consider sick.[34] Even though we could say, almost tautologically, that all dis-eases have been "constructed," what chronic illness owes to its social context is still more decisive. For just as the mere recurrence of symptoms does not deter-mine the presence of a clinical condition, the history of medicine has given us examples of diseases which we now consider non-existent, whose symptoms resemble some of our modern sicknesses. Think, for example, of neurasthenia, which will be discussed below. The symptoms of this debilitating condition, so in fashion in the second half of the nineteenth century, bear a marked resemblance to some symptoms of depression, stress, or more specifically, what we call today chronic fatigue syndrome.[35] The same could be said of hyste-ria, considered an epidemic by the psychiatrists of the mid-nineteenth century. Chronic pain forms no small part of many untreatable or incurable conditions. At the same time, it appears recurrently in long-term nervous illnesses, both if they have a bodily or a psychological origin. This historical evidence suggests that the absence or presence of the expression "chronic pain" does not, by itself, allow us to clarify the nature of the illness. The problem does not depend on the existence of a name – which did not come to be used extensively until the 1970s – but rather on the way in which the patient interprets his or her symptoms and the way in which these symptoms can be framed by a medical and social context that makes them culturally meaningful.[36] The distinction between acute pain and chronic pain, which serves as a basis for the historical explanation of the emergence of pain, or as David B. Morris called it "post-modern pain," is not a prerogative of the twentieth century, nor does it by itself explain the development of palliative medicine.[37] The limited use of the expression "chronic pain" does not allow us to understand the systematic con-cealment of groups of people whose living conditions we would today consider appalling. On the contrary, the "painful uniformity" that Mayhew spoke of, being an involuntary form of objectification of experience, obliges us to answer the question as to why, contrary to what Tolstoy wrote, unhappy families are also so alike.

The account

The social materialization of chronic pain not only depends on the presence of a name, but also on how human beings dialogue, *reiteratively*, with their physical pain.[38] Even when some sick people describe their symptoms with a laconic "I cannot tell you how I feel,"[39] the conceptualization of this silence does not inhibit understanding of their experience through more or less verbalized forms, which maintain a notable historical and geographical uniformity. Along with narrative coherence, which we saw in the previous chapter, what confers emotional credibility and value upon the patient's account is not the correspondence of a theoretical framework that always ends up being insufficient, much less the connection always questioned between lesion and pain, but rather the similarity to other narratives *about the same thing*. While the psycho-physical approach sought to understand the perception of pain through the correspondence between stimuli and responses, pain medicine above all pays attention to narratives' homogeneity. This means that, from the historical point of view, many documents traditionally considered irrelevant for the history of medicine, such as diaries or autobiographies, now take on a leading role. The history of pain, or at least the history of chronic pain, must be anchored in this collective dramatic consideration of homogeneous experiences. The verbalized form of the illness – narrativity, as it is known in medical anthropology – turns this condition into a much more intersubjective experience than acute pain ever was.[40] Let us look at a couple of examples.

Syphilis

Unlike Flaubert, who did not know whether he had gotten it from a Turk or a Christian, the French author Alphonse Daudet [1840–1897] suspected that he had contracted syphilis from a high-born concubine at the age of 17.[41] Although he initially considered the illness a mark of distinction, when it reached the neurodegenerative stage, then known as *tabes dorsalis*, the symptoms already included continuous and untreatable pain. Considered one of the chronic ailments par excellence, syphilis had a very variable duration, sometimes remaining with the patient as long as they lived.[42] This was not Daudet's case. Five years after the first symptoms appeared, Doctor Charcot could only recommend palliative remedies. Nothing and no one could help him regain his health. His story is similar to those of many of the incurably ill, a term used in the nineteenth century for life-threatening conditions like gout, rheumatism, scurvy, tuberculosis, or cancer.[43] Years before his death, Daudet began to write a sort of diary on the progress of his illness, a short text he wanted to call, in Provençal, *La Doulou – Pain.*

His story begins with a routine visit to the urologist: "I went to see Dr. Guyon in the rue Ville-Evêque. He examined me. He found my bladder was somewhat soft; the prostate a little sensitive. In a word: nothing. He found nothing. But this nothing was the beginning of everything."[44] Soon after, he began to notice a tingling sensation in his feet; a burning sensation; excessive sensitivity on the skin linked to loss of sleep. He also started to cough up blood. At the beginning he felt no pain, or at least not very intense pain. As with many other wealthy patients, he visited the best established thermal springs, the best spas, and the best hospitals; he was given the best bath and mud treatments.[45] His continued visits to different specialists reflect just how ineffective the remedies were. Daudet, who no longer wanted to be cured, but just to be able to live with his illness, found no solution. David Gruby – who was also doctor to Chopin, George Sand, and Alexandre Dumas – recommended an emetic diet with such devastating effects that Daudet said he would have preferred death. Brown-Sequard, professor of physiology and neuropathology at Harvard, prescribed injections of extract of bull's testicles, a remedy also used by Émile Zola as a sexual stimulant that, in Daudet's case, only managed to exaggerate his symptoms. The writer combated them with various drugs, especially bromide and morphine. In June 1891, six years before his death, he could reach up to six injections a day. By October of the same year, there was not a single place on his body that didn't bear the mark of the syringe. His tireless search for remedies led him to the so-called Sayre suspension, a technique that was also used for cases of rheumatism and scoliosis. It consisted of hanging the body from a metallic structure, sometimes only by the jaw.

Soon after almost being run down by a carriage on the Boulevard Saint-Michel, when his first suicidal thoughts had begun to flourish, he tried to take strychnine. Once Pain – thus, with a capital P – entered his life, the pharmaceutical remedies began to exhibit some of their most hideous side effects. The nausea caused by the morphine or the bromide was compounded by the tolerance his body demonstrated. To produce the same effect, the doses had to increase in quantity and frequency. On occasions he felt as though a dagger was being stabbed into the soles of his feet; on others, he described his sensation as that of having his fingers devoured by rats with razor-sharp teeth. The pain in his hip and the tendons of his neck was as intolerable as the torments of the medieval wheel. The pain, he wrote, made its way through all parts of his body: "it affects my vision, my feelings, my judgments. It is an infiltrator."[46] Like Illych, Daudet felt that "there are days, long days, when the only part of me alive is my pain."[47] The sensation reappears again at the end of the book: "To my cost I have learned the capacity of simply existing, since I stopped walking, since I stopped being visible."[48]

Phantom limbs

Daudet was 26 when an American newspaper published the simultaneously tragic and comic story of a quadruple amputee. The life of this creature, who claimed to resemble a larva more than a human being, has no shortage of aspects in common with the freak shows which made their appearance in the Victorian world's culture of spectacle.[49] All the misfortunes of this "useless torso," whom the war had punished with the successive loss of all his limbs, are reminiscent of the logic of the circus. The story of George Dedlow begins with his enlisting as a medical officer in an infantry regiment and ends with the imaginary re-composition of his body during a séance. When his legs, under the registration numbers 3486 and 3487 of the Navy Medical Museum, appeared in the room, George recognized them immediately: "Good gracious!" – he exclaimed – "They are my legs! My legs!" While they were present, the amputee had the feeling that he was again a whole person: "It is needless to add that I am not a happy fraction of a man, and that I am eager for the day when I shall rejoin the lost members of my corporeal family in another and a happier world," he wrote.[50]

The story – published anonymously in July 1866 and apparently without the permission of its author, the neurologist and surgeon Silas Weir Mitchell [1829–1914] – obtained a certain notoriety. Its most significant events were constructed upon its protagonist's progressive fragmentation, as well as through the accumulation of unfortunate places to which the tragedy led him. Each amputation corresponded to a new territory where the strangest things coexist with the most extraordinary beings.[51] Deprived of both arms and legs, the soldier survives in a liminal state that incapacitates him from carrying out both his most intimate functions and his most public actions. As if that weren't enough, while he remains dead (to the social world) and alive (to the indeterminate and anomic space of the military hospital), he must bear intense and lacerating pain in the limbs he no longer possesses. What he does have bothers him, but above all what hurts him, and a great deal, is that which he lacks. The story deliberately abounds in the rhetoric of the absurd. This is its only logic. When Dedlow awakes in the field hospital and asks an attendant to rub his calf, he replies: "Calf? You ain't none!" – "I know better," said George, "I have pain in both legs." – "Wall, I never! You ain't got nary legs" – replied the attendant.[52] This is not the only conversation he has with the inhabitants of the underworlds to which his condition, literally, drags him. When complaining in front of a preacher, the cleric rebukes and admonishes him thus: "Such and thus will the wicked be; such will you be if you die in your sins: you will go to where only pain can be felt. For all eternity, all of you will be just like that hand; knowing pain only."[53]

In 1864, already turned into a human remnant, he was sent to a hospital known as the Stump Hospital in Philadelphia, where he lived for three and a half months with other disabled servicemen. Some of his companions had lost an arm, others a leg. There were also those who had lost both arms or an arm and a leg, but not a single patient had all four limbs intact. In Dedlow's next residence, the United States Army Hospital for Injuries and Diseases of the Nervous System in Nashville, the uniformity of the wounded contrasted with the horrible variety of their suffering: one man walked sideways, one had lost his sense of smell, another had gone deaf following an explosion. One patient was given the nickname "Angel" due to the strange condition of the muscles of his back. There were also those who suffered from fits, which were sometimes very frequent. Doctor Neek, one of Dedlow's physicians, told him that on one occasion 150 patients had simultaneous fits that altogether lasted 36 hours. In this Dantesque universe, Dedlow lost the ability to eat and sleep. All his physiological functions diminished, as did his self-awareness: "I was less conscious of myself, of my own existence, than used to be the case," he wrote.[54] During his time in the hospital he also learned that most of the amputees still maintained sensation in their missing limbs for months and that, in some cases, these sensations were accompanied by pain. Before leaving Nashville, he himself began to suffer a similar pain in the little finger of his left hand. The suffering was so great that on some nights he tried to calm one hand with the other, although they were both missing.

The author of this story had been inspired by the experiences he lived through during the Civil War. Partly as an emotional response to a conflict in which more than 600,000 soldiers lost their lives – and also partly as a result of the introduction of spinning conical bullets – Mitchell had to face the material consequences of a national episode from which half a million men returned home mutilated. By the time he began to write his treatise on phantom limbs, causalgia, and ascendant neuritis, some 500,000 men had been injured; many of those who survived returned home in a terminal state.[55] The conflict's exceptional nature gave him, like many other doctors and surgeons, the chance to live alongside an enormous variety of lesions in peripheral nerves. Similar to the history of miracles and prodigies during the early modern period, the growing number of injured soldiers turned the infrequent into the quotidian, so that what one day seemed odd, soon ceased to be so and became commonplace in a short period of time.[56] The same accumulation of cases meant that each one would anticipate the next without any of them being any more than a small exception, an abnormal resistance to the knowledge of the (physiological) and the reconciliation of the (political) body.

His difficulties came from three different places. First of all, Mitchell had to look for clinical precedents to determine whether the phenomenon had been previously described. Secondly, the surgeon considered it absolutely necessary to find a palliative remedy, a treatment that could bring about a significant improvement in the patient's condition. Last, but not least, he had to evaluate the nature of the cases he observed, whether to consider them as examples of psychogenic disorders, organic lesions, or, even worse, a buried desire on the soldier's part to exaggerate his symptoms. This last problem was especially relevant given that the absence of diagnostic elements that could be considered *objective* often made it easier for the symptoms to be framed in the context of mental illness. Even Mitchell occasionally describes the injured in this way: "the soldier becomes a coward and the strongest man is scarcely less nervous than the most hysterical girl."[57] Some time before, Doctor Joinville had said that soldiers "cried out like women giving birth."[58] The patient became hysterical, "if we may use the only term which covers the facts."[59] In the case of causalgia, Mitchell knew well that patients grew progressively more irritable. The sound of a newspaper, a small breath of air, the vibrations produced by a music band or the thumping of feet when walking increased pain and triggered anxiety.[60] Although on occasions this neuralgic pain could be related to the presence of strange objects or to a lesion that could produce inflammation or sclerosis, in most observed cases the surgeon had to return to the metaphysical underworld of irritability or, what seemed then like a defeat, to treat the pain independently of its cause.[61]

At the beginning of the twentieth century, another military surgeon, William Livingston, also asserted that studies on the production, transmission, and reception of nervous signals had made patients' reason disappear to such an extent that their gestures and words could only be understood through the logic of mental illness. The absence of a correlation between the stimulus and the response laid the burden of proof on the sufferer, whose complaints seemed false or excessive in relation to any stimulus that might trigger them: "I knew that the patients sometimes exaggerated their complaints of pain but I assumed that when I had identified the cause of their pain I could tell from the nature of the organic lesion whether their pain complaints were real or due to psychological factors," he wrote.[62] This University of Oregon professor's interest in pain stemmed from his experiments with animal models and, above all, from his experience as a military doctor in the Second World War. As Head of the division on peripheral nerve injury at the Oakland Naval Hospital, he had learned that pain represented a subjective sensorial experience that could only be described by the human being who was living through it.[63] Attempts at objectification, including those that relied on the use of animal models, could account for the physiological sensation, but not for the psychological perception or the clinical symptoms. For the patient, the severity of the pain was much more meaningful than the expert opinions on what the patient *should feel*. Aware of the difficulties, Livingston proposed that pain should not be understood as a scientifically established entity, but rather as a flexible and dynamic concept that should include both psychological and sensorial elements.[64] The conclusion, later accepted by the International Association for the Study of Pain, was obvious: "nothing can be properly called 'pain' unless it can be consciously perceived as such."[65]

Although as late as 1941 some surgeons still defended the idea that the sensations described by amputees had a psychic origin and that consequently the symptoms were manifestations of obsessive neuroses, for Mitchell, the most convincing argument in favor of the reality of painful phantom limb syndrome did not depend on a new definition of pain, or even on a restructuring of medical practice.[66] What made it possible to keep the soldiers' narratives within the schema of clinical rationality, even in the most extraordinary of cases, was the notable similarity between them.[67] As in the stories of Daudet and George Dedlow, the initial condition for subjective discomfort to acquire clinical relevance depended on the ability to frame the patient's extensive suffering in such a way that individual experiences could be compared. For the illness to be established not only as a disease, but also as a socially accepted condition, a sickness and its chronic nature had to be removed from the sphere of private experience and framed within a collective experience capable of adapting to the same narrative structure of another set of illnesses. On its own, mere incurability determined nothing, for there had always existed chronic diseases that were either not medicalized or did not affect the patient's social consideration.[68] For the same reason, not all discomfort has historically corresponded to a meaningful clinical context.[69] Hypertension, for example, is incurable and chronic, but of course is not terminal and is to a certain degree treatable. By the same token, chronic illnesses can be symptomatic or asymptomatic, like, for example, diabetes. When they produce symptoms, pain may be among them, but it need not be the only or even the strongest characteristic. Alphonse Daudet's and George Dedlow's stories exemplify two different forms of facing pain in the second half of the nineteenth century. The first concerns suffering connected to an incurable disease. The second refers to pain that becomes an untreatable syndrome. In the first case, a condition whose cause is unknown will produce an inevitable result: death, along with untreatable pain. In the second, a multiple amputation will cause a pain of unknown cause, for which there is no adequate treatment. The novelist's (autobiographical) tale and the surgeon's (novelistic) story make clear to what degree the new medicine of pain requires the framing of experience, the expressive limitation of life's ebb and flow, as well as the valorizing of an extensive and uniform human group.

Medicalization

Silas Weir Mitchell, an expert in illnesses that we now consider real, such as neuralgia, became famous in his day for writing a book that recommended compulsive rest to treat another disease – neurasthenia – that today we deem imaginary.[70] The most important text published on the subject was the work of George M. Beard, a member of the New York neurological society, who considered that morbid anxiety, chronic fatigue, prolonged suffering and irrational fear formed part of the symptoms of the day. Among the causes of this chronic nervous exhaustion, Beard pointed out, were the social effects of civilization, such as punctuality, the development of the telegraph, train travel, the presence of new ideas, the increase in businesses, emotional repression, and, logically, the freedom that questioned the predictable cycles of socially stratified societies.[71] In her short story *The Yellow Wallpaper*, the American sociologist and writer Charlotte Perkins Gilman developed a harsh critique of therapeutic procedures that Mitchell had recommended to her when she was suffering from what we would today term post-partum depression, but what the neurologist took to be another case of the nervous fatigue epidemic which, according to Beard, gripped the nation.[72] Although Gilman's commentaries have been tied to the male construction of femininity and its attempts to constrain women's activities to the domestic sphere, her doctor did no more than apply what he considered to be the appropriate treatment for an illness, neurasthenia, which we today consider imaginary, despite its close resemblance not only to stress but also to chronic fatigue syndrome.[73] Mitchell, who like Beard contributed to the medicalization of nervous pain in distancing mutilated soldiers from the suspicion of mental illness, also encouraged the symptomatic treatment of some other elusive diseases that many people in his time (and for a long time afterwards) regarded in the light of psychiatry. On the one hand, he diagnosed specific relief methods for illnesses that today are considered to be real, though they were not at the time; on the other hand, he recommended palliative treatment for illnesses that today we deem to be non-existent, though they were somehow *real* in his time. Compared with the famous *Life and Work* in which the Scotsman Samuel Smiles posited that social advances depended upon sobriety and hard work, this American neurologist attempted to turn what until then had belonged to the realm of moral conduct into a problem of a clinical nature. As in the case of Durkheim on suicide, or Munk on euthanasia, the moral evaluation should not interfere with the clinical description. In all cases, the subjective elements of the observed behavior became integrated into cognitive systems that recognized them as comparable and homogeneous social facts.[74]

Although scientific medicine (based on experimentation) and hospital medicine (based on observation) maintained very different methodologies, both conceived of pain in terms of resistance. In the case of chronic pain, suffering showed a resistance that was at once physical and symbolic: physical because it did not correspond to the physiological expectations put forth by different theoretical models, and symbolic because it was built on the patient's isolated testimony. From this standpoint, the appearance of chronic pain sufferers is no less enigmatic than the conceptualization of their harmful syndromes. Those suffering from long-term illnesses open up a process of negotiation through which both the patients and their illnesses acquire social legitimacy and visibility. Only through this mutual redefinition may chronic experience, as the maximum expression of a collective failure, become *an* illness that requires *another* approach and *another* treatment. Depending on its referential framework, the course of life can be transformed into a condition likely to receive medical assistance. At the same time, only in the appropriate context can certain bodily sensations be perceived and expressed as a reality requiring a clinical response.

What distinguished chronic pain from acute pain was not so much its temporal dimension, but rather that this form of suffering did not match up with the standard definitions, didn't fit into taxonomies; it did not have an appropriate name, nor did it behave in accordance with physiological expectations or respond to symptomatic treatment. Its characteristics implied a rupture with the basic structure in which harmful experience had been understood and framed, mostly in relation to the study of cutaneous sensations. This explains why, both in the case of incurable illnesses and intractable harmful syndromes, the proliferation of varieties went hand in hand with a multiplication of treatments, partly as a result of the etiological ignorance of the disease and partly also as a merely empirical approach to the proliferation of symptoms. In 1857, Weldon Fell, of New York University, mentioned various proposed treatments for combating cancer, among them arsenic, jimson weed, hydrocyanic acid, certain animal substances such as cod-liver oil, belladonna poultices, mercury baths, carbonic acid, gastric juices, silver nitrate, zinc chloride, and of course, surgery.[75] For Spender, much more rigorously, therapeutic remedies were classified in accordance with their form of application: either through the digestive system, the respiratory tract, or subcutaneously, as in a hypodermic injection. His treatise combined treatment of acute pain with the symptomatic relief of chronic suffering. In 1908, the surgeon Skene Keith examined different therapeutic approaches from electricity to surgery or radiotherapy wherein "much harm was done at first and the sufferings of many patients were enormously increased by the formation of extensive burns."[76] In all cases, the description of the remedies was accompanied by clinical case histories, that is, observations supported by direct knowledge and the shared experience of the illness's development.

Although in 1965 the physicians Wall and Melzack proposed a new theoretical model which the history of medicine has considered as the culmination of a cognitive process centered on the progressive visibility of harmful syndromes, for sociologists of medicine, however, the most significant reference for the formation of the specialty of pain medicine was not Wall and Melzack's text, but rather the American anesthetist John J. Bonica's book *The Management of Pain*, published in 1953.[77] The book vindicated technical knowledge – the capacity to work almost artisanally with a theoretically elusive phenomenon. The expression "Pain Clinic," introduced by Bonica himself, called attention to the collective effort to transform private suffering into an issue of collective responsibility. A delimited medical practice and a new social cohesion were required to make pain, and especially chronic pain, a matter of public reflection and first aid. Between 1874, when John Kent Spender published *Therapeutic Means for the Relief of Pain*, and 1953, when Bonica's book was published, pain had been transformed into a set of entities susceptible to their own study and treatment. Whether dealing with conditions like causalgia, post-herpetic neuralgia, lumbar pain, or other kinds of chronic pain that, from a theoretical standpoint, languished in a plethora of contradictory hypotheses, many physicians and surgeons did not seek to obtain knowledge through pain, nor even to *cure it*, but to manage, treat, manipulate, and relieve it. Once the laboratory studies had shown themselves to be insufficient, many doctors and surgeons, in part inspired by the cooperative teachings of the Second World War, began to call for transversal actions that, overstepping the parceling out of knowledge, could make the patient's testimony prevail against physiological speculations. The majority of the new clinics, initially created to respond to the suffering associated with terminal cancer, soon began to treat other pains of a non-specific nature, like phantom limbs or facial neuralgias.

There is nothing strange about people coming together in order to separate things. The Latin maxim *divide et impera* (divide and conquer) was also applied to clinical specialties, whose assault on chronic pain had to be carried out in a coordinated manner. For William Livingston, for example, the supposed correlation between the sensorial stimulus and subjective perception, so often questioned by the facts, had to be replaced by a disciplinary cooperation, by the "simplification of medicine" that James Mackenzie spoke of. Writing on the anthropology of experience, the anthropologist Victor Turner observed how social drama requires that its protagonists be bestowed a social value, such that the exceptionality of their status always demands a collective reconciliation.[78] What was never applicable to the segments of the population described by Henry Mayhew did find its place in an itinerant population that already lived in accordance with exceptional parameters. From the time of the Roman emperor Marcus Aurelius, who wrote his *Meditations* with the corpses of the Roman legions still warm, to the military surgeons of the Second World War, the history of pain has always been linked to bloody confrontations and military hospitals. At the beginning of the nineteenth century, the English surgeon Charles Bell left for Belgium, taking with him his surgical instruments and drawing utensils as soon as he learned of the intensity and scope of the conflict. The result was a set of sketches on war wounds that, in the style of Goya, reflected a theatricalized recreation of the experience of dying and killing (see Figure 42). His story is not so very different from those of John Hunter, who had participated in the Seven Years' War, or of Baron Larrey, who did his learning in the military hospitals of the Napoleonic campaigns.[79] Mitchell knew well that the end of the Civil War entailed not only a reconciliation between adversaries, but also the formation of a collective memory starting with the pieces of those injured or disabled. As in the old story of Simonides, to remember it was necessary to count the fragments, put them back in their place of origin, in a word, rememorate them, or more literally, re-member them. Many veterans' resistance to all forms of effective treatment, and the clinical incapacity to free them from their sad condition without, at the same time, being able to classify them under the rubric of mental illness or collective hysteria, constituted an intolerable alteration within the exceptionality of war. Even though the great names related to the emergence of pain medicine were military surgeons or anesthetists (including John Bonica himself, an anesthetist at the Madigan Army Hospital, where the wounded from the Pacific Theater were taken), the relationship between the formation of a new type of pain – untreatable pain – and a new human group – the person ill with incurable chronic pain (represented by the military population, by the hundreds of soldiers injured on the battlefield) – remained uncharted territory. However, the grouping of symptoms related to pain was also connected to the equally essential process of creating a group of previously unclassifiable people. Like the monsters of the Renaissance, they belonged to the rather obscure kind of the un-kind. Chronic untreatable pain and the patient suffering from it became connected to one another in the public space of the military hospital. There, within the dramatic experience of war, the injured *constructed* their illness just as the reiteration of their symptoms allowed them to become patients.

The culture of pain

"A disease does not exist as a social phenomenon until we agree that it does," the historian of medicine Charles E. Rosenberg wrote in 1989.[80] In 1997, he considered that this existence was determined by the way in which the ailment was "named."[81] From the mid-nineteenth to the mid-twentieth century, what we now call chronic or degenerative diseases were often associated with incurability or other life circumstances that prevented the patient's experience from being considered *a disease*. In some cases, medicalization went as far as behaviors that we would not consider illnesses today, for example neurasthenia or homosexuality; in other cases, the same social compartmentalizing of supposedly pathological behavior was regarded as a success in medicine's progress and an effort to secularize the care of incurable and terminal patients. What allowed the emergence of a science of pain was not, however, the internal development of the sciences nor the (poorly named) civilizing process. The scientific and cultural colonization of harmful experience – the entrance of the clinical gaze into the sphere of subjectivity – neither obeyed nor can be explained through a teleological sequence which made the medicine of pain the logical conclusion of the entire suffering of humanity. Chronic pain was able to flourish as a clinical condition once the flow of life that Elliotson's patient described could be transformed into an experience capable of extension over days, weeks, or years. Its appearance as an object of science is not the end of a story, but rather the beginning of another; a story which permitted the materialization of a form of life that until then had been diluted and concealed, with no clinical meaning or cultural value. This is why the medicine of pain corresponds partly with the development of welfare practices related to other long-term illnesses whose appearance in the field of biomedicine is also considered recent.[82] Neither can its appearance be attributed to the culmination of a historical civilizing process; rather, it should be framed by the way in which our contemporary world has been able to transform continuous pain into an experience worthy of scientific research, clinical treatment, and, no less important, cultural meaning.

Although it would be tempting to explain pain's progressive centrality based on a partial and internal reading of the history of science, this experience's cultural materialization does not affect biomedical practices alone. While in 1923, the physiologist Johannes von Kries (mistakenly) insisted that somatization constituted a prior stage to the objectification of pain – and consequently to its study as well – the German philosopher Wilhelm Dilthey sought ways of approximating social research to what he called the sphere of pre-predicative experience; that is, experience prior to all expression and sensation.[83] Unlike Kant, who considered that objects had to be felt through sensitivity prior to being thought of through understanding, Dilthey considered that all experience included a moment of reflexivity; a demand for meaning preceded by a temporal delimiting of the flow of life. In other words, for something to be an experience, it should have a *before* and an *after*. The history of acute pain and cutaneous sensitivity always rested on this sad circumstance. Throughout this book, we have seen sufficient examples of this ritualized form of confronting physical pain, especially with regard to the theatricality of surgical suffering. Dramatization, whether by means of imitation, representation, correspondence, coherence, narrativity, or trust, depended on these ins and outs of experience. The story that Elliotson gives us, however, introduces an unknown dimension, at least inasmuch as there does not seem to be an after that is different from the now, nor a hope for the future distinct from the hell of the present. On the contrary, this space with no perspective dilates in time, into a diffuse boundary that can occupy days, weeks, or years. The area of transit that characterizes the rupture of community, identity, or language turns into a way of life; it is a strangely inhabited and yet inhospitable place.

There is nothing strange in that the emergence of pain medicine depended upon a particular materialization of the flow of life. After all, pain's cultural centrality does not only take place in the biomedical sphere. On the contrary, never before in the history of the West had physical or moral suffering been so visible in all aspects of public life, from the world of the arts, including cinema, to journalism or consumerism. In the twentieth century, suffering was always connected to a collective reflection on the uses and abuses of pain, as well as its visual, literary, or historical representations. From art criticism to anthropology, the New Humanities have turned physical and symbolic violence into an object of academic research, especially with respect to visual culture and the theory of the image.[84] Over the course of the twentieth century, so-called "analytic" philosophy also played its part. The works of Ludwig Wittgenstein, Richard Rorty, Charles S. Peirce, Daniel C. Denett, George Ryle, Hilary Putnam, P. Strawson, John Deway, Paul M. Churchland, John Searle, Saul Kripke, and Willard van Orman Quine were full of references to pain in the context of their investigations into solipsism, the contents of consciousness, private languages, referential opacity, and, in general, the philosophy of language and of the mind.[85] All their research made use of physical suffering to examine the characteristic traits of mental activity, such as consciousness, intentionality, subjectivity, or causation.[86] Pain mattered, but only as an example, as a proof or as evidence of demonstrative reasoning. Enveloped in ontological and epistemic disputes, some philosophers of the mind began to question how we could be sure that others understand our pain or, on the contrary, how we could know about the pain of others. Neither was it clear whether among these "others" to whom we were prepared to attribute meaningful mental states or behavioral patterns we should include superior mammals, nematodes, or computer programs.[87]

Under the wing of critical theory and its reflection on the great genocides of the twentieth century, so-called Continental Philosophy has also grown in relation to the cultural industry of historical memory.[88] Though impregnated with a certain theological aftertaste which prevented, for example, the representation of utopia, the political philosophy derived from the old Frankfurt School understood pain to be the inevitable consequence of reason's autonomy, which had thrown the pilot from the machine as it hurtled uncontrollably through the abyss: "The fact that in the concentration camps it was not an individual who died, but rather an exemplar of a species, also has to affect those who escaped from these measures," wrote the sociologist T. W. Adorno[89] (see Figure 43). Accustomed to thinking outside the scale, we post-moderns count our dead in millions, such that both in content and size, the cultural industry of pain has taken on almost pornographic undertones. The anthropology of memory constitutes yet another phenomenon in the proliferation of studies on the materialization of the emotions or performance practices linked to the rituals of mourning.[90] We can add to this avalanche the studies on visual culture exploring the multiplication of images of extreme violence, either in the arts or journalism (see Figure 44).[91] Finally, the improvement in living conditions, along with aging population pyramids, has a bearing on the reality that not only are we mortal, as we have known from time immemorial, but someday we will also all be ill. The distinction between the hopelessly ill, the chronically ill, the terminally ill, or the incurably ill concerns not only the new geriatric science, but also economics and demographics. Meanwhile, certain expressions like "quality of life," "trust," or "dignity" abound in the media and are extolled in research centers, especially in connection with the treatment of terminal cancer. In all the cases examined, pain's temporal dimension – its duration and not merely its intensity – constitutes one of the crucial aspects overarching among the new forms of objectified experiences or, to use Nietzsche's words, the cultural manifestations of our affects.

Postscriptum

In 1937, deployed by the Republic, a young Spanish sailor painted a self-portrait upon arrival at the military port of Cartagena. He dated it and wrote underneath: "When I arrived, after 37 hours of travel to cover 300 kilometers...the fires caused by the aerial bombardment kept burning. All my thoughts went out to you." During the duration of the Spanish Civil War, this port city in the southeast of Spain, where the Republic's supplies of military material arrived, was the scene of terrible bombings and armed conflicts. This first drawing, however, could not foresee either the development or unfolding of future events. It merely refers to a moment of separation and distancing, to the dramatic circumstances that came between this soldier and his wife and newborn daughter. A full-body portrait with the soldier standing, campaign bedroll in one hand, the drawing depicts a truncated life that is expressed and materialized in a simultaneously pictorial and narrative fashion. During the ensuing years, the same soldier again channeled his experience of the conflict into images. Through his set of illustrations run pain, sorrow, indignation, madness, hunger, love, misery, the absurdity of the military commands, unjustified violence, fear, death, the helplessness of the children that, like dogs, wandered through the streets of Cartagena. In May 1939 he made one of the last of the series. And he wrote again: "The day was breaking...The hours of waiting and of cold had numbed us. Anxious to arrive again, to find ourselves, to daydream. In a scrap of a sailor's blanket, wrapped up and sleeping in that rough dawn, lay the hope and fear of our existence" (see Figure 45). It was not, however, the last of the drawings. The next two depicted beggars and starving children watching the military victory parades of Franco's triumphant troops.

During the time that the Civil War lasted, life was reflected in images that, at the same time, also served to bestow meaning on the experience. Transit through this simultaneously real and imaginary space of the armed conflict, where already no one is nor will ever be again who they once were, made use of ritualized forms and cultural schemas. This young Spaniard's drawings share aesthetic features with Republican murals and propaganda posters. Sometimes, especially in the depiction of women, the lines recall the stylized bodies of Rafael de Penagos, then professor of Drawing in the Workers' Institute (*Instituto Obrero*) in Valencia. But the drawings' value does not depend so much on their artistic quality as on their will and determination to construct a narrative: to make a story that could at the same time serve as fuel for memory. The form of withstanding harm depends on this desire for interpretation that constitutes, in its way, an encoded language. Above the will to live rises the will to order the heterogeneous elements of experience such that the unconnected, the illogical, and the disproportionate acquire the meaningful characteristics of a narrative. Although they are not a military chronicle or a political history, these images rescued from oblivion offer up the experience in the form of its temporal delimitation and its collective meaning. In their way, they reflect the tension between the flow of life and the need to endow this very flow with order, stability, and coherence; they pursue the same thing as always: to bestow meaning upon experience.

The drawings, which remained hidden during the post-war period, were dusted off in the later years of softened Francoism. Around 1960, their author painted his portrait for the last time; alone again, although not now numb with cold, but daydreaming in the shadows of his living room. On this last image he wrote: "The years have passed, but sometimes, when the memories of those days rise up crushed together, we ask ourselves if we have become again the same ones as that yesterday." His work, which has never been published, has no commercial or political value, but it does represent an example of to what extent culture is, as Nietzsche said, the body's symptom, and how experience is materialized, as Dilthey suggests, in legal, literary, scientific, or artistic forms. The 40 or so images that make up the series share the narrative structure of the experience of harm that we have seen throughout the pages of this book. Here too the protagonists wander through imaginary places and impossible spaces. Rupture, separation, and reconciliation meet one another in this form of living and understanding the war. The experience of pain melds with danger or uncertainty. Through their rhetorical and argumentative resources, the pencil and the sanguine explore the public and the private, the body and the soul, one's own pain, the pain of others, physical anguish, and moral suffering.

Throughout the pages of this book, human beings have become present in the half-light. Whether they were virgin martyrs, soldiers in field hospitals, or anesthetized patients, we have seen them wander down the path of shadows and through intermediate spaces. For Don Quixote and the Spanish nuns, the experience of harm took place in a semi-public or semi-private space, in a strange place constructed in the cloisters of convents or on the paths of La Mancha. We ourselves, heirs to the modern culture of the impartial spectator, also inhabit borderlands. Our impartial judgment on world events depends on that middle distance that permits the logic of taste as well as political agreement. Accustomed to sleeping in strangers' beds, we also bear inscribed on our foreheads the indelible mark of liminality, or in a more roundabout fashion, the mark of mediocrity. Within the framework of the clinical practices that we examined in Chapters 4 and 5, there was a great deal of pain, but neither the semiotics of harm, worried by the universality of expressive signs, nor clinical medicine, interested in illness' inscriptions on the bodily geography, vindicated the patient's expression as anything more than an instrument of knowledge; that is, as a means to an end. On the contrary, the sick person always was, as the French historian Michel Foucault wrote so correctly, "between parentheses." This is why the history of pain has been confused on occasions with the history of the progressive liberalization of mechanical models of hospital care. From the perspective of rhetorical forms, however, the sciences and arts constitute nothing more than two different materializations of experience. Cultural history may pursue the emotions in diaries and autobiographies, but it cannot lose sight of the location of these narrative means within other argumentative topics. The correspondent from Berlin who fantasized about submission as a form of sexual arousal found nothing but suffering and misfortune. His public (and false) life was left on one side and his private (and true) existence on the other. He was trapped in the middle. The pain of many of the nervous and mental patients of the nineteenth century shows a similar paradox, although in this case not referring to narrative forms, but the rhetoric of conviction. The suffering of many soldiers wounded by bullets in peripheral nerves was, for a long time, *only mental* whereas that of many of the terminally ill was, until recently, curiously invisible. There resides part of the character of harmful experience that is at the same time paradoxical and resistant. The history of its clinical conceptualization, of its juridical formation, or its artistic materialization does not permit a progressive reading, but a sinuous history of broadening and narrowing of social awareness.

Because history is written for the living and not for the dead, only from the present can the history of pain vindicate as its own the indifferent gestures of the virgin martyrs, the laughter and the mockery that accompanied the misadventures of Spain's most modern character, Don Quixote, or the penitence that took place, in hiding, inside of convents. At the same time, because history is written from the present and not from the past, it is possible to investigate the cultural materializations of past experience, not as a form of valorizing or constructing a memory, but as an intellectual exercise, and also a moral and political one, that allows us to search in history for the crystallizations of the flow of life, whether as a scientific theory, a penal code, a work of art, or the notebook with which a sailor of the Spanish Republic tried to order his experience of pain and war.

Notes

Acknowledgements

1. This research has been carried out with the assistance of the projects MICINN FFI2010-20876: "Epistemología histórica: Historia de las emociones en los siglos XIX y XX," as well as HUM2007-63267: "Epistemología Histórica. Estilos de razonamiento científico y modelos culturales en el Mundo Moderno: El dolor y la Guerra."

Introduction

1. "That is why it is more fitting to judge the quality of a man when he is in doubt and danger, and to observe his manner in adversity, for then at last an honest cry is wrung from the bottom of his heart, the mask of iron is torn off, and the truth stands exposed." (Lucretius, *De rerum natura*, book III) Adapted from Lucretius, *On The Nature Of Things*, translated by Cyril Bailey. Oxford, The Clarendon Press, 1910, Book III.

2. See Peter Burke, "Is there a cultural history of emotions?" in Penelope Gouk and Helen Hills (eds), *Representing Emotions: New Connections in the Histories of Art, Music and Medicine*, London, Ashgate, 2005, p. 35 See also Wilhelm Dilthey, *The Formation of the Historical World in the Human Sciences*, in Rudolf A. Makkreel and Frithjof Rodi (eds), *Selected Works*, vol. III, Princeton and Oxford, Princeton University Press, 2002, p. 169: "History is not something separated from life or remote from the present."

3. See Joanna Bourke, *Fear: A Cultural History*. London, Virago, 2005; by the same author: "Fear and Anxiety: Writing about Emotion in Modern History," *Oxford Journals in the Humanities*, History Workshop Journal, 55, 1 (2003): 111–133. Peter Dinzelbacher, *Angst in Mittelalter. Teufels-, Todes- und Gotteserfahrung: Mentalittsgeschichte und Ikonographie*. München, Wien, Zürich, 1996, Schningh. Peter Gay, *Education of the Senses*, New York, Oxford University Press, 1984. By the same author: *The Tender Passion*, New York, Oxford University Press, 1986 and *The Cultivation of Hatred*, New York, W. W. Norton, 1993. Gail K. Paster, Katherine Rowe and Mary Floyd-Wilson, eds, *Reading the Early Modern Passions: Essays in the Cultural History of Emotion*, Philadelphia, University of Pennsylvania Press, 2004; William M. Reddy, *The navigation of feeling: A framework for the History of Emotions*, Cambridge, Cambridge University Press, 2001; Patricia M. Spacks, *Boredom: the Literary History of a State of Mind*, Chicago, University of Chicago Press, 1995; Carol Z. Stearns and Peter N. Stearns, *Anger: the Struggle for Emotional Control in America's History*, Chicago, University of Chicago Press, 1986. Peter N. Stearns, *Jealousy: The Evolution of an Emotion in American History*, New York, New York University Press, 1989. William James Bouwsma, "Anxiety and the Formation of Early Modern Culture," in William J. Bouwsma (ed.), *A Usable Past: Essays in European Cultural History*, Berkeley, Los Angeles, California, University of California Press, 1990, pp. 157–190.

4. Clifford Geertz, *The Interpretation of Cultures*, London, Basic books 1975, p. 81: "not only ideas, but emotions too, are cultural artefacts in man."
5. Lucien Febvre, "Sensibility and history: How to Reconstitute the Emotional Life of the Past," originally published in 1941, in Lucien Febvre, *A New Kind of History and Other Essays*, edited by Peter Burke, New York, 1973. For a historiographical review of the emotions since the 1940s, see Barbara H. Rosenwein, "Worrying about Emotions in History," *The American Historical Review*, 107 (2002): 821–845. In this article Rosenwein advocates for defending "emotional communities" or "affective systems," an idea she has subsequently developed in her *Emotional Communities in the Early Middle Ages*, Cornell University Press, 2006.
6. This new historiographical approach, which we could legitimately call *inner history*, does not want for precedents. On the contrary, it owes a great deal to the phenomenology of experience of Hegelian idealism, as well as to the vindication of the passions on the part of Nietzschean genealogy. The historian Thomas Dixon has outlined the creation of the emotions as a psychological category; his emblematic text drew from the psychology of William James. Thomas Dixon, *From Passions to Emotions. The Creation of a Secular Psychological Category*. Cambridge, Cambridge University Press, 2003.
7. For a conceptual overview of the history of this concept, see Martin Jay, *Songs of Experience. Modern American and European Variations on a Universal Theme*, Berkeley, Los Angeles, London, University of California Press, 2006. In Spanish, as in English, the word "experience" translates two German terms. The first, *Erlebnis*, which makes reference to life (Leben), is normally translated as "lived experience," while the second, *Erfahrung* – which etymologically refers as much to the journey (Fahrt) as to danger (Gefahrt), to the uncertainties Lucretius spoke about – is interpreted as the result of a process of integration and structuring. This last term is simply translated as "experience." The notion of experience used here comes from Dilthey's so-called Principle of Phenomenality. See Wilhelm Dilthey, *Introduction to the Human Sciences*, vol. II, Princeton, Princeton University Press, 2002, p. 245*ff*.
8. The best example of the first option is Rosalyne Rey, *Histoire de la douleur*, Paris, Éditions La Decouverte, 1993. The best example of the second approach is Thomas Dormandy, *The Worst of Evils: The Fight Against Pain*, New Haven, Yale University Press, 2006. Different aspects of the history of pain have been treated by E. Scarry, *The Body in Pain. The Making and Unmaking of the World*, New York, Oxford, Oxford University Press, 1985; David B. Morris, *The Culture of Pain*, Berkeley and Los Angeles, University of California Press, 1991; David Le Breton, *Anthropologie de la douleur*, París, Métailié, 1995.
9. Some, very uneven, examples would include: Hannes Etzsörfer, ed., *Blutige Geschichten. Ein kulturhistorischer Streifzug durch die Welt der Werbrechen*, Österreichische Nationalbibliothek, Exhibition Catalogue, 2009. David Niremberg, *Communities of Violence, Persecution of Minorities in the Middle Ages*, Princeton, Princeton University Press, 1996; Sean McGlynn, *By Sword and Fire. Cruelty and Atrocity in Medieval Warfare*, London, Cassell Military, 2008.
10. Dilthey, *Selected Works*, Vol. III. *The Formation of the Historical World*, p. 290. On the relevance of Dilthey for this research, as well as the works of Victor Turner, see C. Jason Throop, "Experience, Coherence, and Culture: The Significance of Dilthey's 'Descriptive Psychology' for the Anthropology of Consciousness," *Anthropology of Conciousness*, 13, 1 (2002): 2–26.

11. Edward M. Bruner, "Experience and Its Expressions," in Victor W. Turner and Edward M. Bruner (eds), *The Anthropology of Experience*, Urbana and Chicago, University of Chicago Press, 1986, p. 5. A similar stance in John Dewey, *Art as Experience* [1934].
12. See Reinhart Koselleck, "Transformation of Experience and Methodological Change: A Historical-Anthropological Essay", in Koselleck, *The Practice of Conceptual History. Timing History. Spacing Concepts*, Stanford, California. Stanford University Press, 2002, pp. 45*ff*. In this text, Koselleck also attempts to explore the relationship between "historical modes of experience and historical epistemology", p. 49.
13. Scarry, *The Body in Pain*, p. 4.
14. Ibid. p. 5.
15. Ibid. p. 16.
16. Ludwig Wittgenstein, *Philosophical Investigations*, § 384. English translation by E. G. M. Anscombe, Blackwell Publishing, 2009.
17. The definition was published for the first time in the journal *Pain*, 6, 3 (1979): 249–252. *An unpleasant sensory and emotional experience.* For a discussion of this definition, see David B. Morris, *Illness and Culture in the Postmodern Age*, Berkeley, Los Angeles, London, University of California Press, 1998, pp. 121*ff*.
18. Victor Turner, *From Ritual to Theatre. The Human Seriousness of Play*, New York, Paj Publications, 1982. Kenneth Burke, *The Philosophy of Literary Form*, [1941], Berkeley, Los Angeles, London, University of California Press, 1973.
19. Jody Enders, The Medieval *Theater of Cruelty. Rhetoric, Memory, Violence*, Ithaca and London, Cornell University Press, 1999. See also Anthony Kubiak, *Stages of Terror. Terrorism, Ideology and Coercion as Theatre History*, Bloomington and Indianapolis, Indiana University Press, 1991, p. 22: "The present work suggests a history of pain displayed as theatre before the subject of culture." For the concrete case of contemplating harm, see Jacques Rancière, *The Emancipated Spectator*, London, New York, Verso, 2009.
20. Émile Cioran, *Ese maldito yo*, Barcelona, Tusquets, 1988, p. 77.
21. Aristotle, *Rhetoric* 1355b.
22. Confronting the problem of suffering at a distance, the philosopher Luc Boltanski made reference to the topics (his term, following Aristotle) of denunciation and resignation as general forms of collective response in the face of the spectacle of violence. See Luc Boltanski, *Distant Suffering. Morality, Media and Politics*, Cambridge, Cambridge University Press, 1999, part II: "The Topics of Suffering."

1 Representations

1. On the original display of the altarpiece, see Museo de Bellas Artes de Asturias, *Colección Pedro Masaveu. Pinturas sobre tabla* (SS. XV–XVI). Oviedo, 1999, pp. 40*ff*.
2. Jacobus de Vorágine, *The Golden Legend*. Trans. Christopher Stace. London: Penguin, 1998, pp. 162*ff*.
3. See Jean-Jacques Courtine y Claudine Haroche, *Histoire du visage, xviiième-début xixième siècle*, Paris, Éditions Rivages, 1988.
4. Mark Zborowski, *People in Pain*, San Francisco, Jossey-Bass, 1969. A similar view is defended by John Campbell, "Illness is a Point of View: The Development of Children's Concepts of Illness," *Child Development*, 46 (1975): 92–100.
5. See Wulf Schiefenhövel, "Perception, Expression and Social Function of Pain," *Science in Context*, 8 (1995): 31–46.

6. Tom Lutz, *Crying: The Natural and Cultural History of Tears*, New York, Norton & Co., 1999. Vincent-Buffault, *The History of Tears: Sensibility and Sentimentality in France*, Basingstoke, Macmillan, 1991. On both universal and particular nature of facial expression caused by passions, see Paul Ekman, "Biological and Cultural Contribution to Body and Facial Movement," in John Blacking (ed.), *The Anthropology of the Body*, London, Academic Press, 1977. On representation of emotions and their place in history, see Penelope Gouk and Helen Hills (eds), *Representing Emotions. New Connections in the Histories of Art, Music and Medicine*, Aldershot, Ashgate, 2005.

7. Jérôme Baschet, "Les conceptions de l'enfer en France au XIV siècle: imaginaire et pouvoir," *Annales, économies, sociétés, civilisations*, January–February, 1 (1985): 185–207. On the general context of death, see Philippe Ariès, *The Hour of Our Death*, New York, Random House, 1981, pp. 114–116.

8. Lionello Puppi, *Lo Splendore dei Supplizi. Liturgia delle esecuzioni capitali e iconografia del martirio nell'arte europea dal XII al XIX secolo*, Milán, Berenice Art Books 1990, as well as Lionello Puppi, *Torment in Art. Pain, Violence and Martyrdom*, New York, Rizzoli, 1991. More generally, see: Samuel Y. Edgerton, *Pictures and Punishment: Art and Criminal Prosecution during the Florentine Renaissance*, Ithaca, Cornell University Press, 1985, especially Chapter 4: "Images of Public Execution." By the same author, his "When Even Artists Encouraged the Death Penalty," *Law and Literature*, 15 (2003): 235–265, as well as James Marrow, *Passion Iconography in Northern European Art*, Kortrijk, Van Gheminter Publishing, 1979.

9. See Andrew Cunningham and Ole Peter Grell, *The Four Horsemen of the Apocalypse. Religion, War, Famine and Death in Reformation Europe*, Cambridge, Cambridge University Press, 2000 and Jean Delumeau, *El miedo en Occidente* [1978], Madrid, Taurus, 2002, pp. 368*ff*.

10. Mitchael B. Merback, *The Thief, The Cross and the Wheel*, London, Reaktion Books, 1999, p. 125.

11. On this topic, see especially Richard. J. Evans, *Rituals of Retribution. Capital Punishment in Germany, 1600–1987*, Oxford, Oxford University Press, 1996, particularly Chapter I.

12. See Henry Kamen, *The Spanish Inquisition*, London, Wedenfeld and Nicolson, 1965, pp. 186–196.

13. On this last altarpiece, see Robert Mills, *Suspended Animation. Pain, Pleasure and Punishment in Medieval Culture*, London, Reaktion Books, 2005, Chapter IV: "Invincible Virgins."

14. Katherine J. Lewis, "'Lete me suffre': Reading the Torture of St Margaret of Antioch in Late Medieval England," in J. Wogan-Browne, R. Voaden, A. Diamond, A. M. Hutchison, C. M. Meale and L. Johnson (eds), *Medieval Women: Texts and Contexts in Late Medieval Britain. Essays for Felicity Riddy*, Turnhout, Brepols, 2000, pp. 69–82.

15. Robert Bartlett, *Trial by Fire and Water. The Medieval Judicial Ordeal*, Oxford, Clarendon Press, 1986, pp. 16*ff*.

16. For a complementary view, see Valentin Groebner, *Defaced. The Visual Culture of Violence in the Late Middle Ages*, New York, Zone Books, 2009.

17. Enrique Flórez, *España Sagrada. Theatro Geográfico-Histórico de la Iglesia de España*. Madrid, Pedro Marín, 1763, vol. XVII: *De la Santa Iglesia de Orense*), pp. 209–214. On Marina's life, see also Beato Iácoppo de Varazze, *Flos Santorum* [1520–1521], edition by Félix Juan Cabasés, Madrid, Universidad Pontífica de Comillas, 2007, pp. 311–312.

18. Victor Turner, *From Ritual to Theatre. The Human Seriousness of Play*, New York, PAJ Publications, 1982. Also by the same author, *The Ritual Process*, Chicago, Aldine Publishing Company, 1995. The expression comes from the anthropologist Arnold van Gennep, *Rituals of Passage*, London, Routledge and Kean Paul, 1977, p. 18.

19. On this topic, see Francis Barker, *The Culture of Violence. Essays on Tragedy and History*, Chicago, The University of Chicago Press, 1993.

20. Jody Enders, *The Medieval Theater of Cruelty. Rhetoric, Memory, Violence*, Ithaca, Cornell University Press, 1999, p. 63.

21. On presence and uses of blood see Caroline Walker Bynum, *Wonderful Blood. Theology and Practice in Late Medieval Northern Germany and Beyond*, Philadelphia, University of Pennsylvania Press, 2007.

22. Vorágine, *The Golden Legend*, p. 281. Peter Brown, *The Cult of the Saints. Its Rise and Functions in Latin Christianity*, Chicago, The University of Chicago Press, 1981, pp. 72*ff*.

23. Eckehard Simon, ed., *The Theatre of Medieval Europe. New Research in Early Drama*, Cambridge, Cambridge University Press, 1991.

24. Carmen Torroja Menéndez and María Rivas Palá, *Teatro en Toledo en el siglo* xv*: "Auto de la Pasión" de Alonso del Campo*, Madrid, RAE, 1977.

25. John Spalding Gatton, "'There Must Be Blood': Mutilation and Martyrdom on the Medieval Stage," in James Redmond (ed.), *Violence and Drama*, Cambridge, Cambridge University Press, 1991, pp. 79–92. See also, on the Spanish case, N. D. Shergold, *A History of Spanish Stage from Medieval Times until the End of the Seventeenth Century*, Oxford, Clarendon Press, pp. 63–64. On the French case, Louis Petit de Julleville, *Histoire du Théâtre en France. Les Mystères*, vol. I, Paris, 1880, Chapters 10 and 11.

26. Quoted by Peter Burke, *Popular Culture in Early Modern Europe*. New York: NYU Press, 1978, p. 219.

27. Tertullian, *De Spectaculis*, English translation by T. R. Glover and G. H. Rendall, Harvard, Loeb Classical Library, 1966, p. 271.

28. Emile Mâle, *L'Art religieux de la fin du Moyen Age en France*, Paris, A. Colin, 1938, p. 42. Émile Mâle, *The Gothic Image: Religious art in France of the thirteenth century*, 1961, pp. 176–201. For a critical take on relationships between painting and drama in the Early Modern World see Charlotte Stern, *The Medieval Theater in Castile*, New York, Binghamton, 1996.

29. The term was originally coined by Marc Bloch. See Jean-Claude Schmitt, "The Rationale of Gesture in the West: Third to Thirteenth Centuries," in Jan Bremmer and Herman Roodernburg (eds), *A Cultural History of Gesture*, Ithaca, Cornell University Press, 1991, pp. 59–71. On Jesuit iconography see Leif Holm Monssen, "Rex Gloriose Martyrum: A Contribution to Jesuit Iconography," *The Art Bulletin*, 63 (1981): 130–137.

30. F. Nietzsche, *On the Genealogy of Morality: A Polemic*. Translation and Notes by Maudemarie Clark and Alan Swensen. Indianapolis, Hackett Publishing, 1998, p. 37.

31. Ibid. 38.

32. Enders, *The Medieval Theater of Cruelty*, p. 2. Anthony Kubiak, *Stages of Terror. Terrorism, Ideology and Coercion as Theatre History*, Bloomington and Indianapolis, Indiana University Press, 1991.

33. Esther Cohen has also noted the difficulty of finding written sources on physical pain itself before Erasmus's or Montaigne's works. See Esther Cohen, "The Animated Pain of the Body," *The American Historical Review*, 105 (2000): 36–68, p. 36. See also,

from the same author *The Modulated Scream: Pain in Late Medieval Culture*, Chicago, University of Chicago Press, 2010.

34. See Ernst H. Gombrich, *The Story of Art*. London, Phaidon, 1950. See also Frances Yates, *The Art of Memory* [1966], London, Pimlico, 1994. For a review of the role of images in Renaissance Europe, see Joseph Leo Koerner, *The Reformation of the Image*, London, Reaktion Books, 2004. On the use of images, see Elisabeth Eisenstein, *The Printing Press as an Agent of Change*, Cambridge, Cambridge University Press, 1979. For the Spanish case, see Felipe Pereda, *Las imágenes de la discordia*, Madrid, Marcial Pons, 2008.

35. See Richard Verstegan, *Théâtre des cruautés des hérétiques de notre temps* [1587], in Frank Lestringant (ed.), Paris, Editions Chandeigne, 1995; Bartolomé de las Casas, *Narratio regionum Indicarum per Hispanos quosdam devestarum verisima*, Frankfurt, Theodor de Bry, 1598, as well as Jacques Tortorel and Jean Perrisin, *Histoire diverses qui sont memorables touchant les guerres, massacres et troubles advenus en France en ces derniers annes*, Lyon, 1570.

36. Richard Verstegan, *The Post of the World*, London, Thomas East, 1576. On the veracity attributed to travellers see Juan Pimentel, *Testigos del Mundo*, Madrid, Marcial Pons, 2003. On Verstegan, see Paul Arblaster, *Antwerp and the World: Richard Verstegan and the International Culture of Catholic Reformation*, Leuven, Leuven University Press, 2004.

37. Verstegan, *Théâtre*, pp. 49–50.

38. Quoted by Giuseppe Scavizzi, *The Controversy on Images from Calvin to Baronius*, New York, Peter Lang, 1992, p. 228.

39. See Philip Benedict, "Of Marmites and Martyrs: Images and Polemics in the Wars of Religion," in various authors, *The French Renaissance in Prints from the Bibliothéque Nationale de France*, Los Angeles, Grunwald Center for the Graphic Arts, University of California, 1994, pp. 109–137.

40. Jean Ehrmann, "Massacre and Persecution Pictures in Sixteenth Century France," *Journal of the Warburg and Courtauld Institutes*, 8 (1945): 195–199; p. 195. For similar cases see Alexandra Herz, "Vasari's 'Massacre' Series in the Saga Regia: The Political, Juristic and Religious Background," *Zeitschrift für Kunstgeschichte*, 49 (1986): 41–45; or Todd P. Olson, "Pitiful Relics: Caravaggio's 'Martyrdom of St. Matthew,'" *Representations*, 77 (2002): 107–142.

41. Gauvin Alexander Bailey, *Between Renaissance and Baroque: Jesuit Art in Rome, 1565*, Toronto, University of Toronto Press, 2003.The classic study on this tradition is Émile Mâle, *L'Art religieux après le Concile de Trente*, Paris, Armand Colin, 1932, pp. 109–149 See Monssen, "Rex Gloriose Martyrum: A Contribution to Jesuit Iconography," in *Art Bulletin*, 63 (1981): 130–137 y Thomas Buser, "Jerome Nadal and Early Jesuit Art in Roman," *Art Bulletin*, 47 (1976): 424–433.

42. Antonio Gallonio, *De sanctorum martyrum cruciatibus liber*, Colonia, J. Gymnicus, 1602. On Gallonio see Jetze Touber, "Articulating Pain. Martyrology, Torture and Execution in the Works of Antonio Gallonio (1556–1605)," in *Jan Frans Van Dijkhuizen* (Author, Editor), Karl A. E. Enenkel (ed.), *The Sense of Suffering: Constructions of Physical Pain in Early Modern Culture*, Leiden, Boston, Brill, Intersections; Tearbiij for Early Modern Studies, 2009, pp. 59–90. There is a modern English translation: Rev. Antonio Gallonio, *Tortures and Torments of the Christian Martyrs*, Los Angeles, Feral House, 2004.

43. Verstegan, *Théâtre*, p. 50.

44. Pedro de Bivero, *Sacrum Sanctuarium crucis et patientiae crucifixorum et cruciferorum, emblematicis imaginibus laboratium et agrotantium ornatum: artifices gloriosi novae artis bene vivendi et moriendi,* Antwerp, Officina Plantiniana Balthasaris Moreti, 1634.

45. Jean Crespin, *Histoire des martyrs persecutez et mis à mort pour la vérité de l'Évangile,* Geneva, les héritiers d'Eustache Vignon, 1597.

46. On pain in the Middle Ages, see Françoise Desportes, *Le pain au Moyen Âge,* Paris, Olivier Orban, 1987. On the nineteenth century, see Laurence Guignard, "Les supplices publics au XIXième siècle," in Michel Porret (ed.), *Le corps violenté: du geste à la parole.* Geneva, Droz, 1998, pp. 157–184. Mark Grossman, *Encyclopedia of Capital Punishment,* Santa Barbara, California, ABC-Clio, 1998.

47. Natalie Zemon-Davis, "The Rites of Violence: Religious Riot in Sixteenth-Century France," *Past and Present,* 59 (1973): 51–91.

48. Jacques le Goff, *The Birth of Purgatory,* translation by Arthur Goldhammer, Chicago, Chicago University Press, 1984.

49. On discussions regarding the value and degree of suffering and pain in hell during the early modern period, see Daniel Pickering Walker, *The Decline of Hell. Seventeenth Century Discussions of Eternal Torments,* London, Routledge & Kegan Paul, 1964.

50. See Andrée Hayum, *The Isenheim Altarpiece: God's Medicine and the Painter's Vision,* Princeton, Princeton University Press, 1989, as well as Ruth Mellinkoff, *The Devil at Isenheim: Reflections of Popular Belief in Grünewald's piece,* Berkeley, University of California Press, 1988. On ergotism and Grünewald, see J. García de Yebenes and P. García de Yebenes, "La distonía en la pintura de Matias Grünewald: el ergotismo epidémico en la baja edad media," *Archivos de Neurobiología,* 54, 2 (1991): 37–40. See Isabel Morán Suárez's excellent article: "El fuego de san Antonio: Estudio del ergotismo en la pintura del Bosco," *Asclepio,* 47, 2 (1996): 173–193. On Grünewald's case, see Günter Engel, "Das Antoniusfeuer in der Kunst des Mittelalters: die Antoniter und ihr ganzheitlicher Therapiensatz," *Antoniter Forum,* Heft 7, (1999): 7–35. On hospitals in the medieval world and in the Renaissance, see Vivian Nutton, "Medicine in Late Antiquity and the Early Middle Ages," in Conrad, Neve, Nutton, Porter and Wear (eds), *The Western Medical Tradition, 800 BC to AD 1800,* Cambridge, Cambridge University Press, 1995. As well as John Henderson, *The Renaissance Hospital: Healing the Body and Healing the Soul,* New Haven/London, Yale University Press, 2006. Emmie Donadio, "Painting for Patients: Grünewald's Isenheim Altarpiece," *Medical Heritage,* I, 1 (1985): 448–454. The most detailed study of the relationship between Grünewald's altarpiece and sacred fire was undertaken by Andrée Hayum, "The meaning and function of the Isenheim Altarpiece: The Hospital Context Revisited," *Art Bulletin,* 59, 507 (1977), 27. Mitchell B. Merback has shown the symbolic nature of Christ's tranquility in his torment in opposition to the figures of thieves that accompanied him in many medieval and early modern representations. Merback, *The Thief,* 1999.

51. See Judith Perkins, *The Suffering Self. Pain and Narrative Representation in the Early Christian Era,* London, Routledge, 1995. The quotes appropriated from the *Phaedon* are found in 80b–81c.

52. Vorágine, *The Golden Legend,* p. 45.

53. Matthew, 26: 39.

54. The reality and unreality of the altar has been observed by Gottfried Richter in a small book entitled *The Isenheim Altar. Suffering and Salvation in the Art of Grünewald.* Edinburgh, Floris Books, 1997.

55. On monsters in the Modern World, see Jean Céard, *La Nature et les prodiges. L'insolite au XVI siècle en France*, Geneva, Libraire Droz, 1977; see also Katharine Park and Lorraine Daston, *Wonders and the Order of Nature*, New York, Zone Books, 1998.

56. John, 3: 30.

57. Matthew, 4: 25–4. See also Leviticus. 6: 20–26. Isaiah, 61: 1–3.

58. On the relationship between art and anatomy, see Deanna Petherbridge, Claude Ritschard and Andrea Carlino, *Corps à vif. Art et anatomie*, Geneva, Musée d'art et d'histoire, 1998.

59. The canvases are on display in the Museo Nacional del Prado in Madrid. Painted by Botticelli circa 1483 for the illustrious Florentine Pucci family, the set illustrates one of Boccaccio's *Decameron* tales; the eighth story of the fifth day, entitled "The Hell of Cruel Lovers."

60. See Jonathan Sawday, "The fate of Marsyas: Dissecting the Rennaisance Body," in Lucy Gent and Nigel Llewellyn (eds), *Renaissance Bodies. The Human Figure in English Culture, c. 1540–1660*, London, Reaktion Books, 1990, pp. 111–135. For a criticism of Sawday's view, see Katharine Park, "The Life of the Corpse: Division and Dissection in Late Medieval Europe," *Journal of the History of Medicine and Allied Sciences*, 50, (1995): 111–132.

61. Ovid, *Metamorphoses*, book vi, pp. 383ff. Edith Wyss, *The Myth of Apollo and Marsyas in the Art of the Italian Renaissance. An Inquiry into the Meaning of Images*, London, University of Delaware Press, 1996. Wyss explains and reproduces more than a hundred images produced on this matter during the Renaissance.

62. See Katharine Park, "The Criminal and the Saintly Body: Autopsy and Dissection in Renaissance Italy," *Renaissance Quarterly* 47 (1994): 1–33, and Roger French, *Dissection and Vivisection in the European Renaissance*, Aldershot, Ashgate, 1999, pp. 41–54.

2 Imitation

1. Michel Foucault, *The Order of Things: An Archaeology of the Human Sciences* [1966], New York, Routledge, 1989, Chapter 3.

2. Ian Watt, *The Rise of the Novel* [1957], Berkeley and Los Angeles, University of California Press, 1984.

3. See Anne Vincent-Buffault, *The History of Tears. Sensibility and Sentimentality in France* [1986], English translation by Teresa Bridgeman, London, The Macmillan Press, 1991.

4. Quoted by David B. Morris, *The Culture of Pain*, Berkeley and Los Angeles, University of California Press, 1991, p. 90.

5. All quotations come from Edith Grossman's translation of *Don Quixote*, New York, Harper Collins, 2003, p. 706.

6. Grossman, *Quixote*, p. 190.

7. Ibid. p. 266.

8. Regarding possible classifications of pain, see Javier Moscoso, "Historia del dolor," *Claves de razón práctica*, 139 (2004): 34–40.

9. On the relationship between Don Quixote and melancholy, see Roger Bartra, *Cultura y melancolía. Las enfermedades del alma en la España del Siglo de Oro*, Barcelona, Anagrama, 2001. English version, *Melancholy and Culture: Diseases of the Soul in Golden Age Spain*, Cardiff, University of Wales Press, 2008.

10. Mikhail Bakhtin, *Rabelais and His World* [1965], Bloomington, Indiana University Press, 1984, pp. 22*ff.*
11. Bartra, Cultura *y melancolía*, 2001.
12. Grossman, *Quixote*, p. 520.
13. Ibid. p. 937.
14. Ibid. p. 196.
15. Ibid. p. 380.
16. Ibid. p. 147.
17. Ibid. p. 156.
18. Ibid. p. 114.
19. Ibid. p. 673.
20. Ibid. p. 89.
21. Ibid. p. 40.
22. Ibid. p. 63.
23. Ibid. p. 104.
24. Ibid. p. 118.
25. Ibid. p. 114.
26. Ibid. p. 130.
27. Ibid. p. 130.
28. Ibid. p. 383.
29. Ibid. p. 842.
30. Ibid. p. 765.
31. Ibid. p. 519.
32. Ibid. p. 476.
33. Morris, *The Culture of Pain*, p. 97.
34. Grossman, *Quixote*, Part 1 book 9.
35. Ibid. p. 119.
36. Esther Cohen, "Towards a History of Physical Sensibility: Pain in the Later Middle Ages" *Science in Context*, 8 (1995): 47–74, p. 53.
37. Grossman, *Quixote*, p. 89.
38. Ibid. 107.
39. Ibid. p. 108.
40. Ibid. p. 117.
41. Ibid. p. 671.
42. Ibid. p. 836.
43. Ibid. p. 832.
44. Ibid. p. 702.
45. Ibid. p. 397.
46. Ibid. p. 422.
47. Bartra, *Cultura y melancolía*, p. 180.
48. Bakhtin, *Rabelais*, p. 124.
49. Erving Goffman, *The Presentation of Self in Everyday Life*, University of Edinburgh Social Sciences Research Centre, 1956, revised and expanded edition, Anchor Books, 1959.
50. Grossman, *Quixote*, p. 899.
51. Jean Louis de Lolme and Jacques Boileau, *The History of the Flagellants, or the Advantages of Discipline; being a Paraphrase and Commentary on the Historia Flagellantium of the Abbé Boileau, Doctor of the Sorbonne … By somebody who is not Doctor of the Sorbonne (i.e. Jean Louis de Lolme)*, London, Fielding & Walker, 1777, p. 242: *In almost*

every place [in Spain] *there is constantly some good friar, who makes his posteriors answerable for the sins of the whole Parish; and who, according as he has been fee'd for that purpuse, flogs himself, or at least tells his customers he has done so.*

52. Grossman, *Quixote*, p. 922.

53. See Judith Perkins, *The Suffering Self: Pain and Narratives Representation in the Early Christian Era*, New York, Routledge, 1995.

54. Grossman, *Quixote*, Chapter xxv.

55. On these matters, see Erwin Goffman, "On Face-Work. An Analysis of Ritual Elements in Social Interaction," in E. Goffman, *Interaction Ritual. Essays on Face-to-Face Behaviour*, New York, Pantheon Books, 1967, pp. 5–45.

56. A similar argument is found in Roger Bartra's "Doce historias de melancolía en la Nueva España," *Frenia*, vol. IV, fascículo 1 (2004): 31–52.

57. Joseph Vela del Sagrado Orden, *Idea de la Perfecta Religiosa en la vida de la Ven. Madre sor Josepha María García, capuchina de la villa de Castellón de la Plana en el Reyno de Valencia*, Valencia, Imprenta de la Viuda de Antonio Bordazar, 1750, p. 150.

58. Cohen, "Pain in the Later Middle Ages," p. 52. Cohen made a correct distinction between *impassivity* and *impassibility*. In the latter case, it is not a question of supporting pain impassibly, but being able to transcend it entirely, to the point of freeing oneself from the sensations themselves.

59. *Vita di S. Giuseppe di Copertino*, Florence, 1768, pp. 20–21. Quoted by Piero Camporesi, *The Incorruptible Flesh: Bodily Mutation and Mortification in Religion and Folklore*, English translation by Tania Croft-Murray, Cambridge and New York, Cambridge University Press, 1983, p. 56.

60. Padre Longazo degli Oddi, *Vita del B. Francesco di Girolamo sacerdote professo della Compagnia di Gésu*, Roma, 1761.

61. Richard Kieckhefer, *Unquiet Souls: Fourteenth-Century Saints and their Religious Milieu*, Chicago and London, University of Chicago Press, 1984, p. 26.

62. Quoted by Morris, *The Culture of Pain*, p. 132.

63. Padre Longaro degli Oddi, *Vita del B. Francesco di Girolamo sacerdote professo della Compagnia di Gésu*, Roma, 1806, p. 68. Quoted by Camporesi, *The Incorruptible Flesh*, p. 61.

64. Cfr. Pierre Groult, *Anthologie de la littérature spirituelle au XVIe siècle*, Paris, Klincksieck, 1959. William A. Christian, Jr, *Local Religion in Sixteenth-Century Spain*, Princeton, Princeton University Press, 1981.

65. Ignatius of Loyola, *Spiritual Exercises*, Rome, Antonio Bladio, 1548. On Ignatius of Loyola, see Terence O'Reilly, From Ignatius Loyola to John of the Cross: *Sprituality and Literature in Sixteenth-Century Spain*, Aldershot, Variorum, 1995. See also the classic and very antiquated study by E. Allison Peers, *Spanish Mysticism: A Preliminary Survey*, London, Methuen and Co. Ltd, 1924, p. 11.

66. Joseph Vela, *Idea de la Perfecta Religiosa*, p. 15.

67. Ibid. p. 306.

68. Carolyne Walker Bynum, *Holy Feast and Holy Fast: The Religious Significance of Food to Medieval Women*, Berkeley, University of California Press, 1987. See also Judith Perkins, *The Suffering Self*.

69. Joseph Vela, *Idea de la Perfecta Religiosa*, p. 26.

70. Miguel González Vaquero, *La mujer fuerte. Por otro título, la vida de doña María Vela, monja de san Bernardo en el convento de santa Ana de Ávila*, Madrid, Imprenta Real, 1674, p. 10.

71. Ibid.

72. Jacques Gélis, "El cuerpo, la Iglesia y lo sagrado," in A. Corbin, J. J. Courtine and G. Vigarello (eds), *Historia del cuerpo*, vol. I, Madrid, Taurus, 2005: pp. 27–112, p. 70.

73. Lisa Silverman, *Tortured Subjects. Pain, Truth, and the Body in Early Modern France*, Chicago and London, The University of Chicago Press, 2001, Chapter IV. On confraternities, see John Henderson, "The Flagellant Movement and Flagellant Confraternities in Central Italy, 1260–1400," in Derek Baker (ed.), *Religious Motivation: Biographical and Sociological Problems for the Church Historian*, Oxford, Basil Blackwell, 1978. For a study on confraternities in Florence, see John Henderson, *Piety and Charity in Late Medieval Florence*, Oxford, Clarendon Press, 1994.

74. Vicenzo Puccini, *The Life of the Holly and Venerable Mother suor Maria Maddlanea de Patsi* [1619], Scholar Press, 1970, p. 9.

75. Joseph Vela, *Idea de la Perfecta Religiosa*, p. 26.

76. *Cf*. Esther Cohen, "The Animated Pain Body," *The American Historical Review*, 105 (2000): 36–68.

77. See Pierro Camporesi, *The Incorruptible Flesh*. See also Katharine Park, *Secrets of Women. Gender, Generation, and the Origins of Human Dissection*, New York, Zone Books, 2006.

78. All references are taken from Camporesi. In this case, cited on page 4.

79. Battista Piergili's words, who wrote "*Vita Della B. Chiara della Croce da Montefalco dell'ordine di S. Agostino*" [1640], Foligno, 1663.

80. Niklaus Largier, *In Praise of the Whip: A Cultural History of Arousal*, New York, Zone Books, 2007, pp. 52*ff*.

81. See also Isabelle Poutrin, *Le Voile et la Plume. Autobiographie et sainteté féminine dans l'Espagne moderne*, Madrid, Casa de Velázquez, 1996.

82. *Mariana de Jesús, Autobiographía Resumida en Beata Mariana de Jesús, Mercedaria Madrileña*, Elías Gómez Domínguez, Rome, Instituto Histórico de la Orden de la Merced, 1991; José Esteban Noriega, *La Pecadora arrepentida. Vida y Conversión de la venerable María del Santísimo Sacramento, llamada La Quintana* [1737], summarized edition in *Confesión y trayectoria femenina: vida de la venerable Quintana*, por María Helena Sánchez Ortega, Madrid, CSIC, 1996.

83. Marcos Torres, *Noticias de la vida y virtudes de doña María de Pol*, Málaga, 1660; María Vela y Cueto, *Autobiografía y Libro de las Mercedes*, edited by Olegario González Hernández, Barcelona, Juan Flors, 1961.

84. Matthew, 25: 4–5 and Luke 6: 21. See *El evangelio de Mateo*, annotated reading by J. Mateos and F. Camacho, Madrid, Ediciones Cristiandad, p. 51; and *El evangelio según san Lucas*, edited by François Bovon, Salamanca, Sígueme, vol. I, p. 418.

85. On the Augustinian Isabel de Jesús, see, Jodi Bilinkoff, *Related Lives: Confessors and their Female Penitents, 1450–1750*, Ithaca, Cornell University Press; Bristol, University Presses Marketing, 2005, pp. 54–58.

86. Isabel de Jesús, *Tesoro del Carmelo escondido, Vida de la venerable madre Isabel de Jesús*; Madrid, Ivlian de Paredes, Imp. de Libros, 1685.

87. Quoted by Sherry M. Velasco, *Demons, Nausea and Resistance in the autobiography of Isabel de Jesús: 1611–1682*, Albuquerque, University of New Mexico Press, 1996, p. 4.

88. Joseph Vela, *Idea de la Perfecta Religiosa*, p. 16.

89. Patrick Vandermeersch, *Carne de la pasión. Flagelantes y disciplinantes. Contexto histórico-psicológico*, Madrid, Trotta, 2004. This history of flagellation takes the *Cofradía de la Vera Cruz*, in La Rioja, as its starting point.

90. On biographies written by women during the seventeenth century, regarding to pain and suffering gender, see Jacques Le Brun, "L'institutition et le corps, lieux de la mémoire, d'après les biographies spirituelles féminines du XVIIe siècle," *Corps écrit*, 11, *La mémoire*, Paris, 1984: 111–121. See also by the same author "Mutations de la notion de martyre au xviie siècle d'apres les biographies féminines," in Jacques Marx (dir), *Sainteté et martyre dans les religions du livre*, Bruselas, Université Libre, 1991, pp. 77–90. By the same author: "Cancer serpit. Recherches sur la représentation du cancer dans les biographies spirituelles féminines du XVIIe siècle," *Sciences sociales et santé*, June, 1984: 9–31.

91. Margaret Ann Ress, *Doña María Vela y Cueto. Cistercian Mystic of Spain's Golden Age*, in *Spanish Studies*, 27 (2004). See also, *The Spiritual Diaries of doña María Vela y Cueto*, edition and introduction by Margaret A. Ress, Lewiston, Lampeter, Edwin Mellen Press, 2007.

92. Vaquero, *La mujer fuerte*, pp. 18–i.

93. Ibid. p. 45.

94. Ibid. p. 57.

95. The expression comes from Joseph Vela, *Idea de la Perfecta Religiosa*, p. 16: "para quebrantar totalmente su amor propio" ("to completely break her self-esteem").

96. Vaquero, *La mujer fuerte*, p. 6. In this edition only the even pages are numbered. The pages are divided into two columns.

97. Joseph Vela, *Idea de la Perfecta Religiosa*, p. 301.

98. Corinthians 9 v. 27.

99. Joanna Bourke, *An Intimate History of Killing. Face-to-Face Killing in Twentieth Century Warfare*, London, Basic Books, 2000.

100. On the history of mimesis in the world of the arts see Wladyslaw Tatarkiewicz, *Historia de seis ideas*, Barcelona, Tecnos, 1976, Chapter 9.

101. Plato, *Republic,* Book X. This is not, by the way, Aristotle's position, in *Poetics* 1448^a. The body becomes the material on which mimetic representation is inscribed.

102. René Girard, *To Double Business Bound: Essays in Literature, Mimesis and Anthropology*, Baltimore, Johns Hopkins University Press, 1978.

3   Sympathy

1. Adam Smith, *The Theory of Moral Sentiments*, edited by D. D. Raphael and A. L. Macfie, Indianapolis, Liberty Fund, 1984, p.13.

2. David Hume, *A Treatise of Human Nature* [1739–1740], Oxford, Clarendon Press, 1978, pp. 385–386. Edmund Burke, *A Philosophical Enquiry into the Origin of our Ideas of the Sublime and Beautiful* [1757], London, Penguin, 1998, p. 91.

3. Smith, *Theory of Moral Sentiments*, p. 9. See also Norman S. Fiering, "Irresistible compassion: An aspect of eighteenth century sympathy and humanitarianism," *Journal of the History of Ideas*, 37 (1976): 200–202.

4. Smith, *Theory of Moral Sentiments*, p. 9. For a biological anchoring of sympathy, see Jean Decety and Philip L. Jackson, "The Functional Architecture of Human Empathy," *Behavioral and Cognitive Neuroscience Reviews*, 3 (2004): 71–100. The universality of empathetic emotions has been also defended through image theory. David Freedberg and Vittorio Gallese, "Motion, Emotion and Empathy in Aesthetic Experience," *Trends in Cognitive Science*, 11, 5 (2007): 197–203, see also Freedberg's classic book, *The Power of Images: Studies in the History and Theory of*

Response, Chicago, Chicago University Press, 1989. On the development of humanitarianism and its connections with lubricity, see Karen Halttunen, "Humanitarism and the Pornography of Pain in Anglo-American Culture," *The American Historical Review*, 100, 2 (1995): 303–334. On the development of humanitarianism in relation to capitalism, Thomas L. Haskell, "Capitalism and the Origins of the Humanitarian Sensibility, part 1," *The American Historical Review*, 90, 2 (1985): 339–361.

5. Malebranche, *La recherche de la vérité* had five French editions between 1721 and 1772 and was one of the most popular works of the French Enlightenment. Cf. Désiré Roustan's critical edition, Paris, Revue Philosophique, 1938, pp. 120 and 121.

6. John Mullan, *Sentiment and Sociability: The Language of Feeling in the Eighteenth Century*, Oxford, Clarendon Press, 1988. See also Roselyne Rey, *The History of Pain*, Cambridge, MA and London, Harvard University Press, 1995, pp. 137*ff*; Janet Todd, *Sensibility: An Introduction*, New York, London, Methuen, 1986; G. S. Rousseau, "Nerves, Spirits and Fibres: Towards Defining the Origins of Sensibility," *Enlightenment Crossings: Pre- and Post-Modern Discourses Anthropological*, Manchester, Manchester University Press, 1991, pp. 122–141; and see David Marshall, *The Surprising Effects of Sympathy. Marivaux, Diderot, Rousseau and Mary Shelley*, London, Chicago, University of Chicago Press, 1988.

7. See Keath Thomas, *Man and the Natural World. Changing Attitudes in England. 1500–1800*, London, Penguin, 1984, pp. 143*ff*.

8. William Hogarth, "Autobiographical notes," in Joseph Burke (ed.), *The Analysis of Beauty*, Oxford, Clarendon Press, 1955.

9. Humphrey Primatt, *A Dissertation on the Duty of Mercy and Sin of Cruelty to Brute Animals*, London, R. Hett, 1776, p. 7. Quoted also by James Turner, *Reckoning with the Beast: Animals, Pain and Humanity in the Victorian Mind*, Baltimore and London, Johns Hopkins University Press, 1980, p. 11.

10. Quoted by H. Moehle and U. Throler, "Animal experimentation from Antiquity to the End of the Eighteenth Century," in N. A. Rupke (ed.), *Vivisection in Historical Perspective*, London, Routledge. 1990, p. 26.

11. On the problem of animals' souls in the seventeenth and eighteenth centuries, see Hester Hastings, *Man and Beast in French Thought of the Seventeenth Century*, Baltimore, John Hopkins University Press,1936; Leonora Cohen, *From Beast-Machine to Man-Machine: Animal Soul in French Letters from Descartes to La Mettrie*, New York, Oxford University Press, 1941; Aram Vartanian, *Diderot and Descartes*, Princeton, Princeton University Press, 1953; George Boas, *The Happy Beast in French Thought of the Seventeenth Century*, Baltimore, John Hopkins Press, 1933.

12. Cf. Thomas, *Man and the Natural World*, pp. 122*ff*.

13. Charles Bonnet, *Contemplation de la nature*, en *Oeuvres*, Neufchâtel, Faulche, 1779–1783, IV, pp. 38–115.

14. Joseph Addison, Spectator, num. 419 (1 July 1712), in D. F. Bond (ed.), *The Spectator*, 5 vols, Oxford, Oxford Clarendon Press, 1965, vol. I, pp. 490–491. Quoted by Holger Maehle, "Literary responses to animal experimentation in 17th and 18th century Britain," *Medical History*, 34 (1990): 27–51, p. 33.

15. This has been emphasized by Luc Boltanski, *Distant Suffering. Morality, Media and Politics*, Cambridge, Cambridge University Press, 1999.

16. The term comes from Rousseau, *Discurso sobre el origen y los fundamentos de la desigualdad entre los hombres*, Spanish edition by Antonio Pintor, Madrid, Tecnos, 1995, p. 151.

17. Smith calls the impartial spectator "the great inmate of the breast." Smith, *Theory*, p. 134.

18. Fonna Forman-Barzilai, "Sympathy in Space(s). Adam Smith on Proximity," *Political Theory*, 33 (2005): 189–217, p. 192.

19. See Peter Gay, *The Enlightenment. An Interpretation of the Science of Freedom*, London, Norton Library, 1977, pp. 437 and *ff.* Jacques Revel (*et alia*), "Forms of Privatization" in Ariès and Duby (eds), *History of Private Life* vol. 3, Cambridge, Belknap Press of Harvard University Press, 1993, p. 161.

20. D'Alembert, *Preliminary Discourse to the Encyclopedia of Diderot* [1751], translation by Richard N. Schwab, University of Chicago Press, 1995 (1963), p. 11: "The necessity of protecting our own bodies from pain and destruction causes us to examine which among the external objects can be useful or harmful to us, in order to seek out some and shun others." See Paul Hazard, *European Thought in the Eighteenth Century*, New Haven, Yale University Press, 1954, Chapter II.

21. Juan Pablo Forner, *Tratado contra la tortura* [1793], edited by Santiago Mollfulleda Barcelona, Crítica, 1990.

22. Richard Evans, *Rituals of Retribution. Capital Punishment in Germany, 1600–1987*, Oxford, Oxford University Press, 1996, p. 122.

23. Cesare Beccaria, *Dei delitti* [1764], Chapter 12. English translation, *On Crimes and Punishments and Other Writings*, Cambridge, Cambridge University Press, 1995.

24. Michael Ignatieff, *A Just Measure of Pain: The Penitentiary and the Industrial Revolution, 1750–1850*, New York, Pantheon Books, 1978.

25. See Edward Peters, *Torture*, Oxford, Oxford University Press, 1985, pp. 166–167, as well as Pieter Spierenburg, *The Spectacle of Suffering. Executions and the Evolution of Repression: From a Preindustrial Metropolis to the European Experience*, Cambridge, Cambridge University Press, 1984. p. 188.

26. See Thomas Lacqueur, "Bodies, Details, and the Humanitarian Narrative," in Hunt (ed.), *The New Cultural History*, Berkeley, California, 1989, pp. 176–204. On the case of the progressive elimination of corporal punishment in schools, see J. H. Plumb, "The New World of Children in Eighteenth Century England," *Past and Present*, 67 (1974): 64–95.

27. On an interpretation of the history of torture linked to the ideology of progress, see for instance Marcello T. Maestro, *Voltaire and Beccaria as Reformers of the Criminal Law*, New York, Columbia University Press, 1942. For a refutation, see Peter Edwards's classic, *Torture*, Oxford, Penguin, 1985, pp. 103–140. See also Elaine Scarry's now classic text, *The Body in Pain. The Making and Unmaking of the World*, New York and London, Oxford University Press, 1985.

28. Martin Dinges, "The Reception of Michel Foucault's Ideas on Social Discipline, Mental Asylums, Hospitals and the Medical Profession in German Historiography," in Colin Jones and Roy Porter (eds), *Reassessing Foucault: Power, Medicine and the Body*, London, Routledge, 1993.

29. Michel Foucault, *Discipline and Punish. The Birth of Prison*, London, Penguin. 1977, p. 82.

30. Beccaria, *Dei delitti*, Chapter 45.

31. The expression "culture of sensibility" was coined by Graham John Barker-Benfield, *The Culture of Sensibility. Sex and Society in Eighteenth-Century Britain*, Chicago, Chicago University Press, 1992. On the French case, see J. Moscoso, *Materialismo y Religión. Ciencias de la vida en la Europa Ilustrada*, Barcelona, Serbal, 2000.

32. Norbert Elias, *Über den Prozess der Zivilisation* [1939], English translation *The Civilizing Process: Sociogenetic and Psychogenetic Investigations*. Translation Edmund Jephcott. Oxford, Blackwell, 1994.

33. Nicolas Andry, *L'Orthopédie*, Paris, la Veuve Alix, 1741, 2 vols; vol. I., pp. xxvi–xxvii.

34. See J. Moscoso, "Los efectos de la imaginación: ciencia, medicina y sociedad en el siglo XVIII," *Asclepio*, 53 (2001): 141–171.

35. Gérard Tilles, *La Naissance de la dermatologie (1776–1880)*, Paris, Les Editions Roger Dacosta, 1989; by the same author: "In Praise of Make-up," in Eric Warner and Graham Hough (eds), *Strangeness and Beauty: An Anthology of Aesthetic Criticism 1840–1910*, 2 vols, Cambridge, Cambridge University Press, 1983.

36. Choderlos de Laclos, *Les liaisons dangereuses* [1782], Paris, Livre de Poche, letter CLXXXV, p. 446.

37. David Hume, "On Polygamy and Divorces," [1777] published in D. Hume, *Essays Moral, Political and Literary*, edited by Eugene F. Miller, Indianapolis, Liberty Fund, 1987, pp. 186–187.

38. François Fénelon [1689], *De l'éducation des filles*, Paris, Editions d'aujourh'hui, 1983.

39. Smith, *Theory*, p. 24.

40. Ibid. pp. 49 and 47: "It is always miserable to complain, even when we are oppressed by the most dreadful calamities."

41. Ibid. p. 22.

42. Ibid. p. 110.

43. Ibid. p. 113: "The first of these personalities corresponds to the spectator, "whose sentiments with regard to my own conduct I endeavour to enter into, by placing myself in his situation, and by considering how it would appear to me, when seen from that particular point of view. The second is the agent, the person whom I properly call myself, and whose conduct, under the character of a spectator, I was endeavour to judge."

44. Spierenburg, *The Spectacle of Suffering*, p. 190. See also Spierenburg, *Broken Spell: A Cultural and Anthropological History of Preindustrial Europe*, Basingstoke, Macmillan Education, 1991 and Arlette Farge, *Fragile Lives: Violence, Power and Solidarity in Eighteenth-Century Paris*, Oxford, Oxford University Press, 1993.

45. See Robert Muchembled, *L'invention de l'homme moderne. Sensibilités, moeurs et comportement collectifs sous l'Ancien Régime*, Paris, Fayard, 1988.

46. Spierenburg, *The Spectacle of Suffering*, pp. 184–185.

47. On Enlightenment imagination, see John Brewer, *The Pleasures of the Imagination: English Culture in the Eighteenth Century*, Bath, Harper Collins, 1997. See also Lynn Hunt, *Inventing Human Rights: A History*, London, W. W. Norton and Co., 2008, Chapter 1.

48. Ian Watt, *The Rise of the Novel* [1957], Berkeley and Los Angeles, University of California Press, 1984.

49. Alexandre Wenger, *La fibre littéraire. Le discours médical sur la lecture au xviiie siècle*. Geneva, Droz, 2007.

50. Smith, *Theory*, p. 21.

51. Quoted by Anne Vincent-Buffault, *A History of Tears: Sensibility and Sentimentality in France*; English translation by Teresa Bridgeman, Basingstoke, Macmillan, 1990, p. 37.

52. See Carolyne D. Williams, " 'The Luxury of Doing Good': Benevolence, Sensibility and the Royal Human Society," in Roy Porter and Mary M. Roberts (eds), *Pleasure in the Eighteenth Century*, Basingstoke, Macmillan, 1996, pp. 77–107.

53. See, for example, V. A. C. Gatrell, *The Hanging Tree. Execution and the English People 1770–1868*. Oxford, Oxford University Press, 1996, pp. 242*ff*.

54. Addison, *The Spectator*, p. 571. Cited by E. J. Clery, "The Pleasure of Terror: Paradox in Edmund Burke's Theory of the Sublime," en Porter y Roberts, *Pleasure in the Eighteenth Century*, p. 167.

55. Cesare Beccaria, *On Crimes and Punishments and Other Writings*, Cambridge, Cambridge University Press, 1995, Chapter 47, p. 113.

56. Hunt, *Inventing Human Rights*.

57. Boltanski, *Distant Suffering*, p. 116.

58. Michael L. Frazer, *The Enlightenment of Sympathy: Justice and the Moral Sentiments in the Eighteenth Century and Today*, Oxford, OUP, 2010, p. 104. This work by Smith, along with Burke's work, continues the tradition started by Hutchenson in his *Inquiry into the Original of Our Ideas of Beauty and Virtue*. See also Boltanski, *Distant Suffering*, p. 124: "Now what maintain contact or, to use an anachronistic term, an interface between aesthetic and politics, was nothing other than the idea of objectivity in the sense of perception without a particular perspective [...]"

59. The gradual liberation from the empire of disease and war, as well as improved living conditions, enabled that "*spectatorial sympathy*" particular to the Enlightenment. The expression is used by Halttunen, "Humanitarism and the Pornography of Pain." See also George Sebastian Rousseau, "Cultural History in a New Key: Towards a Semiotics of the Nerve," in Pittock and Wear (eds), *Interpretation and Cultural History*, London, Macmillan, 1991, pp. 25–81; and Jessica Riskin, *Science in the Age of Sensibility. The Sentimental Empiricists of the French Enlightenment*, Chicago, University of Chicago Press, 2007.

60. The expression "ideal presence" comes from Lord Kames, *Elements of Criticism*, 1762. Cited by Hunt, *Inventing Human Rights*, pp. 56*ff*.

61. Diderot, *Oeuvres esthétiques*, edited by Paul Verniére, Paris, Garnier Frères, 1968, p. 230. See M. Fried, *Absorption and Theatricality: Painting and Beholder in the Age of Diderot*, Berkeley and London, University of California Press, 1980.

62. Frazer uses the expression "projective empathy" in *The Enlightenment of Sympathy*, pp. 97*ff*.

63. M. Foucault, *Truth and Juridical Forms*, in *Power: Essential Works of Foucault, 1954–1984*: vol. 3. Translated by Robert Hurley. New York, The New Press, 2001.

64. Voltaire, *Candide* [1759], Chapter 6: "How the Portuguese Made a Beautiful Auto-Da-Fé, to Prevent Any Further Earthquakes; and How Candide Was Publically Whipped." English translation by Boni and Liveright, Inc, Introduction by Philip Litell, New York, Boni and Liveright, 1918. Various books have recently been published on the Lisbon earthquake. See, for example, Nicholas Shrady, *The Last Day: Wrath, Ruin and Reason in the Great Lisbon Earthquake of 1755*, London, Penguin, 2009, and Edward Paice, *The Wrath of God: The Great Lisbon Earthquake of 1755*, London, Quercus, 2010.

65. Alessa Johns (ed.), *Dreadful Visitations. Confronting Natural Catastrophe in the Age of the Enlightenment*, Routledge, London and New York, 1999.

66. Shrady, *The Last Day*, p. 53.

67. Adam Smith, *Essays on Philosophical Subjects*, W. P. D. Wightman and J. C. Bryce (ed.), vol. III of the *Glasgow Edition of the Works and Correspondence of Adam Smith* vol. III, History of Astronomy, Indianapolis, Liberty Fund, 1982.
68. See Ian Hacking, *The Emergence of Probability*, Cambridge, Cambridge University Press, 1975.
69. Burke, *A Philosophical Enquiry*, p. 92.
70. Hans Blumenberg, *Schiffbruch mit Zuschauer: Paradigma einer Dasainmetaphor*, 1979, English translation by Steven Rendall, Shipwreck with Spectator, Cambridge, MIT University Press, 1996, Chapter 3: "Aesthetics and Ethics of the Spectator." On the metaphor of the theatre in connection with sympathy, see David Marshall, "Adam Smith and the Theatricality of Moral Sentiments," *Critical Inquiry*, 10 (1984): 592–613; Marshall, *The Surprising Effects of Sympathy*. On the critique of the theatrical model, see J. Barish, *The Antitheatrical Prejudice*, Berkeley, University of California Press, 1981.
71. Diderot, *Correspondence*, compiled by G. Roth and annotated by G. Roth and J. Varloot, Paris, Editions de Minuit, 1955–61, vol. III, p. 171.
72. For an interesting discussion on the spaces of proximity in Smith, see Forman-Barzilai, "Sympathy in Space(s): Adam Smith on Proximity," 189–217.
73. Carlo Ginzburg, "Killing a Chinese Mandarin: On the Moral Implications of Distance," *Critical Inquiry*, 21 (1994), 46–60. See also Eric Hayot, *The Hypothetical Mandarin: Sympathy, Modernity, and Chinese pain*, Oxford, OUP, 2009.
74. Smith, *Theory*, p. 136.
75. Burke, *A Philosophical Inquiry*, pp. 93–94.
76. Ibid. p. 92: "for terror is a passion which always produces delight when it does not press too close."
77. For Smith, almost everything happens "in some measure," without indicating in what measure we are dealing with or how it could be established. That is also, partially, Burke's and Beccaria's difficulty.

4 Correspondence

1. Marcel Proust, *A Remembrance of Things Past*, vol. 6, *The Sweet Cheat Gone*, translation by C. K. Scott Moncrieff, New York, Random House, 1934, p. 1.
2. On these issues, see Peter Gay, *The Tender Passion*, New York, Oxford University Press, 1986.
3. See Peter Stanley, *For Fear of Pain. British Surgery 1790–1850*, Amsterdam/New York, Rodopi, 2003; André Soubiran, *Le baron Larrey, chirurgien de Napoléon*, Paris, Fayard, 1966. Also Rosalyne Rey, *Histoire de la douleur*, Paris, La Découverte, pp. 162*ff*.
4. Pat Hodgson, *Early War Photographs, 50 Years of War Photographs from the Nineteenth Century*, Boston, New York Graphic Society, 1974. On the uses of the photography of pain, see Susan Sontag, *Regarding the Pain of Others*, New York, Farrar, Straus, and Giroux, 2003. In relation to the American Civil War and the uses of photography, see Timothy Sweet, *Traces of War: Poetry, Photography, and the Crisis of the Union*, Baltimore, Johns Hopkins University Press, 1990.
5. On the history of flagellation, see Ernst Kern, "Cultural-Historical Aspects of Pain." in *Pain: A Medical and Anthropological Challenge*, J. Brihate, F. Loew, and H. W. Pia (eds), *Acta Nerochirurgica*, 38, suppl. (1987), pp. 187–188. John K. Noyes, *The Mastery of Submission. Inventions of Masochism*, Ithaca, Cornell University Press, 1997.

6. Thomas Jefferson, *Notes on the State of Virginia*, Query XIV [1785]. New York, Penguin, 1999, p. 146.

7. See Ann Dally, "Pain Disorders. Social Sections," in Berrios and Porter, (eds), *A History of Clinical Psychiatry: The Origin and History of Psychiatric Disorders*, London, Athlone, 1995.

8. See Roy Porter, "Pain and Suffering," in W. F. Bynum and R. Porter (eds), *Companion Encyclopaedia to the History of Medicine*, London, Routledge, 1993, vol. II, and Olivier Fauré, *Histoire sociale de la médecine, XVIII–XX*, Paris, Anthropos, 1994, p. 107.

9. John D. Lesch, *Science and Medicine in France. The Emergence of Experimental Physiology, 1790–1855*, Cambridge, MA/London, Harvard University Press, 1984. Antoine Louis, *Mémoire sur une question anatomique relative à la jurisprudence*, Paris, P. G. Cavelier, 1763. The connection between passion for science, respect for animals, and disdain for pain in the Victorian nineteenth century has been demonstrated by James Turner, *Reckoning with the Beast. Animals, Pain and Humanity in the Victorian Mind*, Baltimore/London, The Johns Hopkins University Press, 1980. In the English-speaking world, see Diana Manuel, "Marshall Hall [1790–1857]: Vivisection and the Development of Experimental Physiology," in N. Rupke (ed.), *Vivisection in Historical Perspective*, London, Routledge, 1990, 78–104. On different procedures of researching the nervous system during the first decades of the nineteenth century, see Edwin Clarke y L. S. Jacyna, *Nineteenth-Century Origins of Neuroscientific Concepts*, Berkeley, University of California Press, 1987, 1–28. On the pain of animals, see Bernard E. Rollin, *The Unheeded Cry: Animal Consciousness, Animal Pain and Science*, Oxford, OUP, 1989. Also James Turner, *Reckoning with the Beast: Animals, Pain, and Humanity in the Victorian Mind*, Baltimore, Johns Hopkins University Press, 1982, and Anita Guerrini, *Experimenting with Humans and Animals. From Galen to Animal Rights*, Baltimore, Johns Hopkins University Press, 2003, especially Chapter 4.

10. See Mirko D. Grmek (ed.), *De la Renaissance aux Lumiéres*, 1997, vol. II and III, in *Histoire de la pensée médicale en Occident*, 4 vols, Paris, Seuil, 1995–1999. Fauré, *Histoire sociale de la médecine*, p. 35.

11. Stanley Reiser, *Medicine and the Reign of Technology*, Cambridge, Cambridge University Press, 1978. See also Kurt Danziger, *Constructing the Subject: Historical Origins of Psychological Research*, Cambridge, Cambridge University Press, 1990. Alain Ségal, "Les moyens d'exploration du corps," in Mirko Grmek (ed.), *Histoire de la pensée médicale*, Paris, Seuil, 1999, vol. III, p. 169–186 and Soraya de Chadarevian, "Graphical Method and Discipline: Self-Recording Instruments in Nineteenth-Century Physiology," *Studies in the History and Philosophy of Science*, 35 (1999): 35–57.

12. Etienne-Jules Marey, *La Méthode graphique dans les sciences expérimentales et particulièrement en physiologie et en médecine*, Paris, G. Masson, 1878. Quoted by Daston, "Scientific Objectivity and the Ineffable," in L. Krüger and B. Falkenburg (eds), *Physik, Philosophie und die Einheit der Wissenschaften*. Heidelberg, Spektrum Akademischer Verlag, 1995, p. 325.

13. See Lorraine Daston and Peter Galison, "The Image of Objectivity," *Representations*, 40 (1992): 81–128.

14. See Edwin G. Boring, *Sensation and Perception in the History of Experimental Psychology* [1942], New York, Irvington, 1970.

15. John Keats, *The Letters of John Keats*, edited by Jack Stillinger, Cambridge, MA, Harvard University Press, 1958, p. 102 (21 April 1819). Quoted by David D. Morris, *The Culture of Pain*, Berkeley, University of California Press, 1991, p. 208.
16. Steven Bruhn, *Gothic Bodies, The Politics of Pain in Romantic Fiction*, Philadelphia, University of Pennsylvania Press, 1994, p. xxi.
17. John B. Lyon, " 'You can kill, but you cannot bring to life:' Aesthetic Education and the Instrumentalization of Pain in Schiller and Hölderlin," *Literature and Medicine*, 24 (2005): 31–50.
18. Yrjö Hirn, *The Origins of Art: A Psychological and Sociological Inquiry*, New York, Macmillan, 1900, "The Enjoyment of Pain;" quoted by Havelock Ellis, "Pain and Love", in *Studies in the Psychology of Sex*, vol. III, Philadelphia, F. A. Davis, 1904, p. 78.
19. Friedrich Nietzsche, "Schopenhauer as Educator", in *Untimely Mediations*, edited by Daniel Breazeale, Cambridge, Cambridge University Press, 2007, p. 153.
20. On these issues, see Patrick Kiley, *Making Sense of Pain: Reading the Sensible Body of Late Eighteenth- and Early Nineteenth-Century France*. Purdue University, West Lafayette, Indiana. University Microfilms International, 2003; Jean Pierre Peter, *Silence et cris. La médecine devant la douleur ou l'histoire d'une élision*, Le Genre Humanine, autumn, 1988.
21. Marc-Antoine Petit, *Discours sur la douleur prononcé à l'ouverture des cours d'anatomie et de chirurgie de l'hospice général des malades de Lyon*, 1799, in Jean Pierre Peter (ed.), *De la douleur. Observations sur les attitudes de la médecine prémoderne envers la douleur, suivis de traités* de A. Sassard, M. A. Petit y J. A. Salgues. Paris, Quai Voltaire, 1993.
22. Petit, *Discours sur la douleur*, p. 75.
23. On Lyon during the Revolution, see William D. Edmonds, *Jacobinism and the Revolt of Lyon, 1789–1793*, Oxford, Clarendon Press, 1990.
24. Marc Antoine Petit, *Discours sur l'influence de la Révolution française sur la santé publique* [1796], in Marc-Antoine Petit (ed.), *Essai sur la médecine du coeur*, Paris, Garnier, Reymann, 1806, pp. 116–157; p. 116.
25. Jacques-Alexandre Salgues, *De la douleur considérée sous le point de vue de son utilité en médecine, et dans ses rapports avec la physiologie, l'hygiène, la pathologie et la thérapeutique* [1823], in Jean Pierre Peter (ed.), *De la douleur*, 1993.
26. See J. Ph. Hamel, *De la néuralgie faciale, communément tic douloureux de la face. Dissertation présentée et soutenue à l'École de Médecine de Paris, le an II*. (J. Ph. Hamel is a doctoral student at the medical school of Paris, and surgeon at the Charity Hospital), Paris, Valade, 1803. See Boissier de Sauvages, *Theoria Doloris, Dissertation*, Montpellier, Apud Joannem Martel, 1757; F.-Émile Vivier-Brunelière, *Esquisse physiologique de la douleur*, doctoral thesis, Paris, 1851; Victor Alexandre Guénébaud, *Du Symptôme douleur dans les maladies*, doctoral thesis, 1853.
27. Benedetto Mojon, *Sull'utilità del dolore*, Genova, Y. Gravier, 1818.
28. William Griffin [1794–1796], a member of the Royal College of Surgeons, in Edinburgh, published *An Essay on the Nature of Pain; with Some Considerations on Its Principal Varieties and Connected with Disease, and Remarks on the Treatment*, Edinburgh, J. Moir, 1826.
29. Griffin, *An Essay on the Nature of Pain*, p. 8.
30. François Marie Hippolyte Bilon, *Dissertation sur la douleur*, Paris, Feugueray, 1803, p. 12.
31. Quoted by Salgues, *De la douleur*, p. 127.

32. Charles Robert Richet, *Recherches expérimentales et cliniques sur la sensibilité*, Paris, G. Masson, 1877, p. 247.
33. *Gravative*, that consists of a kind of heaviness; the *tensive*, that seems to tense parts of the body, the *pulsative*, which is characterized by more or less strong and frequent pulsations, or the *pongitive*, where a kind of stabbing seems to penetrate the skin or the organs.
34. François Magendie, *An Elementary Treatise on Human Physiology. On the basis of the Précis Élémentaire de Physiologie*, New York, Harper & Brothers, 1844, p. vi.
35. Petit, *Discours sur l'influence de la Révolution française*, p. 77.
36. Magendie, *Précis Elémentaire de Physiologie*, translation of the fifth French edition by John Revere, *An Elementary Treatise on Human Physiology*, New York, Harper and Brothers, 1844, p. vi.
37. See William Schupbach, "A Select Iconography of Animal Experiment," in N. Rupke (ed.), *Vivisection in Historical Perspective*, pp. 340–360.
38. Bilon, *Dissertation sur la douleur*, p. 40.
39. Ibid. p. 39.
40. Ibid. p. 40, and Charles Delucena Meigs, *Obstetrics: The Science and the Arts*, Philadelphia, Lea & Blanchard, 1849, pp. 254–255.
41. Richet, *Recherches sur la sensibilité*, p. 237.
42. P. Mantegazza, *Atlante delle espressioni del dolore. Fotografie prese dal vero e da molte altre opere d'arte*, Florence, Brogi, 1876.
43. P. Mantegazza, *Fisiologia del dolore*, Florence, Felize Paggi, 1880. See also P. Mantegazza, *La Physionomie et l'expression des sentiments* [1885], Paris, Félix Alcan, 1889, ChapterVIII: "Classification des expressions" and Chapter X: "Mimique de la douleur."
44. Salgues, *De la douleur* [1823], in Jean-Pierre Peter, *De la douleur. Observations sur les attitudes de la médecine prémoderne envers la douleur, suivis de traités de A. Sassard*, M. A. Petit y J. A. Salgues, Paris, Quai Voltaire, 1993, pp. 125–202.
45. Salgues, *De la douleur*, p. 132. Griffin, *An Essay on the Nature of Pain*, p. 1; Bilon, *Dissertation sur la douleur*, pp. 10–11.
46. Pierre-Jean Cabanis, *Rapport de physique et de morale de l'homme* [1798], Paris, Fortin et Masson, 1843, p. 157. Quoted by Rey, *Histoire de la douleur*, p. 130. On Cabanis, see Martin S. Staum, *Cabanis: Enlightenment and Medical Philosophy in the French Revolution*, Princeton, Princeton University Press, 1980. See François Picavet, *Les Ideologues. Essai sur l'Histoire des idées et des théories scientifiques, philosophiques, religieuses, etc. en France depuis 1789*, Paris, Félix Alcan, 1891. Reprinted in New York, Arno Press, 1975.
47. On this subject, see especially John Hilton, *On Rest and Pain; a Course of Lectures on the Influence of Mechanical and Physiological Rest in the Treatment of Accidents and Surgical Diseases*, London, George Bell, 1877, p. 58.
48. Stanley, *For Fear of Pain*, p. 55.
49. William Balfour, *Observations with Cases Illustrative of the Sedative and Febrifugue Powers of Emetic Tartar*, Edinburgh, P. Hill, 1818, p. 7.
50. See Stanley, *For Fear of Pain*, p. 54.
51. Petit, *Discours sur l'influence de la Révolution française*, p. 102.
52. Jean-Baptiste Bonnefoy, *De l'application de l'électricité à l'art de guérir*, Lyon, De l'imprimerie d'Aimé de la Roche, 1782.

53. See Pierre Rodamel, *Essai pratique sur l'emploi des vésicatoires dans les inflamma-tions internes, éclairé par les résultats de leur application sur les inflammations externes*, Montpellier, G. Izar et A. Ricard, 1798.

54. François Gondret, *Considérations sur l'emploi du feu en médecine, suivies de l'exposé d'un moyen épispatique propre à suppléer la cautérisation, et à remplacer l'usage des cantharides*, Paris, Gondret & Blaise, 1819, p. 14.

55. Gondret, *Considérations sur l'emploi du feu*, pp. 19 and 77.

56. Robert Dunglison, "Introduction," in Baron Dominique Jean Larrey (ed.), *On the Use of Moxa, as a Therapeutical Agent, Translated from the French, with Notes, and an Introduction Containing a History of the Substance*, London, Thomas and George Underwood, 1822, p. lxx.

57. Rey, *Histoire de la douleur*, pp. 164*ff.*

58. Dunglison, "Introduction," p. lvi.

59. See William Balfour, *Illustrations of the Power of Emetic Tartar, in the Cure of Inflam-mation, and Asthma, and in Preventing Consumption and Apoplexy*, Edinburgh, P. Hill, 1819. By the same author, Balfour, *Observations with Cases Illustrative.* Previously a certain doctor James, *Considerations on the Use and Abuse of the Antimonial Medicines in Fevers, and Other Disorders*, London, John Murray, 1773.

60. Griffin, *An Essay on the Nature of Pain*, p. 63.

61. Paul Dubé, *Le Medecin des pauvres. Qui enseigne le moyen de guérir les maladies par des remèdes faciles à trouver dans les Païs et préparer à peu de frais par toutes sortes de personnes*, Lyon, François Sarrazin, 1693.

62. On the ineffectiveness of *spongia*, see Plinio Prioreschi, "Medieval Anesthesia – The Spongia Somnifera," *Medical Hypotheses*, 61, 2 (August 2003): 213–219.

63. Michel Dechaume et Pierre Huard, *Histoire illustrée de l'art dentaire*, Paris, R. Dacosta, 1977, p. 11.

64. Quoted by J. -L. André Bonnet, *Histoire Générale de la Chirurgie Dentaire*, Paris, Société des Auteurs Modernes: P. -C. Ash, 1910, pp. 12 and 138.

65. Quoted by Ibid. pp. 138–139.

66. Quoted by Ibid. p. 145.

67. Pierre Dionis, *Cours d'opérations de chirurgie, démontrées au Jardin du Roi*, Paris, Méquignon l'aîne, 1782. Upon examining these efforts, Dionis recognizes that pain is inevitable, 616.

68. Bonnet, *Histoire Générale*, p. 16.

69. Quoted by James Wynbrandt, *The Excruciating History of Dentistry. Toothsome Tales and Oral Oddities from Babylon to Braces*, New York, St. Martin's Press, 1998, p. 59. See also, for an intellectual history of dentistry, Walter Hoffman-Axthelm, *History of Dentistry*, Chicago, Quintessence Pub. Co., 1981.

70. John Hunter, *The Natural History of the Human Teeth* [1771], London, W. Spilsbury for J. Johnson, 1803, p. 150.

71. Salgues, *De la douleur*, p. 131.

72. Marquis de Sade, *Justine*, quoted by Morris, *The Culture of Pain*, p. 229. For a cor-respondence between the new physiology and Sade's literature, see Kiley, *Making Sense of Pain*.

73. Albrecht von Haller, *Mémoires sur la nature sensible et irritable des parties du corps animal*, Lausana, M. M. Bousquet (-S. d'Arnay), 1756–1760, vol. I, p. 109. Quoted also by Rey, *Histoire de la douleur*, p. 127. Rey, however, confuses the volume with the memoire. This is vol. I., but of the second memoire. The same applies to the next footnote.

74. Haller, *Mémoires sur la nature*, p. 108. Quoted also by Rey, *Histoire de la douleur*, p. 127.
75. Marie Francois Xavier Bichat, *Physiological Recherches on Life and Death*, English translation by Gold, London, Longman, Hurst, Rees, Orme and Browne, 1815, p. 56.
76. Bichat, *Physiological Researches*, p. 54.
77. Ibid. p. 57.
78. Griffin, *An Essay on the Nature of Pain*, pp. 53–55.
79. Charles D. Meigs, *Females and their Diseases*, Philadelphia: Lea & Blanchard, 1848, p. 49.
80. Charles D. Meigs, *Obstetrics: the Science and the Art*, Filadelphia, Lea and Blanchard, 1849, p. 253.
81. William Osborn, *An Essay on Laborious Parturition: In which the Division of the Symphysis is Particularly Considered*, London, 1783, p. ix. Quoted by Helen King, *Midwifery, Obstetrics and the Rise of Gynaecology: The Uses of a Sixteenth-Century Compendium*. Aldershot, Ashgate Pub., 2007, p. 184.
82. Adrian Wilson, "The Perils of Early-Modern Procreation: Childbirth with or without Fear?" *British Journal for Eighteenth-Century Studies*, 16 (1993): 1–19, p. 3.
83. Brudenel Exton, *A New and General System of Midwifery. In four parts*, London, W. Owen, 1751, p. 43.
84. Michael Stolberg, "The Monthly Malady: A History of Premenstrual Suffering," *Medical History*, 44 (2000): 301–322. Regarding menopause, Michael Stolberg, "A Woman's Hell? Medical Perceptions of Menopause in Preindustrial Europe," *Bulletin of the History of Medicine*, 73 (1999): 404–428.
85. Pierre Dionis, *Traité général des accouchements, qui instruit de tout ce qu'il faut faire pour être habile accoucheur* [1718], Paris, C. M. d'Houry, 1724, p. 209.
86. James Young Simpson, *On the Early History and Progress of an Aesthetic Midwifery*, Edinburgh, 1848, p. 6.
87. Quoted by Howard Riley Raper, *Man Against Pain. The Epic of Anaesthesia*, London, Victor Gollancz Ltd, 1947, p. 11.
88. Adrian Wilson, "Participant or patient? Seventeenth-Century Childbirth from the Mother's point of view," in Roy Porter (ed.), *Patients and Practitioners. Lay Perceptions of Medicine in Pre-Industrial Society*, Cambridge, Cambridge University Press, 1985, pp. 129–145; p. 134.
89. See Katharina Park, *Secrets of Women. Gender, Generation and the Origins of Human Dissection*, New York, Zone Books, 2006. On William Hunter's illustrations, see Ludmilla J. Jordanova, "Gender, Generation and Science: William Hunter's Obstetrics Atlas," in W. F. Bynum and R. Porter (eds), *William Hunter and the Eighteenth Century Medical World*, Cambridge, Cambridge University Press, 1985, pp. 385–413. Jordanova writes in terms of relationships and cultural assumptions present in the images of Hunter's *The Anatomy of the Human Gravid Uterus*, also, but to a lesser extent in William Smelie's work, *A Sett of Anatomical Tables*. See William Shorter, "The Management of the Normal Deliveries and the Generation of William Hunter," in W. F. Bynum and R. Porter (eds), *William Hunter and the Eighteenth Century Medical World*, Cambridge, Cambridge University Press, 1985, pp. 371–383. For an alternative view, Adrian Wilson, "William Hunter and the Varieties of Man-Midwifery," in W. F. Bynum and R. Porter (eds), *William Hunter*, pp. 323–343. For a more general view, Adrian Wilson, *The Making of Man-Midwifery. Childbirth in England 1660–1770*, London, UCL Press, 1995.
90. See Gillaume Mauquest de la Motte, *Traité complet des accouchements naturels, non naturels, et contre nature*, Paris, L. d'Houry, 1722, p. 6; and François Mauriceau, *Elements of the Practice of Midwifery*, London, 1775, p. 65.

91. Quoted by Jacques Gélis, *L'arbre et le fruit. La naissance dans l'Occident moderne XVI-XIX siècle*, Fayard, Evreux, 1984, p. 313. The Spanish does not maintain the Latin term *labor, -oris*, "I labor" to refer to the birth, although it does continue referring to "laborious births;" the English "*to be in labor*" retains this sense, especially for the period in which uterine contractions occur to bring about the expulsion of the fetus.
92. W. Tyler Smith, *A Manuel of Obstetrics*, London, Churchill, 1858, p. 305.
93. Dionis, *Traité général des accouchemens*, pp. 124 and 152.
94. Ibid., pp. 126–127.
95. Paulin Cazeaux, *Traité théorique et pratique de l'art des accouchements* [1840], Paris, Chamerot, 1853, pp. 508–509.
96. Dionis, *Traité général des accouchemens*, p. 217.Edmund Chapman, *A Treatise of the Improvement of Midwifery, Chiefly with Regard to the Operation*, London, John Brindley, 1753, p. 151.
97. Cazeaux, *Traité*, p. 418.
98. Ibid. p. 430.
99. Ibid. pp. 414–432.
100. Charles Darwin, *The Expression of the Emotions in Man and Animals* [1872], London, Fontana Press, 1999, p. 73.
101. Chapman, *A Treatise of the Improvement of Midwifery*, p. xxxii.
102. Ibid. p. 430.
103. Simpson, *On the Early History and Progress*, p. 6.
104. On the question of whether the anesthetized body may or may not feel pain, see infra, Chapter 5.
105. Helen King, Midwifery, *Obstetrics and the Rise of Gynaecology. The Uses of a Sixteenth-Century Compendium*, Aldershot, Ashgate, 2007, p. 183.
106. Simpson, *History*, p. 11.
107. Quoted by Ibid. p. 43.
108. Samuel William John Merriman, *Arguments against the Indiscriminatory Employment of Chloroform in Midwifery*, London, Churchill, 1848.
109. Meigs, *Obstetrics*, p. 316.
110. Ibid. 318.
111. William Tyler Smith, "A lecture on the Utility and Safety on the Inhalation of Ether in Obstetric Practice," *Lancet* (March 1847). See also Stephanie J. Snow, *Operations Without Pain. The Practice and Science of Anaesthesia in Victorian Britain*, New York, Macmillan, Palgrave, 2006.
112. Dionis, *Traité général des accouchemens*, pp. 206–207 and 215.
113. Simpson, *History*, p. 20.
114. Alastair Masson, "Crime and Anaesthesia: Rape and Abduction," *History of Medicine*, 9 (1981): 8–25.
115. See Bram Dijkstra, *Idols of Perversity. Fantasies of Feminine Evil in Fin-de-Siècle Culture*, New York, Oxford University Press, 1986.
116. Smith, "A Lecture," p. 383.
117. Nancy Cartwright, *Nature's Capacities and Their Measurement*, Oxford, Clarendon Press, 1989.
118. On these issues, see Danziger, *Constructing the Subject*. See also Joel Michell, *Measurement in Psychology. A Critical History of a Methodological Concept*, Cambridge, Cambridge University Press, 1999.
119. R. Steven Turner, "Helmholtz, Sensory Physiology and the Disciplinary Development of German Psychology," *The Problematic Science*, pp. 147–166. See also

Lorraine Daston and Peter Galison, *Objectivity*, New York, Zone Books, 2007, pp. 262 and 22.

120. Wilhelm Wundt, *Grundzüge der physiologischen Phychologie*, Leipzig, Engelmann, 1874, pp. 2–3. Quoted by Danziger, *Constructing the Subject*, p. 206. Wundt's position received the support and the influence of the generation of scientists immediately following Johannes Müller—who, after all, maintained a very sporadic experimental position. Together with Du Bois-Reymond, Ludwig, and Helmolhtz, he allowed himself to feel the powerful influence of French physiology and especially the work of François Magendie. This explains Wundt's emphasis on the physiology of sensations and, more specifically, on problems related to the intensity, duration, and location of the stimulus.

121. Strictly speaking, the sensation is proportional to the logarithm of the physical magnitude of the stimulus.

122. Gustav Theodor Fechner [1860], *Elements of psychophysics*, English translation by Helmut E. Adler, New York/London, Holt, Rinehart & Winston, 1966, p. 7. On Fechner, see Michael Heidelberg, *Nature from Within. Gustav Theodor Fechner And His Psychophysical Worldview*, University of Pittsburgh Press, 2004, especially Chapter VI.

123. Quoted by Edwin G. Boring, *A History of Experimental Psychology* [1929], New York, Appleton-Century-Crofts, 1950.

124. Weber's book was later reprinted in 1851. On the translation of the German term "Gemaingefühl," see Jean Starobinski, *Razones del cuerpo*, Valladolid, Ediciones Cuatro, 1999, Chapter II: "El concepto de cenestesia."

125. G. Gigerenzer, "From Metaphysics to Psychophysics and Statics," *The Behavioral and Brain Sciences*, 16 (1993): 139–140. Pierre Bourguer, *Traité d'Optique sur la gradation de la lumière*, Paris, printed by H.-L. Guérin, 1760. While the physiologist Johannes Müller had unsuccessfully attempted to measure the velocity of nerve impulses, von Helmoltz managed to establish a parameter that received experimental confirmation by Bernstein in 1871. See Kathryn M. Olesko and Frederic L. Holmes: "Experiment, Quantification, and Discovery: Helmholtz's Early Physiological Researches, 1843–1850," in David Cahan (ed.), *Hermann von Helmholtz: Scientist and Philosopher*, Berkeley and London, University of California Press, 2000.

126. David J. Murray, "A Perspective for Viewing the History of Psychophysics," *Behavioral and Brain Sciences*, 16 (1993): 115–186.

127. This law, called *Weber's* law, should really be called "Fechner's law." See Boring, *Sensation and Perception in the History*, pp. 34–45 and 50–52.

128. See M. E. Marshall, "Physics, Metaphysics, and Fechner's Psychophysics," in W. R. Woodward and M. G. Ash (eds), *The Problematic Science*, New York, Praeger, 1982, pp. 65–87.

129. J. D. Hardy, H. G. Wolff and H. Goodell, *Pain Sensation and Reactions*, Baltimore, Williams & Wilkins, 1952.

130. Ronald Melzack y Patrick D. Wall, *The Challenge of Pain* [1982], London, Penguin, 1996, pp. 7–9.

131. Quoted by Peter Fairley, *The Conquest of Pain*, London, Joseph, 1978, p. 32.

132. H. K. Beecher, "Pain in Men Wounded in Battle," *Annals of Surgery*, 123 (1946). See also his *Measurement of Subjective Responses*, New York, Oxford University Press, 1959.

133. Robert Richet, *Recherches expérimentales et cliniques sur la sensibilité*, Paris, G. Masson, 1877, p. 314.

134. See Carl G. Hempel, *Fundamentals of Concept Formation in Empirical Science*, Chicago, University of Chicago Press, 1952.

135. By identifying ontological objectivity with realism we only mean to suggest that there exist as many varieties of the first as of the second. On varieties of scientific realism see A. Díeguez Lucena, *Realismo científico. Una introducción al debate actual en filosofía de la ciencia*, Málaga, Universidad de Málaga, 1998; W. González, "El realismo y sus variedades: el debate actual sobre las bases filosóficas de la ciencia," in Alberto Carreras (ed.), *Conocimiento, ciencia y realidad*, Zaragoza, Universidad de Zaragoza, SIUZ, 1993. Ilkka Niinililuoto, *Critical Scientific Realism*, Oxford, Oxford University Press, 1999.

136. Bill Noble *et al.*, "The Measurement of Pain, 1945–2000," *Journal of Pain and Symptom Management*, 29 (2005): 14–21.

137. See Charles Gillispie, *The Edge of Objectivity, An Essay in the History of Scientific Ideas*, Princeton, Princeton University Press, 1960; Theodore Porter, *Trust in Numbers. The Pursuit of Objectivity in Science and Public Life*, Princeton, Princeton University Press, 1995, Cartwright, *Nature's Capacities*. See also Daston and Galison, *Objectivity*.

138. See Lorraine Daston, "Objectivity and the Escape from Perspective" in Mario Biagioli, (ed.), *The Sciences Studies Reader*, New York and London, Routledge, 1999, 110–124 and Thomas Nagel, *The View from Nowhere*, Oxford, Oxford University Press, 1986.

139. The term *"unforced agreement"* was coined by Richard Rorty in "Solidarity or objectivity?" *Objectivity, Relativism and Truth*, Philosophical Papers, vol. I, Cambridge, Cambridge University Press, 1991.

140. The objectivity I am referring to is that that could be denominated *epistemic or epistemological objectivity*. Other authors maintain the idea of an *ontological objectivity*. These forms of metaphysical realism do not form a part of our subject. For some of these considerations in the early modern period see Yolton, *Perceptual Acquaintance from Descartes to Reid*, Minneapolis, University of Minnesota Press, 1984; and Daston and Galison, *Objectivity*.

5 Trust

1. Grace Steel Woodward, *The Man Who Conquered Surgical Pain: A Biography of William Thomas Green Morton*, Boston, Beacon Press, 1962.

2. Denis Brindell Fradin, *"We Have Conquered Pain," The Discovery of Anaesthesia*, New York, Margaret K. McElderry Books, 1996.

3. Richard Manning Hodges, *A Narrative of Events, Connected with the Introduction of Sulphuric Ether into Surgical Use*, Boston, Little Brown, 1891, pp. 25–26.

4. Ibid. p. 34.

5. Ibid. p. 36.

6. The history of medicine has produced some works on the development of anaesthesiology. One of these is Donald Caton's *What a Blessing She Had Chloroform. The Medical and Social Response to the Pain of Childbirth from 1800 to the Present*, New Haven/London, Yale University Press, 1999. More general is Martin S. Pernick's *A Calculus of Suffering. Pain, Professionalism and Anesthesia in Nineteenth-Century America*, New York, Columbia University Press, 1985. Other works deal with the history of anesthesia from a very general point of view, for instance, Howard Riley Raper, *Man Against Pain. The Epic of Anaesthesia*, London, Victor Gollancz, 1947. Betty MacQuitty, *The Battle of Oblivion: The Discovery of Anaesthesia*, London, Harrap, 1969; George Bankoff, *The Conquest of Pain: The Story*

of Anaesthesia, London, Macdonald, 1939–1945; Victor Robinson, *Victory over Pain: A History of Anaesthesia*, London, Sigma, 1947; René Fülop-Miller, *Triumph over Pain*, New York, The Literary Guild of America, 1938; Frederick Fox Carwright, *The English Pioneers of Anaesthesia: Beddoes, Davy and Hickman*, Bristol, John Wright/London, Simpkin Marshall, 1952. A good Spanish introduction is Juan Riera Palmero's *Breve historia de la anestesiología*, Valladolid, Universidad de Valladolid, 1997.

7. John Aitkin, *A Probationary Essay on Stone in the Bladder and Lithotomy*, Edinburgh, 1816, p. 2. Quoted by Peter Stanley, *For Fear of Pain. British Surgery 1790–1850*, Amsterdam/New York, Rodopi, 2003, p. 85.

8. Quoted by Daniel H. Tuke, *Illustrations of the influence of the mind upon the body in health and disease, designed to elucidate the action of the imagination*. London, J. & A. Churchill, 1872, p. 36: "I have considerable doubt of the propriety of putting a patient into so unnatural a condition as results from inhaling ether, which seems scarcely different from severe intoxication, a state in which no surgeon would be desirous of having a patient who was about to be submitted to a serious of operations." See also J. Robison, *A Treatise on the Inhalation of the Vapour of Ether for the Prevention of Pain in Surgical Operations*, London, Webster & Co., 1847.

9. Nikolai Ivanovich Pigorov, *Researches Practical and Physiological on Etherization*, Park Ridge, Ill., Wood Library Museum of Anesthesiology, 1992. Quoted by Caton, *What a Blessing She had Chloroform*, 1999, p. 28.

10. François Marie Hippolyte Bilon, *Dissertation sur la doleur*, Paris, Feugueray, 1803, p. 38.

11. John Elliotson, *Numerous Cases of Surgical Operations without Pain in the Mesmeric State*, London, Ballière, 1843, p. 59.

12. Cases quoted by Tuke, *Illustrations*, pp. 36 and 37.

13. "On the Injurious Effects of the Inhalation of Ether," *Edinburgh Medical and Surgical Journal*, July, 1847, p. 258. Quoted by J. Y Simpson, *Answer to the Religious Objections advanced against the Employment of Anaesthetic Agents in Midwifery and Surgery*, Edinburgh, Sutherland and Knox, 1848, p. 3.

14. On these topics, see Pernick, *A Calculus of Suffering*.

15. James Moore, *A Method of Preventing or Diminishing Pain in Several Operations of Surgery*, London, T. Cadell, 1784, p. 2.

16. Henry-Froçois Le Dran, *The Operations in Surgery*, English translation by W. Cheldesen, London, C. Hitch & R. Dodsley, 1752, p. 1.

17. Edmund Chapman, *A Treatise of the Improvement of Midwifery, Chiefly with Regard to the Operation*, London, John Brindley, 1753.

18. See Astley Cooper, *The Principles and Practice of Surgery*, London, E. Cox, 3 vols, 1837; vol. I, p. 3, and Pierre Dionis, *Cours d'opérations de chirurgie, démontrées au Jardin du Roi*, Paris, Méquignon l'aîne, 1782, p. 11.

19. See David Kunzle, "The Art of Pulling Teeth in the 17th and 19th Centuries: From Public Martyrdom to Private Nightmare and Political Struggle," in Michel Feher, Ramona Nadaff and Nadia Tazi (eds), *Fragments for the History of the Human Body*, Berkeley, 1989, vol. 3, pp. 28–89.

20. On dental pain in the Early Modern period, see N. W. Kerr, "Dental Pain and Suffering prior to the Advent of Modern Dentistry," *British Dental Journal*, 184 (1998): 397–399, as well as Roger King, *The Making of the "Dentiste" in France, 1650–1780*, London, 1999 and, by the same author: "John Hunter and 'The Natural History of the Teeth':

Dentistry, Digestion and the Living Principle," *Journal of History of Medicine and Allied Sciences*, 1994.

21. Pierre Fauchard, *Le Chirurgien-dentiste, ou Traité des dents* [1728], Paris, P. -J. Mariette, 1746, 2 vols. There is also a modern English translation: *The Surgeon Dentist: or, Treatise of the Teeth*, London, Butterworth, 1946. On Hunter, see David E. Postillo, "John Hunter's Contribution to Dentistry," *Dental Historian*, 38 (2001): 13–17. Hunter's book referenced here is *The Natural History of the Human Teeth, Explaining their Structure, Use, Formation, Growth, and Diseases*, London, J. Johnson, 1771.

22. See Michel Dechaume, *Histoire Illustrée de l'art dentaire: stomatologie et odontologie*, Paris, R. Dacosta, 1977. See also Malvin E. Ring, *Dentistry: An Illustrated History*, New York, Abrams, 1985, as well as Colin Jones's excellent article: "Pulling Teeth in Eighteenth Century Paris," *Past and Present*, 166 (2000): 100–145. Colin Jones hits the nail on the head when he asserts that "itinerant tooth-drawers have as rightful a place in the history of theatre as of dentistry;" p. 126.

23. For an interpretation of these changes, see Roy Porter y Colin Jones, *Reassessing Foucault: Power, Medicine, and the Body*, London, Routledge, 1994.

24. See Ian A. Burney, *Bodies of Evidence: Medicine and the Politics of the English Inquest, 1830–1926*, Baltimore, Johns Hopkins University Press, 2000.

25. Quoted by Robert Hanham Collyer, *Early History of Anaesthetic Discovery or Painless Surgical Operations*. London, Vickers, 1877, p. 7: "to do away with pain in Surgical Operations is a visionary impossibility [...] the cutting instrument and pain in Surgical Operations, are two things which cannot be presented to the mind of the one without the other."

26. Benjamin Bell, *Cours complet de chirurgie*, fourth edition, Paris, Barroiss, 1796, vol. VI, Chapter XIV. Quoted by Joyn Kirkup, "Surgery Before General Anaesthesia," in Ronald D. Mann (ed.), *The History of the Management of Pain*, Casterton Hall, Carnforth, The Parthenon Publishing Group, 1988, pp. 17–18.

27. See D. N. Phear, "Thomas Dover 1662–1742: Physician, Privateering Captain, and Inventor of Dover's Powder," *Journal of the History of Medicine and Allied Sciences*, 9 (1954): 139–156.

28. Dionis, *Cours d'opérations de chirurgie*, p. 747; Charles Robert Richet, *Recherches expérimentales et cliniques sur la sensibilité*, Paris, G. Masson, 1877, p. 253.

29. Moore, *A Method*, p. 22.

30. Astley Cooper, *A Treatise on Dislocations and Fractures of the Joints*, London, Longman, 1831, pp. 24–25. Quoted by Kirkup, "Surgery Before Anaesthesia," pp. 20–21. See also Ambroise Tranquille Sassard, "Essai et dissertation sur un moyen à employer avant quelques opérations pour en diminuer la douleur," *Observation sur la physique, sur l'histoire naturelle et sur les arts*, 1780. Included in Jean Pierre Peter, *De la douleur*, Paris, Quai Voltaire, 1993.

31. Moore, *A Method*, p. 31.

32. Griffin, *Dissertatio physiologica inauguralis de dolore*, Edinburgh, J. Moir, 1826, p. 21.

33. Ibid. p. 32.

34. James Wardrop, "Some Observations on a mode of performing operations on irritable patients, with a case where the practice was successfully employed," *Medico-Chirurgical Transactions*, 18 (1819): 273–277.

35. Quoted by Lloyd G. Stevenson, "Suspended Animation and the History of Anaesthesia," *Bulletin of the History of Medicine*, 49 (1975): 482–511, p. 487.

36. S. W. Mitchell, *The Autobiography of a Quack and the Case of George Dedlow*, New York, The Century Co., 1900, p. 124.

37. Alexander Turnbull, *A Treatise on Painful and Nervous Diseases, and on a New Mode of Treatment for diseases of the Eye and Ear*, London, John Churchill, 1837, p. 32.

38. John Hunter, *A Treatise on the Blood, Inflammation and Gun-Shot Wounds*, London, John Richardson, 1794, p. 556.

39. Larrey, *Mémoire sur les amputations des membres à la suite des coups de feu*, Paris, du Pont, An V, 1797.

40. Miller, *of Chloroform*, Edinburgh, Sutherland and Knox, 1848, p. 29.

41. James Miller, *Surgical Experience of Chloroform*, Edinburgh, Sutherland and Knox, 1848, p. 58.

42. See Steven Shapin, *Social History of Truth*, Chicago, University of Chicago Press, 1994. Regarding elaborations of Cartesian methodical doubt in early modern Europe, see Javier Moscoso, *Materialismo y religión. Ciencias de la vida en la Europa Ilustrada*. Barcelona, Serbal, 2000, Chapter II: "Sectas cartesianas."

43. See Taylor Stoehr, "Robert H. Collyer's Technology of the Soul," in Arthur Wrobel (ed.), *Pseudo-Science and Society in 19th Century America*, Lexington, University Press of Kentucky, 1987.

44. Collyer, *Early History*.

45. "The History of Anaesthetic Discovery," *Lancet*, June 11 (1870): 840–844, p. 842.

46. See Alison Winter, "Ethereal Epidemic: Mesmerism and the Introduction of Inhalation Anaesthesia to Early Victoria London," *The Society for the Social History of Science*, (1991): 1–27.

47. Winter, "Ethereal Epidemic," p. 1. See also Stephanie J. Snow's, *Operations Without Pain, The Practice and Science of Anaesthesia in Victorian Britain*, London, Palgrave Macmillan, 2006.

48. George K. Behlmer, "Grave Doubts: Victorian Medicine, Moral Panic, and the Signs of Death," *Journal of British Studies*, 42 (2003): 206–235.

49. See Alison Winter, *Mesmerized: Powers of Mind in Victorian Britain*, Chicago, University of Chicago Press, 1998.

50. See Stevenson, "Suspended Animation and the History of Anaesthesia."

51. Collyer, *Early History*, p. 3.

52. See Thomas L. Haskell, "Capitalism and the Origins of the Humanitarian Sensibility," *American Historical Review*, 90 (June 1985): 547–566. See also, Thomas W. Laqueur, "Bodies, Details, and the Humanitarian Narrative," in Lynn Hunt (ed.), *The New Cultural History*, Berkeley, University of California Press, 1989: 176–204.

53. Collyer, *Early History*, p. 8.

54. *Lancet*, p. 842.

55. F. F. Cartwright, *The English Pioneers of Anesthesia: Beddoes, Davy and Hickman*, Bristol, John Wright, London, Simpkin Marshall, 1952.

56. See Stevenson, "Suspended Animation and the History of Anaesthesia," 482–511.

57. Hodges, *A Narrative*, p. 127.

58. *American Journal of Dental Science*, vol. 7, N 2, December 1846. Quoted in Malvin E. Ring, "Surprise!: The Leaders of Dentistry were not that Pleased with Morton's Discovery," *Bulletin of the History of Dentistry*, 42, 3 (1994): 127–128.

59. Christine Hillam, "The Development of Dental Practice Before 1850," *Medical Historian*, 1 (1988): 10–16. See also H. Berton McCauley, "The First Dental College: Emergence of Dentistry as an Autonomous Profession," *Journal of the History of Dentistry*, 51 (2003): 41–45.

60. Robert Darnton, *Mesmerism and the End of the Enlightenment in France*, Cambridge, MA, Harvard University Press, 1968, See also Alan Gauld, *A History of Hypnotism*,

Cambridge, Cambridge University Press, 1995. Adam Crabtree, *From Mesmer to Freud: Magnetic Sleep and the Roots of Psychological Healing*, New Haven/London, Yale University Press, 1993.

61. Simon Mialle, for instance, published two volumes on animal magnetism in which there were far from rare cases of pain relief. Mialle, *Exposé par ordre alphabétique des cures opérées en France par le magnétisme animal, depuis Mesmer jusqu'a nos jours (1774–1826)*, Paris, J. G. Dentu, 1826.

62. James Braid, *Neurypnology; or The Rationale of Nervous Sleep Considered in Relation with Animal Magnetism*, London, J. Churchill, 1843.

63. *The Lancet*, June 11, 1870, p. 841.

64. Elliotson, *Numerous Cases*, p. 8. On Elliotson, see Roger Cooter, *The Cultural Meaning of Popular Science: Phrenology and the Organization of Consent in the Nineteenth Century*, Cambridge, Cambridge University Press, 1984.

65. James Esdaile, *Mesmerism in India and Its Practical Application in Surgery and Medicine*, London, Longman, 1846.

66. Tuke, *Illustrations*, p. 35.

67. Elliotson, *Numerous Cases*, p. 16.

68. Ludwig Wittgenstein, *Philosophical Investigations*, Oxford, Basil Blackwell, 1953.

69. See David B. Morris, *Cultures of Pain*, Berkeley, University of California Press, 1991. For a contrary view: Elaine Scarry, *The Body in Pain: the Making and Unmaking of the World*, New York/Oxford, Oxford University Press, 1985.

70. Charles Bell, *Idea of New Anatomy of the Brain: Submitted for the Observation of his Friends* [1811], *Journal of Anatomical Physiology*, 3 (1869): 153–166.

71. Richet, *Recherches*, p. 237.

72. William Griffin, *An Essay on the Nature of Pain; with some Considerations on its Principal Varieties and Connected with Disease, and Remarks on the Treatment*, Edinburgh, J. Moir, 1826 , p. 43.

73. John Brown, *Horea Subsecivae*, Edinburgh, Constable, 1859, pp. 308–309, quoted by Kirkup, "Surgery Before Anaesthesia," pp. 25–26.

74. On these issues, see Pernick, *A Calculus of Suffering*, Chapter 7, pp. 148–167.

75. Griffin, *An Essay*, p. 42.

76. Richet, *Recherches*, p. 235.

77. Ibid. p. 243.

78. Pernick, *A Calculus of Suffering*.

79. J. B. Bonnefoy, *De l'influence des passions de l'âme dans les maladies chirurgicales*, Dissertation. Paris, Académie Royale de Chirurgie, 1786, pp. 69–70.

80. William Fergusson, *The Introductory Lecture Delivered at King's College, London, on Opening the Medical Session of 1848–49*, London, John Churchill, 1848, quoted by Collyer, *Early History*, p. 4.

81. Sean M. Quinlan, "Apparent Death in Eighteenth Century France and England," *French History*, 9 (1995): 27–47.

82. London Association for the Prevention of Premature Burial (LAPPB). Behlmer, "Grave Doubts: Victorian Medicine, Moral Panic, and the Signs of Death," *Journal of British Studies*, 42 (2003): 206–235.

83. Daniel Arasse, *La Guillotine et l'imaginaire de la Terreur*, Paris, Flammarion, 1993.

84. *Opinion du Cen. Sue, professeur de médecine et de botanique, sur le supplice de la guillotine*, [sl] [sd]. Paris, 1796.

85. Anonymous, *Anecdotes sur les décapites*, in the form of a letter to M. B..., Membre de l'Institut national, et du Conseil de santé. Paris anné V de la république.
86. J. J. Sue, *Recherches physiologiques et expériences sur la vitalité*, Paris, an VI (1797) "Suivies d'une nouvelle Edition de son Opinion sur le supplice de la guillotine ou sur la douleur qui survit à la décolation." Lues à l'Institut national de France le ii Messidor, an V de la République.
87. See J. J. Sue, *Recherches expérimentales faites sur différents animaux, [...] pour reconnaître quelle est dans les nerfs et dans les fibres musculaires la durée de la force vitale, soit par des effets spontanés, soit par des excitemens produits par le contact de substances métalliques.*
88. Billon, *Dissertation sur la doleur*, Paris, Feugueray, 1803, p. 32.
89. J. Y. Simpson, *On the Inhalation of Vapour of Ether in Surgical Operations*, London, Churchill, 1847, p. 11.
90. Ann Taves, *Fits, Trances, and Visions: Experiencing Religion and Explaining Experience from Wesley to James*. Princeton, Princeton University Press, 1999.
91. William James, *The Varieties of Religious Experience: A Study in Human Nature*. Twentieth Impression. London, New York, Bombay and Calcutta: Longmans, Green, and Co., 1911, p. 387.
92. Ibid.
93. Richet, *Recherches*, pp. 238–239.
94. Vigoroux, *Comptes-rendus de l'Académie des Sciences*, Bachelier, Gauthier-Villars, 1861, p. 202.
95. Simpson, *On the Inhalation of vapour of Ether*, 6ff; see also by the same author *History*, p. 19.
96. Richet, *Recherches*, p. 258.
97. Ibid. p. 262.

6 Narrativity

1. For a general review, see C. Tilley, W. Keane *et al.* (eds), *Handbook of Material Culture*, London, Sage Publications, 2006, Part I, as well as Christopher Tilley, *Metaphor and Material Culture*, First part.
2. See Gerald M. Ackerman, *La vie et l'oeuvre de Jean-Léon Gérôme*, Paris, ACR Édition, 1986, pp. 55–56.
3. Bram Dijkstra, *Idols of Perversity. Fantasies of Feminine Evil in Fin-de-Siècle Culture*, New York, Oxford University Press, 1986.
4. Ackerman, *La vie et l'oeuvre de Gérôme*, p. 142. On Fuchs, see Walter Benjamin, "Eduard Fuchs: Collector and Historian," *New German Critique* 5 (Spring, 1975), 27–58.
5. Émile Zola, *Nana*, [1879] English Translation by Burton Rascoe, Forgotten Books, 1963, p. 9.
6. John K. Noyes, *The Mastery of Submission. Inventions of Masochism*, Ithaca, Cornell Studies in the History of Psychiatry, Cornell University Press, 1997, p. 9. See Theodor Reik, *Masochism in Modern Man* [1941], translation by Margaret H. Biegel and G. Kurth, New York, Farrar, Straus, 1949, p. 383. Reik, a disciple of Freud, wrote the first major book entirely dedicated to masochism. Sigmund Freud [1915], "Instincts and their Vicissitudes." *The Standard Edition of the Complete Psychological Works of Sigmund Freud*, Volume XIV [1914–1916]: On the History of the Psycho-Analytic Movement, Papers on Metapsychology and Other Works, 109–140. See also Freud, [1924] "The Economic Problem of Masochism." *The Standard Edition of the Complete*

Psychological Works of Sigmund Freud, Volume XIX [1923–1925]: The Ego and the Id and Other Works, 155–170. For a study of the general climate, see Peter Gay, *The Cultivation of Hatred: The Bourgeois Experience, from Victoria to Freud*, New York, Norton, 1993, as well as Elaine Showalter, *Sexual Anarchy: Gender and Culture at the Fin de Siècle*, New York, Viking, 1990.

7. Reik, *Masochism in Modern Man*, p. 10.
8. Gilles Deleuze, *Masochism: Coldness and Cruelty*, New York, Zone Books, 1991, p. 22.
9. See Arjurn Appadurai, *The Social Life of Things. Commodities in Cultural Perspective*, [1986], Cambridge, Cambridge University Press, 2006. See José Miguel Marinas, *La fábula del bazar. Orígenes de la Cultura del Consumo*. Madrid, La Balsa de la Medusa, 2001, pp. 39 and *ff.*
10. Richard von Krafft-Ebing, *Psychopathia Sexualis: With Especial Reference to Antipathic Sexual Instinct. A Medico-Forensic Study*, English translation by Francis J. Rebman, London, Rebman, 1899. Unless otherwise specified, all quotations come from this edition. See also Arnold Davidson, "Closing up the Corpses," in A. Davidson, *The Emergence of Sexuality: Historical Epistemology and the Formation of Concepts*, Cambridge, MA/London, Harvard University Press, 2001.
11. Michel Foucault, *The History of Sexuality*, Vol. I, *An Introduction* [1978], New York, Vintage Books, 1990. part 2, Chapter 2, "The Perverse Implantation," p. 43.
12. Krafft-Ebing, *Psychopathia Sexualis*, p. 47.
13. Karl Marx, "The Fetishism of Commodities and the Secret Thereof," in *Capital: A Critique of Political Economy*. Translation by Samuel Moore and Edward Aveling, New York, Modern Library, 1904, pp. 81*ff.*
14. Ibid. p. 95.
15. Sigmund Freud, "Fetishism" [1927], *The Standard Edition of the Complete Psychological Works of Sigmund Freud*, Volume XXI [1927–1931]: The Future of an Illusion, Civilization and its Discontents, and Other Works, 147–158.
16. Sigmund Freud, *Three Essays on the Theory of Sexuality*. [1905] Translation by James Strachey (ed.), New York, Basic Books, p. 26.
17. Cases quoted by Kraft-Ebbing, *Psychopathia Sexualis*, collected by Renate Hauser, "Kraft-Ebbing's Psychological Understanding of Sexual Behaviour," in Roy Porter and Mikulas Teich (eds), *Sexual Knowledge. Sexual Science*, Cambridge, Cambridge University Press, 1994, pp. 210–227, p. 222. See also Alfred Binet, "Le fetichisme dans l'amour," *Études de psychologie expérimentale* [1888], Paris, Octave Doin, 1981.
18. Charles Féré, *The Evolution and Dissolution of the Sexual Instinct* [1899], Paris, Charles Carrington, English translation of the second edition, 1904, p. 177.
19. On the Pygmalion myth, see Facundo Tomás and Isabel Justo (eds), *Pigmalión o el amor por lo creado*. Barcelona, Anthropos, Universidad de Valencia, 2005.
20. Ackerman, *La vie et l'oeuvre de Gérôme*, p. 84.
21. Binet, "Le fétichisme dans l'amour," p. 36.
22. Ibid. p. 84.
23. Denis Diderot, *Le rêve de d'Alembert* [1769] *in Oeuvres philosophiques*, classical Edition by P. Vernière, Paris, Garnier, 1990, pp. 257 and *ff.*
24. Binet, "Le fétichisme," p. 49.
25. Igof Kopytoff, "The Cultural Biography of Things: Commoditization as Process," in A. Appadurai (ed.), *The Social Life of Things*, Cambridge, Cambridge University Press, pp. 65–95. See also Daniel Miller, *Material Culture and Mass Consumption*, Oxford, Basil Blackwell, 1987.

26. Thomas Wetzstein *et al.*, *Sadomasochismus: Szenen und Rituale*, Hamburg, Rowolt, 1993. In relation to the formation of sadomasochistic subcultures and images, see Andreas Spengler, *Sadomasochisten und ihre Subkultur*, Frankfurt, Campus, 1979.
27. Gilles Deleuze, *Difference and Repetition [1968]*, English translation, London, The Athlone Press, 2004.
28. Féré, *Sexual Instinct*, p. 138, called it *algophilia*.
29. For a discussion of these authors, see Ivan Crozier, "Philosophy in the English Boudoir: Havelock Ellis, *Love and Pain*, and Sexological Discourses on Algophilia," *Journal of the History of Sexuality*, 13 (2004): 275–305.
30. Havelock Ellis, *Love and Pain*, in *Studies on the Psychology of Sex*, vol. III, Philadelphia, F. A. Davis, 1904.
31. Ellis, *Love and Pain*, p. 67.
32. Féré, *Sexual Instinct*, p. 165.
33. Ellis, *Love and Pain*, p. 68. Cesare Lombroso and Guglielmo Ferrero, in their *La donna delincuente, la prostitute e la donna normale*, originally published in 1895, tried to relate the imaginary recreation of pain to a supposed variation in female sensitivity to pain. English translation: *Criminal Woman, the Prostitute and the Normal Woman*, Durham/London, Duke University Press, 2004.
34. Ellis, *Love and Pain*, p. 70.
35. Ibid. p. 67.
36. Cf Robert Tobin, "Masochism and Identity," in Michael C. Finke and Carl Niekerk (eds.), *One Hundred Years of Masochism*, Amsterdam/Atlanta, Rodopi, 2000, pp. 33–52, and Michael C. Finke, "An Introduction," in the same book.
37. Charles Féré, "Le sadisme aux courses de Taureaux," *Revue de Médecine*, August, 1900. Quoted by Ellis, *Love and Pain*, pp. 134–135.
38. Féré, *Sexual Instinct*, pp. 156*ff*.
39. Giovanni Giacomo Casanova, *Mémoires du vénitien J. Casanova de Seingalt*, vol. VIII, Paris, Tournachon-Molin, 1825–1829, pp. 74–76.
40. On the use of flagellation in England, see Iwan Bloch, *Sexual Life in England*, London, Corgi Books, 1965, Chapter 12: "Flagellomania," pp. 270–322.
41. Krafft-Ebing, *Psychopathia Sexualis*, p. 135.
42. Noyes, *The Mastery of Submission*, p. 53.
43. Féré, *Sexual Instinct*, p. 163.
44. Ellis, *Love and Pain*, p. 72.
45. Noyes, *The Mastery of Submission*, p. 8. John K. Noyes considers that a proper understanding of Sacher-Masoch's work should also include his "fascination with gross social injustice and violence in Eastern Europe." See also Larry Wolff, *Inventing Eastern Europe: The Map of Civilization on the Mind of the Enlightenment*, Stanford, California, Stanford University Press, 1994; especially Chapter 2: "Possessing Eastern Europe: Sexuality, Slavery, and Corporal Punishment."
46. Walter Hough, "A Bayanzi Execution," *Science*, 9 [1887]: 615.
47. Robert Howard Russell, "Glave's Career," *The Century, a Popular Quarterly*, 50, 6 [1895]: 864–868. Both expeditionists were quoted by the anthropologist Lévy-Bruhl in *La mentalidad primitiva* [1922], Buenos Aires, La Pléyade, 1972. For a review of the historical-political events in the last decades of the nineteenth century, see E. J. Hobsbawm, *The Age of Empire, 1875–1914*, London, Weidenfeld and Nicolson, 1987.
48. The first reference where I have found similar Chinese models of dwellings was in the universal exhibition in St Louis, in Missouri, in 1904.

49. George Henry Mason, *The Punishment of China. Illustrated by Twenty-Two Engravings: With Explanations in English and French*, London, W. Bulmer, 1801.
50. Krafft-Ebing, *Psychopathia Sexualis*, p. 76. Krafft-Ebing distinguishes between *perversion*, that is a disease, and *perversity*, that he considers a vice.
51. Ellis, *Love and Pain*, p. 149.
52. Novalis quoted by Féré, *Sexual Instinct*, p. 169.
53. William James, *The Varieties of Religious Experience*, London: Longmans, Green, & Co., 1902. The book was published after James's lectures in Edinburgh between 1901 and 1902.
54. Louis-Émile Bougaud, *Histoire de la bienhereuse Marguerite Marie*, Paris, C. Poussielgue, 1894, pp. 265–271. Quoted by James, *Varieties of Religious Experience*, "Lectures", xi, xii and xiii.
55. James Kiernan, "Responsibility in Sexual Perversion," *Chicago Medical Recorder* (March, 1892): 185–210.
56. Sor Jeanne des Anges, *Soeur Jeanne des Anges, autobiographie d'une hystérique possédée*. Paris, Delahaye et Lecrosnier, 1886.
57. Gilles de la Tourette, *Traité clinique et thérapeutique de l'hystérie, d'après l'enseignement de la Salpêtrière*, Paris, E. Plon, Nourrit et Cie, 1891–1895, p. 223.
58. Teresa de Ávila, *Vie de sainte Thérese écrite par elle-mème*, French translation by M. Bouix, 1889, vol. I, p. 364. See also, P. G. Hahn, "Les phénomenes hystériques et les révélations de sainte Thérése," *Revue des Questions scientifiques de Bruxelles*, vol. XIII, 1883.
59. Jacques Lacan, "God and the Jouissance of The Woman," in *Feminine Studies*, Juliet Mitchell and Jacqueline Rose (eds), New York, Norton, 1982, p. 147. Gian Lorenzo Bernini's sculpture [1598–1680], at Cappella Cornaro, Chiesa di Santa Maria della Vittoria (Roma), was made between 1647 and 1652.
60. Krafft-Ebing, *Psychopathia Sexualis*, p. 36.
61. Anonymous, *History of Flagellation*, London, 1888, p. 53.
62. Piero Camporesi, *The Incorruptible Flesh: Bodily Mutilation and Mortification in Religion and Folklore*, Cambridge, Cambridge University Press, 1988, p. 61.
63. See Niklaus Largier, *In Praise of the Whip: A Cultural History of Arousal*, New York, Zone Books, 2007. See also, George Ryley Scott, *The History of Corporal Punishment* [1968], London, Senate, 1996.
64. Ian Gibson, *The English Vice: Beating, Sex, and Shame in Victorian England and after*, London, Duckworth, 1978.
65. Ellis, *Love and Pain*, p. 107.
66. John Cleland, *Fanny Hill. Or Memoirs of a Woman of Pleasure* [1749], London, Penguin, 1985, pp. 180–190.
67. Johann Heinrich Meibom, *Tractatus de usu flagrorum in re medica et veneria*, Lübeck, 1639.
68. Franz Christian Paullini, *Flagellum salutis*, Frankfurt, In Verlegung Friederich Knochens, 1698; [Amédé Doppet], *Aphrodisiaque externe, ou traité du fouet et de ses effets sur le physique de l'amour, ouvrage médico-philosophique*, [sl., sn], 1788. p. 26.
69. Benedetto Mojon, *Sull'utilità del dolore*, Genoa, Y. Gravier, 1818, p. 11.
70. Jacques Alexandre Salgues, *De la douleur considérée sous le point de vue de son utilité en médecine et dans ses rapports avec la physiologie, l'hygiène, la pathologie et la thérapeutique*, Dijon, V. Lagier, 1823, p. 151. On history of flagellation, see Ernst Kern, "Cultural-Historical Aspects of Pain," in *Pain: A Medical and Anthropological Challenge*, J. Brihate, F. Loew, and H. W. Pia (eds), *Acta Nerochirurgica*, 38, suppl. [1987]: 187–188.
71. Ellis, *Love and Pain*, 108.

72. Cleland, *Fanny Hill*, p. 182.
73. Here I follow Lucy Bending's book, *The Representation of Bodily Pain in Late Nineteenth-Century English Culture*, Oxford, Oxford University Press, 2000.
74. William Acton, *Functions and Disorders of the Reproductive Organs*, Philadelphia, Lindsay and Blakiston, 1867. See Ivan Crozier, " 'Rough Winds do Shake the Darling Buds of May': A Note on William Acton and the Sexuality of the (Male) Child," *Journal of Family History*, 26 (2001): 411–420, p. 414.
75. Ellis, *Love and Pain*, p. 109. Curiously, Ellis refers here to an article devoted to Udall in the *Dictionary of National Biography*.
76. Acton, *Functions and Disorders*, p. 23.
77. The same considerations had already been made by Krafft-Ebing, *Psychopathia Sexualis*, p. 35.
78. [Anonymous], *History of Flagellation among Different Nations*, London, 1888.
79. Alexander Bain, *Mind and Body. The Theories and their Relation*, second edition, Henry S. King, 1873, p. 175. Also quoted by Bending, *The Representation of Bodily Pain*, pp. 272–273.
80. Krafft-Ebing, *Psychopathia Sexualis*, p. 201.
81. Leopold von Sacher-Masoch, *Venus in Furs*, translated by J. Neugroschel, New York/London, Penguin Books, 2000, p. 42.
82. Krafft-Ebing, *"Detailed autobiography of a masochist,"* case 41 of the 10th edition of *Psychopathia Sexualis*, pp. 117*ff*. According to Oosterhuis, even the term "masochist" was suggested to Krafft-Ebing by this correspondent. See Harry Oosterhuis, *Stepchildren of Nature. Krafft-Ebing, Psychiatry and the Making of Sexual Identity*, Chicago/London, University of Chicago Press, 2000, pp. 174–175.
83. Roy F. Baumeister, *Masochism and the Self*, Hillsdale, NJ, Erlbaum, 1989, p. 53. Also quoted by John Noyes, *The Mastery of Submission*, p. 9. See also Gerd Falk and Thomas S. Weinberg, "Sadomasochism and Popular Western Culture", in Thomas Weinberg and Levi Kamel (eds), *S and M: Studies in Sadomasochism*, New York, Prometheus, 1983, p. 137.
84. Sacher-Masoch, *Venus in Furs*, pp. 117.
85. On this matter in Rousseau's case, see Jean Starobinksi, *Rousseau, La transparencia y el obstáculo*, Madrid, Taurus, 1983.
86. See Michael Finke, "Sacher-Masoch, Turgenev and Other Russians"; see also Daniel Rancour-Laferriere, "Lev Tolstoy's Moral Masochism in the Late 1880's," pp. 155–171, in Michael M. Finke and Carl Niekert (eds), *One Hundred Years of Masochism. Literary Texts, Social and Cultural Contexts*, Amsterdam, Atlanta, GA, Rodopi, 2000, pp. 119–139.
87. Jean-Jacques Rousseau, *Confessions*, book I, part I. Quoted by Ellis, *Love and Pain*, p. 112.
88. Harry Oosterhuis, *Stepchildren of Nature*, especially Chapter 15: "Autobiography and Sexual Identity." Also Ian Hacking, "Making up People," in Thomas Haller *et al.* (eds), *Reconstructing Individualism*, Stanford, Stanford University Press, 1986.
89. Krafft-Ebing, *Psychopathia Sexualis*, p. 124.
90. Ibid. p. 121.
91. Ibid. p. 122.
92. The boundaries between reality and fiction belonging to sadomasochism permeate the film world. See Gaylyn Studlar, *In the Realm of Pleasure: Von Sternberg, Dietrich and the Masochistic Aesthetic*, Urbana, University of Illinois Press, 1988. For

an overview of Dietrich's films, see Carol Siegel, *Male Masochism: Modern Revisions of the Story of Love*, Bloomington, Indiana University Press, 1995; especially regarding Cavani's *The Night Porter*, pp. 81–87.
93. Krafft-Ebing, *Psychopathia Sexualis*, p. 138.
94. Ibid. p. 124.
95. Ibid. p. 131.
96. On the construction of a similar model in the case of *eonism* (or transvestism) in Havelock Ellis's case, see Ivan Crozier, "Havelock Ellis, Eonism and the Patient's Discourse; or Writing a Book About Sex," *History of Psychiatry*, 9 (2000): 125–154.
97. For a study on background of psychoanalysis, see Gay, *The Cultivation of Hatred*.

7 Coherence

1. Charles Robert Richet, *Recherches expérimentales et cliniques sur la sensibilité*, Paris, G. Masson, 1877, p. 251.
2. J. Strachey, "Notes Upon a Case of Obsessional Neurosis," *The Standard Edition of the Complete Psychological Works of Sigmund Freud, Volume X (1909): Two Case Histories ("Little Hans" and the "Rat Man")*, 1909: 151–318.
3. George Berkeley, *Three Dialogues Between Hylas and Philonous* [1713], edited by Jonathan Dancy, Oxford, Oxford University Press, 1999, p. 65.
4. This is not exactly Berkeley's view.
5. Arthrur Kleinman, *Illness Narratives, Suffering, Healing and the Human Condition*, New York, Basic Books, 1988, Chapters 1 and 2.
6. M. Foucault, *The Birth of the Clinic: An Archeology of Medical Perception* (1963), translation by A. M. Sheridan. London, Tavistock Publications, 1973.
7. Edward Shorter, *From Paralysis to Fatigue: A History of Psychosomatic Illness in the Modern Era*, New York, Free Press; Toronto, Maxwell Macmillan Canada; New York, Maxwell Macmillan International, 1992, p 290.
8. J. P. Williams, "Psychical Research and Psychiatry in Late Victorian Britain," in W. F. Bynum, Roy Porter and Michael Sheperd (eds), *The Anatomy of Madness*, vol. I, London, Tavistock, 1985.
9. Quoted by Xavier Bichat, *Physiological Researches on Life and Death*, English translation by Gold, London, Longman, Hurst, Rees, Orme and Browne, 1815, pp. 62*ff.*
10. See Henri Ellenberger, *The Discovery of the Unconscious. The History and Evolution of Dynamic Psychiatry*, New York, Basic Books, 1970.
11. On this topic see Chris Alma and H. Merskey, "Changes in the Meaning of Neuralgia," *History of Psychiatry*, 5 (1994): 429–474.
12. George M. Beard, *A Practical Treatise on Nervous Exhaustion (Neurasthenia)*, New York, William Wood, 1880, See Edward Shorter, *From Paralysis to Fatigue. A History of Psychosomatic Illness in the Modern Era*, New York, Free Press, 1993, pp. 220*ff.* George Frederick Drinka, *The Birth of Neurosis. Myth, Malady, and the Victorians*, New York, Simon and Schuster, 1984, 184*ff.* Martin Stone, "Shell Shock and the Psychologists," in R. Porter, W. F. Bynum and M. Shepherd (eds), *The Anatomy of Madness: Essays in the History of Psychiatry. The Asylum and its Psychiatry*, vol. III, London, Routledge, 1988.
13. Andrew Hodgkiss, *From Lesion to Metaphor: Chronic Pain in British, French and German Medical Writings, 1800–1914*. Amsterdam, Atlanta, GA, Rodopi, 2000. Bichat, did, in

fact, recognize pain with no lesion: "Doctors have not given too much attention to this cause of pain that is often developed in a considerable extension, with no apparent lesion," in Bichat, *Anatomie générale, précédée des recherches physiologiques sur la vie et la mort*, Paris, Ladrange, 1818, vol. 1, p. 184.

14. On the history of somatization, see Edward Shorter, *From the Mind to the Body: The Cultural Origins of Psychosomatic Symptoms*, New York, Free Press, 1994.
15. G. W. F. Hegel, *Phenomenology of Spirit*. Translation by A. V. Miller. Oxford, Clarendon Press, 1977, B. Self-Consciousness.
16. Leo Tolstoy, *The Death of Ivan Ilyich*, London, Penguin Books, 1960, p. 109.
17. Ibid. p. 113.
18. See A. D. Hodgkiss, "Chronic Pain in Nineteenth-Century British Medical Writings," *History of Psychiatry*, ii (1991): 27–40.
19. Benjamin Collins Brodie, *Lectures Illustrative of Certain Local Nervous Affections*, London, Longman, 1837, p. 14.
20. Ibid. pp. 44–45.
21. Alexander Turnbull, *A Treatise on Painful and Nervous Diseases, and on a New Mode of Treatment for diseases of the Eye and Ear*, London, John Churchill, 1837.
22. Brodie, *Lectures*, p. 37.
23. John Hilton, *On Rest and Pain: A Course on the Influence of Mechanical and Physiological Rest in the Treatment of Accidents and Surgical Diseases*, London, George Bell, second edition, 1877, p. 62.
24. Ibid. pp. 63–64.
25. François Louis Isidore Valleix, *Traité des néuralgies ou affections douloureuses des nerfs*, Paris, J. B. Baillière, 1841, p. 653.
26. Herbert W. Page, *Injuries of the Spine and Spinal Cord without Apparent Mechanical Lesion, and Nervous Shock, in their Surgical and Medico-Legal Aspects*, London, J. & A. Churchill, 1883. John E. Erichsen, *On Concussion of the Spine: Nervous Shock and other Obscure Injuries of the Nervous System in their Clinical and Medico-Legal Aspects*, p. 287. For the notion of "railway spine," see Ralph Harrington, *The Neuroses of the Railway: Trains, Travel and Trauma in Britain, c. 1850 – c. 1900*, PhD, Dissertation, 1998, especially Chapter 4: "Railway spine." See also Michael R. Trimble, *Post-Traumatic Neuroses: from Railway Spine to Whiplash*, Chichester, John Wiley, 1981. Ralph Harrington, "The Railway Accident: Trains, Trauma and Technological Crisis in Nineteenth Century Britain," in Mark S. Micale and Paul Lerner (eds), *Traumatic Past: History and Trauma in the Modern Age, 1870–1930*, New Haven, Conn, Yale University Press, 1998. See also Allan Young, *The Harmony of Illusions: Inventing Post-Traumatic Stress Disorder*, Princeton, Princeton University Press, 1995.
27. John Eric Erichsen, "Six Lectures on certain obscure Injuries of the Nervous System commonly met with as the Result of Shocks to the Body received in Collisions on Railways" [1866], *On Concussion of the Spine*.
28. Page, *Injuries of the Spine*, p. 3.
29. Harrington, "The Railway Accident." See also Wolfgang Schivelbush, *The Railway Journey: The Industrialization of Time and Space in the Nineteenth Century*, Oxford, Blackwell, 1977.
30. Harrington, "The Railway Accident," p. 21. See also E. J. Hobsbawm, *The Ages of Empire: 1875–1914*, London, Weidenfeld and Nicholson, 1987, especially p. 27ff.
31. Eric Caplan, "Trains, Brains, and Sprains: Railway Spine and the Origins of Psychoneuroses," *Bulletin of the History of Medicine* 69, 3 (1995): 387–419.

32. Herbert Page, *Railway Injuries: with Special Reference to those of the Back and the Nervous System, in their Medico-Legal and Clinical Aspects*, London, Charles Griffin & Co, 1891, pp. 151–152.
33. Alfred Ogan, *Railway Collisions Prevented*, London, G. J. Pope, 1855, p. vii.
34. *The Lancet*, 11 January 1862, p. 151. Quoted by Harrington, "The Railway Accident," p. 114.
35. Page, *Railway Injuries*, p. 153.
36. Ibid. p. 103.
37. Ibid. p. 226.
38. Samuel Wilks, *Lectures on Diseases of the Nervous System*, London, J. & A. Churchill, 1878, p. 374.
39. Not for nothing, the chapter title is "Malingering."
40. Page, *Railway Injuries*, p. 157.
41. Ibid. p. 236.
42. Ibid. p. 255.
43. Pierre Janet, *The Mental State of Hystericals. A Study of Mental Stigmata and Mental Accidents; with a Preface by Professor J. M. Charcot*, translation by Caroline Rollin Corson, New York and London, G. P. Putnam's Sons, 1901, p. 32.
44. On the continuity of war trauma, see Stone: "Shell Shock and the Psychologists;" as well as Joanna Bourke, *Dismembering the Male: Men's Bodies, Britain and the Great War*, London, Reaktion Books, 1996.
45. Allan Young, "Suffering and the Origins of Traumatic Memory," in A. Kleinman, V. Das and M. M. Lock (eds), *Social Suffering*, Berkeley, University of California Press, 1997, p. 246. See also Henri F. Ellenberger, "The pathogenic Secret and its Theraupetics," in Mark Micale (ed.), *Beyond the Unconscious: Essays of Henry F. Ellenberger in the History of Psychiatry*, Princeton, Princeton University Press, 1993, pp. 341–359.
46. Janet, *The Mental State*, 1901, p. x.
47. Peter Gay, *Freud: A Life for Our Time*, New York, W. W. Norton and Co., 1988, p. 50. On pain in Freud, see Annie Aubert, *La douleur. Originalité d'une théorie freudienne*, Paris, PUF, 1996.
48. Quoted by Gay, *Freud*, p. 74.
49. Freud, *On the Psychical Mechanism of Hysterical Phenomena* [1893], in Freud, *The Standard Edition of the Complete Psychological Works*, English translation by James Strachey, London, Hogarth Press, 1955, vol. II.
50. Ibid. pp. 116–117.
51. Ibid. p. 118. Emphasis in the original.
52. On the history of the unconscious, see Ellenberger, *The Discovery of the Unconscious*, see also Ronald Melzack, *The Puzzle of Pain*, Harmondsworth, Penguin Education, 1973, pp. 147–162.
53. Peter Smith and O. R. Jones, *The Philosophy of the Mind: An Introduction*. Cambridge, Cambridge University Press, 1986.
54. Paul Briquet, *Traité clinique et thérapeutique de l'hystérie*, Paris, J. B. Baillière, 1859, p. 205.
55. José María López Piñero, *Orígenes históricos del concepto de neurosis*, Valencia, Cátedra e Instituto de Historia de la Medicina, 1963. An important part of the definition of these new functional diseases, what the Spanish historian López Piñero called the "*principle of negative lesion*," comes from Georget.
56. Étienne-Jean Georget, *De la Physiologie du système nerveux et spécialement du cerveau, recherches sur les maladies nerveuses en général et en particulier sur le siège, la nature*

et le traitement de l'hystérie, de l'hypochondrie, de l'épilepsie et de l'asthme convulsif, Paris, Baillière, 1821, vol. II, pp. 187–188. See Mark S. Micale, *Approaching Hysteria: Disease and its Interpretations*, Princeton, NJ, Princeton University Press, 1995.

57. Georget, *De la Physiologie*, pp. 317–318.
58. Ibid. pp. 319–320.
59. Ibid. pp. 268–269.
60. See Freud, Strachey, J. (1890). Psychical (or Mental) Treatment (1890). *The Standard Edition of the Complete Psychological Works of Sigmund Freud*, Volume VII *(1901–1905): A Case of Hysteria, Three Essays on Sexuality and Other Works*, 281–302, p. 287: "However pains may be caused—even by imagination—they themselves are no less real and no less violent on that account."
61. Georget, *De la Physiologie du système nerveux*, pp. 268–269.
62. Sophocles, *Philoctetes*, Trans. Carl Phillips, Oxford, Oxford University Press, 2003.
63. Daniel Hack Tuke, *Illustrations of the Influence of the Mind upon the Body in Health and Disease, designed to Elucidate the Action of the Imagination*, London, J. & A. Churchill, 1872, p. 127.
64. Louis Basile Carré de Montgeron, *La Vérité des miracles opérés à l'intercession de M. de Pâris et autres appellans démontrée contre M. l'archevêque de Sens*, Utrecht, chez les libraires de la Compagnie, 1737. Quoted by Tuke, *Illustrations*, p. 128.
65. Pierre Janet, *L'automatisme psychologique: essai de psychologie expérimentale sur les formes inférieures de l'activité humaine* [1889], Paris, Félix Alcan, 1903 (fourth edition), p. 442.
66. Philippe Hecquet, *Le naturalisme des convulsions dans les maladies de l'épidémie convulsionnaire*, Rouen, Jorre, 1733.
67. See Jacques Fontaine, *Des marques des sorciers et de la réelle possession que le diable prend sur le corps des hommes*, Lyon, Calude Larjot, 1611, p. 7.
68. Janet, *L'automatisme*, p. viii.
69. Wilhelm Max Wundt, *Éléments de psychologie physiologique. Précédés d'une nouvelle préface de l'auteur et d'une introduction par M. D. Nolen*, French translation by É. Rouvier, Paris, F. Alcan, 1886, vol. I, p. 305.
70. Janet, *The Mental State of Hystericals*, p. 40.
71. See also A. Binet, "Contribution à l'étude de la douleur chez les hystériques," *Revue Philosophique*, ii (1889): 169ff.
72. Albert Pitres, *Leçons cliniques sur l'hystérie et hypnotisme: faites à l'Hôpital Saint-André de Bordeaux*, Paris, O. Doin, 1891, vol. I, pp. 181–188; Georges Gilles de la Tourette, *Traité clinique et thérapeutique de l'hystérie, d'après l'enseignement de la Salpêtrière*, Paris, E. Plon, Nourrit et Cie, 1891, p. 222.
73. Janet, *The Mental State of Hystericals*, p. 314.
74. Ibid. p. xvi.
75. Allan Young, *The Harmony of Illusions: Inventing Post-Traumatic Stress Disorder*, Princeton, NJ, Princeton University Press, 1997, pp. 36–38 and 77–81. Also Kenneth Levin, *Freud's Early Psychology of the Neuroses: a Historical Perspective*, Pittsburgh, Pittsburgh University Press, 1978.
76. Briquet, *Traité clinique et thérapeutique*, p. 310: "the remembrance, the image of a past pain, seems to be associated with a particular sensation and reproduces itself as soon as this signal is given."
77. S. Freud and J. Breuer, *On the Psychical Mechanism of Hysterical Phenomena* [1893], in Freud, The Standard Edition of the complete Psychological Works, English translation by James Strachey, London, Hogarth Press, 1955, vol II, p. 3: "*the connection*

between the provocation and the symptom may be symbolical: A moral pain may engender neuralgia, a moral disgust start vomiting."
78. Ibid. pp. 9 and 10.
79. Ibid. p. 304.
80. S. Freud, *The Psychotherapy of Hysteria* [1895], in Freud, The Standard Edition of the complete Psychological Works, vol. II, p. 269. "distressing nature, calculated to arouse the affects of shame, of self-reproach and of psychical pain, and the feeling of being harmed; they were all of a kind that one would have preferred not to have experienced, that one would rather forget." The relationship between memory and forgetting is mediated by pain. If forgetting produces pain, memory does too. That is the reason why pain comes to be present again in the so-called transference mechanisms.
81. S. Freud and J. Breuer. Preface to the Second Edition of Studies on Hysteria. *The Standard Edition of the Complete Psychological Works of Sigmund Freud, Volume II (1893–1895): Studies on Hysteria*, 1908.On these issues, see Aubert, *La douleur.*
82. See Immanuel Kant, *Transición de los principios metafísicos de la ciencia natural a la física.* Spanish edition by Félix Duque, Madrid, Editora Nacional, 1983.

8 Reiteration

1. Adam Smith, *The Theory of Moral Sentiments*, Indianapolis, Liberty Fund, 1984, p. 29.
2. The case appears collected in Alexander Turnbull, *A Treatise on Painful and Nervous Diseases, and on a New Mode of Treatment for Diseases of the Eye and Ear*, London, John Churchill, 1837, p. 96ff.
3. Ibid. p. 106.
4. Jean Pierre Falret, *De l'hypochondrie et du suicide. Considérations sur les causes, sur le siege et le traitement de ces maladies, sur les moyens d'en arrêter les progress et d'en prevenir le développement*, Paris, Croullebois, 1822, p. 157.
5. Émile Durkheim, *Le Suicide. Etude de sociologie* [1897]. Translated by John A. Spaulding and George Simpson. Glencoe, IL, The Free Press of Glencoe, 1997.
6. Isabelle Baszanger, *Inventing Pain Medicine. From the Laboratory to the Clinic*, London, Rutgers University Press, 1998. English translation of original French edition, published in 1995, p. 3. Jennifer Beinart, " 'The Snowball effect': The growth of the treatment of intractable pain in postwar Britain," in Ronald D. Mann (ed.), *The History of the Management of Pain*, New Jersey, The Parthenon Publishing Group, 1988, pp. 179–186. See also Jason Szabo, *Incurable and Intolerable. Chronic Disease and Slow Death in Nineteenth-Century France*, New Brunswick, New Jersey and London, Rutgers University Press, 2009, especially, Chapter 10.
7. Sarah Natas, *The Relief of Pain: The Birth and Development of the Journal* Pain *from 1975 to 1985 and its Place within Changing Concepts of Pain*, B.Sc. Dissertation, University College, 1996.
8. Herbert Snow, *The Palliative Treatment of Incurable Cancer, with an Appendix of the Use of the Opium-Pipe*, London, J. & A. Churchill, 1890. On these matters, see also David Clark, "The Rise and Demise of the Brompton Cocktail" and Christina Faull and Alexander Nicholson, "Taking Myths out of the Magic: Establishing the Use of Opioids in the Management of Cancer Pain," in Marcia L. Meldrum (ed.), *Opioids and Pain Relief: A Historical Perspective*, Seattle, IASP Press, 2003, pp. 111–129.
9. William Munk, *Medical Treatment in Aid of Easy Death*, London, Longmans, Green, and Co., 1887.

10. Ronald Melzack and Patrick D. Wall, *The Challenge of Pain* (1982), London, Penguin, 1996, pp. 36*ff.*

11. J. J. Bonica, *Proceedings on the First World Congress on Pain*, Raven Books, New York, 1976, p. 17. Quoted by Natas, *The Relief of Pain*. p. 22.

12. Marcia L. Meldrum, "A Capsule History of Pain Management," *Journal of the American Medical Association*, 290 (2003): 2470–2475. On the development of aspirin, see Diarmuid Jeffreys, *Aspirin: The Remarkable Story of a Wonder Drug*, London, Bloomsbury, 2004.

13. On the one hand, throughout the nineteenth century, living conditions fostered increased life expectancy, leading to more people with chronic diseases. Cancer, for instance, known since time immemorial, began to be perceived as a problem requiring serious scientific attention only at the beginning of the twentieth century. Regarding breast cancer, see Daniel de Moulin, *A Short History of Breast Cancer*, Boston, The Hague, Dordrecht, Martines Nijhoff Publishers, 1983; Robert A. Aronowitz, *Unnatural History. Breast Cancer and American Society*, Cambridge, Cambridge University Press, 2007. Equally interesting in relation to the social nature of the disease, see Barron H. Lerner, *The Breast Cancer Wars. Hope, Fear, and the Pursuit of a Cure in Twentieth-Century America*, Oxford, Oxford University Press, 2001. For a general history of cancer, see Siddhartha Mukherjee, *The Emperor of All Maladies: A Biography of Cancer*, London, Fourth State, 2011.

14. Arthur Kleinman, Paul E. Brodwin, Byron J. Good and Mary-Jo DelVecchio Good: "Pain as Human Experience. An introduction," in Mary-Jo Delvecchio *et al.* (eds), *Pain as Human Experience: An Anthropological Perspective*. London and Los Angeles, University of California Press, 1992, p. 3.

15. AISP provides a definition of pain which is worth quoting at length:

> *An unpleasant sensory and emotional experience associated with actual or potential tissue damage, or described in terms of such damage. Note: The inability to communicate verbally does not negate the possibility that an individual is experiencing pain and is in need of appropriate pain-relieving treatment. Pain is always subjective. Each individual learns the application of the word through experiences related to injury in early life. Biologists recognize that those stimuli which cause pain are liable to damage tissue. Accordingly, pain is that experience we associate with actual or potential tissue damage. It is unquestionably a sensation in a part or parts of the body, but it is also always unpleasant and therefore also an emotional experience. Experiences which resemble pain but are not unpleasant, e.g., pricking, should not be called pain. Unpleasant abnormal experiences (dysesthesias) may also be pain but are not necessarily so because, subjectively, they may not have the usual sensory qualities of pain.*
>
> *Many people report pain in the absence of tissue damage or any likely pathophysiological cause; usually this happens for psychological reasons. There is usually no way to distinguish their experience from that due to tissue damage if we take the subjective report. If they regard their experience as pain and if they report it in the same ways as pain caused by tissue damage, it should be accepted as pain. This definition avoids tying pain to the stimulus. Activity induced in the nociceptor and nociceptive pathways by a noxious stimulus is not pain, which is always a psychological state, even though we may well appreciate that pain most often has a proximate physical cause.*

16. See J. Moscoso, "Volkomene Monstren und unheilvole Gestalten. Zur Naturalisierung der Monstrosität im 18 Jahrhundert," in Michael Hagner, (ed.), *Der Falsche Korper*, pp. 56–72, Göttingen, Wallstein Verlag, Second edition, 2005.

17. Wall and Melzack, *The Challenge of Pain*, pp. 284*ff.*

18. W. K. Livingston, *Pain Mechanisms: A Physiologic Interpretation of Causalgia and Its Related States*, New York, The Macmillan Company, 1943.

19. John Kent Spender, *Therapeutic Means for the Relief of Pain*, London, Macmillan and Co., 1874, p. 7, 17–18. See David Sinclair, *Cutaneous Sensation*, London, Oxford University Press, 1967, p. 8*ff*. Henri Piéron, *The Sensations. Their Functions, Processes and Mechanisms*, London, 1952, especially Chapter 6: "Algic Excitation." For a history of the critiques of the theory of specificity, see William Livingston, *Pain and Suffering* (1957), Seattle, IASP Press, 1998.

20. This first classification was published in the journal *Pain*. H. Merskey, ed., "Classification of Chronic Pain: Descriptions of Chronic Pain Syndromes and Definitions of Pain Terms," *Pain*, supplement, 3 (1986) 1–225. Reprinted in 2002, by IASP Press.

21. René Lériche, *La chirurgie de douleur*, [1937], Paris, Masson and Cie, 1949, p. 30.

22. Martha Stoddard Holmes, " 'The Grandest Badge of His Art': Three Victorian Doctors, Pain Relief, and the Art of Medicine," in Marcia L. Meldrum (ed.), *Opioids and Pain Relief: A Historical Perspective*, Seattle, IASP Press, 2003, pp. 21–34.

23. Weldon Fell, *Treatise on Cancer, and Its Treatment*, London, John Churchill, 1857, pp. 13*ff*. For a classification of types of cancers, see H. Snow, *Cancers and the Cancer-Process*, London, J. & Churchill, 1893, pp. 28*ff*, as well as J. Bland-Sutton, *Tumors. Innocent and Malignant. Their Clinical Characters and Appropriate Treatment*, London, Paris, New York, Casswell and Company [1893], 1903.

24. N. D. Jewson, "The Disappearance of the sick man from the medical cosmology, 1770–1870," *Sociology*, 10 (1979): 225–244.

25. James Mackenzie, *The Future of Medicine*, London, Oxford University Press, 1919, pp. 31–32. Mackenzie, 1919, p. 67.

26. John Ryle, *The Natural History of Disease*, [1928], second edition, London, New York, Toronto, Oxford University Press, 1948, especially Chapter 3: "The Clinical Study of Pain. With Special Reference to the Pains of Visceral Disease" p. 438, as well as John Ryle, *The Aims and Methods of Medical Science*, Cambridge, Cambridge University Press, 1935, pp. 35–36. On Ryle, Dorothy Porter, "John Ryle: of Revolution?" in D. Porter and R. Porter, (eds), *Doctors, Politics and Society*, Amsterdam, Rodopi, 1993, pp. 247–274. See also Linda G. Garro, "Chronic Illness and the Construction of Narratives," in Mary-Jo Delvecchio Good, *et al.* (eds), *Pain as Human Experience. An Anthropological Perspective*, Berkeley, Los Angeles, London, 1992, pp. 100–137.

27. See Shirley du Boulay, *Ciceley Saunders. Founder of the Modern Hospice Movement*, London, Hodder and Stoughton, 1984, especially pp. 172*ff*.

28. John Kent Spender, *Therapeutics Means for the Relief of Pain*, London, Macmillan and Co., 1874, p. 7, pp. 17–18.

29. Lériche, *La chirurgie de douleur*, pp. 13–14. On Lériche, see Rosalyne Rosalyne Rey, *History of Pain*, translated by Louise Elliott Wallace and by J. A. and S. W. Cadden, Paris, La Découverte, 1993. pp. 331*ff*.

30. K. D. Keele, *Anatomies of Pain*, Oxford, Blackwell Scientific Publications, 1957, p. v.

31. On polyneuritis, particularly linked to alcoholism, see Jean-Charles Sournia, *Histoire de l'alcoolisme*, Paris, Flammarion, 1986. See also Caroline Moriceau, *Les Douleurs de l'industrie. L'hygiénisme industriel en France, 1860–1914*, doctoral thesis, EHESS, 2002.

32. Liza Picard, *Victorian London, The Life of a City 1840–1870*, London, Phoenix, 2006, p. 232.

33. Henry Mayhew, *London Labour and the London Poor*, London, Penguin, 1985, p. 213. Friedrich Engels, *The Condition of the Working Class in England: From Personal Observation and Authentic Sources*, Moscow, Progress Publishers, 1973.

34. On elusive diseases, see Ian Hacking, *Mad Travelers: Reflections on the Reality of Transient Mental Illnesses*, London, University of Virginia Press, 1998; and *Rewriting the Soul: Multiple Personality and the Sciences of Memory*, Princeton, NJ, Princeton University Press, 1995.

35. On neurasthenia, see G. F. Drinka, *The Birth of Neurosis: Myth, Malady and the Victorians*, New York, Simon and Schuster, 1984. On post-traumatic stress, see Chris R. Brewin, *Post-Traumatic Stress Disorder. Malady or Myth?* New Haven and London, Yale University Press, 2003; Marijke Gijswijt-Hofstra and Roy Porter, *Cultures of Neurasthenia. From Beard to the First World War*, Amsterdam, New York, Rodopi Editions, 2001, especially Chapter 1, Roy Porter, "Nervousness, Eighteenth and Nineteenth Century Style: From Luxury to Labour," pp. 31–49. On chronic fatigue syndrome, which appears in the 1980s, see, Robert A. Aronowitz, *Making Sense of Illness. Science, Society and Disease*, Cambridge, Cambridge University Press, 1998, Chapter 1: "From Myalgic Encephalitis to Yuppie Flu. A History of Chronic Fatigue Syndromes," pp. 19–38.

36. Baszenger, Chapter 2: "The Creation of World of Pain," pp. 63*ff.*

37. David B. Morris, *Illness and Culture in the Postmodern Age*, Berkeley, Los Angeles, London, University of California Press, 1998, especially Chapter 4: "Reinventing Pain."

38. On the experience and the voice of the patient, see Philip Rieder, "Patients and Words: A Lay Medical Culture," in G. S. Rousseau, Miranda Gill and David B. Haycock, (eds), *Framing and Imagining Disease in Cultural History*, London, Palgrave Macmillan, 2003, pp. 215–230. In this same book, regarding anorexia, see Catherina Albano, "Within the Frame: Self-Extarvation and the Making of Culture," pp. 51–67. David Shuttleton, "A Culture of Disfigurement: Imagining Smallpox in the Long Eighteenth Century," in George Sebastian Rousseau (ed.), *Framing and Imagining Disease in Cultural History*. London, Palgrave Macmillan, 2003, pp. 68–91.

39. George M. Beard, *A Practical Treatise on Nervous Exhaustion (Neurasthenia)*, New York, William Wood and Company, 1880, p. 17.

40. Arthur Kleinman, Paul E. Brodwin, Byron J. Good and Mary-Jo DelVecchio Good, *"Pain as Human Experience."* p. 9.

41. Julian Barnes (editor and translator), *In the Land of Pain* by Alphonse Daudet, New York, Alfred A. Knopf, 2002.

42. See E. Lanceraux, *Traité Historique et pratique de la syphilis*, Paris, J. B. Baillière, 1866, p. 524.

43. Szabo, *Incurable and Intolerable*. Milton J. Lewis, *Medicine and the Care of the Dying, A Modern History*, Oxford, OUP, 2007.

44. Daudet, *In the Land of Pain*, New York, Alfred A. Knopf, 2002, p. 6.

45. Szabo, *Incurable and Intolerable*, Chapter 3: "I Told You So."

46. Daudet, *In the Land of Pain*, p. 23.

47. Ibid. p. 29.

48. Ibid. p. 48.

49. Nadja Durbach, *The Spectacle of Deformity: Freak Shows and Modern British Culture*, Berkeley, University of California Press, 2009, and Lilian E. Craton, *The Victorian Freak Show: The Significance of Disability and Physical Differences in 19th-Century Fiction*, 2009, as well as Robert Bogdan's classic *Freak Show. Presenting Human Oddities for Amusement and Profit*, Chicago and London, The University of Chicago Press, 1990.

50. [Silas Weir Mitchell], *The Autobiography of a Quack* and *The Case of George Dedlow*, New York, The Century Co., 1900, pp. 148–149.

51. V. Turner, "Liminal to Liminoid, in Play, Flow, and Ritual," in V. Turner (ed.), *From Ritual to Theatre*, New York, PAJ Publications, 1982, p. 25.
52. [Mitchell], *George Dedlow*, p. 128.
53. Ibid. p. 122.
54. Ibid. p. 137.
55. On George Dedlow's case, see Robert I. Goler's excellent article, "Loos and the Persistence of Memory: 'The Case of George Dedlow' and Disabled Civil War Veterans," *Literature and Medicine*, 23 (2004): 160–183. On the historical context, see Drew Gilpin Faust, *This Republic of Suffering. Death and the American Civil War*, New York, Vintage Books, 2009.
56. Weir Mitchell, *et al. Gunshot Wounds, and Other Injuries of the Nerves*, Philadelphia, Lippincott, 1864, p. 9. On S. W. Mitchell, see Nancy Cervetti, "S. Weir Mitchell: The Early Years," *American Pain Association Bulletin*, 13 (2003): 7–9.
57. Mitchell, *Gunshot Wounds*; quoted by Meldrum, "History of Pain Management," p. 2471.
58. P. E. Dauzat, "Regards médicaux sur la douleur: histoire d'un deni," *Psycho-Oncologie* 2 (2007): 71–75, p. 73.
59. Mitchell, *Gunshot Wounds*, p. 103. Mitchell, Morehouse and Keen, 1864, *Gunshot Wounds*, quoted by Cervetti, "S. Weir Mitchell: The Early Years:"

> As the pain increases, the general sympathy becomes more marked. The temper changes and grows irritable, the face becomes anxious, and has a look or weariness and suffering. The sleep is restless, and the constitutional condition, reacting on the wounded limb, exasperates the hypersthetic state, so that the rattling of a newspaper, a breath of air, another's step across the ward, the vibrations caused by a military band, or the shock of the feet in walking, give rise to increase pain. At last the patient grows hysterical, if we may use the only term which covers the facts.

60. Mitchell, *Gunshot Wounds*, pp. 102–103.
61. S. Weir Mitchell, *Injuries of the Nerves and their Consequences*, [1872], New York, Dover Publications, 1965, p. 266. On the term *causalgia*, see R. L. Richards (1967), "The Term Causalgia," *Medical History* 11, 1 (1967): 97–99.
62. Livingston, *Pain and Suffering*, p. 4. See also p. 87:

> The complaints of these patients seemed to be excessive in relation to any cause I could identify. Their symptoms did not remain confined to the distribution of any single somatic nerve or spinal segment, and in some cases they spread beyond the injured limb to other extremities or distant internal organs.

Also p. 4:

> I knew that patients sometimes exaggerated their complaints of pain but I assumed that when I had identified the cause of their pain I could tell from the nature of the organic lesion whether their pain complaints were real or due to psychological factors.

63. Livingston, *Pain and Suffering*, p. 1: "*each pain represents a unique, subjective sensory experience that can be described only by the conscious human being who is experiencing it.*"
64. Livingston, *Pain Mechanisms*, p. 62.
65. Livingston, *Pain and Suffering*, [1957], p. 207:

> We also agreed that what was most important to the patient was the severity of the pain he felt as opposed to what we thought he ought to be feeling or even what nerve impulses might be ascending his central nervous system when his tissues were being cut by the

surgeon's knife while he was deeply anesthetized. So we subscribed to the proposition that nothing can be properly called 'pain' unless it can consciously perceived as such.

66. A. A. Bailey and F. P. Moersch, "Phantom Limb Pain," *Canadian Medical Association Journal*, 45 (1943): 37–42.

67. Livingston, *Pain Mechanisms*, p. 9. Later on, Wall and Melzack considered a mistake the division between the pain belonging to the phantom limb into organic or psychological, see Wall and Melzack, *The Challenge of Pain*, p. 62.

68. See G. S. Rousseau, *et al.* eds, *Framing and Imagining Disease in Cultural History*, New York, Macmillan, Palgrave, 2003. See also the classic text of Charles E. Rosenberg and Janet Golden (eds), *Framing Disease. Studies in Cultural History*, New Brunswick, New Jersey, Rutgers University Press, 1997 and Eric J. Cassell, *The Nature of Suffering and the Goals of Medicine*, Oxford, Oxford University Press, [1991], second edition, 2004, p. 47. Diabetics or those suffering hypertension are not permanently ill.

69. Szabo, *Incurable and Intolerable*. See also Lewis, *Medicine and Care of the Dying*.

70. S. W. Mitchell, *Wear and Tear: or Hints for the Overworked*, edition and introduction by Michael Kimmel, Lanham, MD, Altamira Press, 2004.

71. George M. Beard, *American Nervousness: Its Causes and Consequences. A Supplement to Nervous Exhaustion (Neurasthenia)*, New York, G. P. Putnam's Sons, 1881. On the chronic nature of neurasthenia, see pp. 90 and *ff*. On the causes of this disease, see pp. 96 and *ff*.

72. Quoted by Kimmel, "Introduction" to Mitchell, *Wear and Tear*, p. viii. "*Live as domestic a life as possible* [...] *Have but two hours' intellectual life a day and never touch pen, brush or pencil as long as you live.*" For a positive assessment of Weir Mitchell's methods regarding the treatment of female neurasthenia, see Adrien Proust and Gilbert Ballet, *The Treatment of Neurasthenia*, New York, Edward R. Pelton, 1903, pp. 183*ff*. For a critique of the "*dramatic story of Saint Charlotte and the evil Dr. Mitchell,*" see Julie Bates Dock, compiler and editor, *Charlotte Perkins Gilman's "The Yellow Wall-Paper" and the History of Its Publication and Reception*, Pennsylvania, The Pennsylvania State University Press, 1998.

73. Cary L. Cooper and Philipe Dewey, *Stress. A Brief History*, Victoria, Blackwell Publishing, 2004.

74. Michael MacDonald, "The Medicalization of Suicide in England: Laymen, Physicians, and Cultural Change, 1500–1870," in Charles E. Rosenberg and Janet Golden, (eds), *Framing Disease. Studies in Cultural History*, New Brunswick, New Jersey, Rutgers University Press, 1997, pp. 85–104.

75. Fell, *Treatise on Cancer*, also proposes the use of a plant called *puccoon*, which he had heard tell of from the American Indians, and he considered an infallible cure, pp. 56*ff*.

76. Skene Keith, *Cancer. Relief of Pain and Possible Cure*, London, Adam and Charles Black, 1908, pp. 14–15.

77. John J. Bonica, *The Management of Pain*, London, Henry Kimpton, 1953.

78. Turner, *From Ritual to Theater*, p. 69: "*The main actors* [of a social drama] *are persons for whom the group which constitutes the field of dramatic action has a high value priority.*"

79. Marcus Aurelius, *Meditations*, Book VII, epigraph 28.

80. C. Rosenberg, "Disease in History: Frames and Framers," *Milbank Quarterly*, 67, 1 (1989): 1–15.

81. Rosenberg and Golden (eds), *Framing Disease*, p. xiii.

82. William Ray Arney and Bernard J. Bergen, "The Anomaly, the Chronic Patient and the Play of Medical Power," *Sociology of Health and Illness*, 5, 1 (1983): 1–24.

83. Johannes von Kries, *Allgemeine Sinnesphysiologie*, Leipzig, F. C. W. Vogel, 1923, pp. 15 and *ff*. Quoted by Frederic Jacobus Johannes Buytendijk, *El dolor. Fenomenología. Psicología. Metafísica*, Madrid, Revista de Occidente, 1958, pp. 68–69. C. Jason Troop, "Experience, Coherence, and Culture: The Significance of Dilthey's 'Descriptive Psychology' for the Anthropology of Consciousness," *Anthropology of Consciousness*, 13, 1 (2002): 2–26.

84. Veena Das, Arthur Kleinman, Mamphela Ramphele and Pamela Reynolds, *Violence and Subjectivity*. Berkeley, Los Angeles, London, University of California Press, 2000; Veena Das, Arthur Kleinman, Margaret Lock, Mamphela Ramphele and Pamela Reynolds, *Remaking a World. Violence, Social Suffering and Recovery*, Berkeley, Los Angeles, London, University of California Press, 2001. Interest in violence has also reached historical research. See for instance: David Nieremberg, *Communities of Violence. Persecution of Minorities in the Middle Ages*, Princeton, Princeton University Press, 1996.

85. See Donald Davidson, "Thought and Talk," in S. Guttenplan (ed.), *Mind and Language*, Oxford, Oxford University Press, 1974, pp. 7–24. John Dewey, *Experience and Nature*, Dover, Dover Publications, 1958. Daniel C. Dennet, "Why you can't make a computer that feels pain," in *Brain Storms. Philosophical Essays on Mind and Psychology*, London, Penguin Books, 1978. Paul M. Churchland, [1988] *Matter and Consciousness: A Contemporary Introduction to the Philosophy of Mind*, Cambridge, MA, MIT Press, 1999.

86. John Searle, *Minds, Brains, and Science*. Cambridge, MA: Harvard University Press, 1984.

87. See John Searle, *The Rediscovery of the Mind*, Cambridge, MA, MIT University Press, 1992, pp. 154*ff*. and Hilary Putnam, "The nature of mental states," [1968] in Hilary Putnam, *Mind, Language and Reality, Philosophical Papers*, vol. II, Cambridge, Cambridge University Press, 1997. pp. 429–440. Putnam, "The nature of mental states," p. 429. For a current analysis of some of these issues, see, Murat Aydede, *Pain. New Essays on Its Narratives and the Methodology of Its Study*, Cambridge, MA, MIT, 2005, as well as Nikola Grahek, *Feeling Pain and Being in Pain*, Cambridge, MA, and London, The MIT Press, 2001. In an article in 1967, Putnam argued that pain was not a physical-chemical state of the brain or nervous system as a whole, but a functional state of an organism in its entirety. A position later taken up and expanded by his disciple, Jerry Fodor, even after Putnam himself reneged on his initial position and replaced it with a form of socio-functionalism. For a critique by Putnam himself regarding his functionalist stage, see Putnam, *Representation and Reality*, [1988]. See also Daniel Dennet: "Why You Can't Make a Computer that Feels Pain" in *Brainstorms. Philosophical Essays on Mind and Psychology* [1978], London, Penguin Books, 1997, pp. 190–229; Thomas Nagel, "What Is It Like to Be a Bat?" [1974], reprinted in *Mortal Questions*, Cambridge, Cambridge University Press, 1979; Hilary Putnam, *Reason, Truth and History*, [1981]. For an introduction to some of these texts, Pascual Martínez-Freire, *La nueva filosofía de la mente*, Barcelona, Gedisa, 1995.

88. Barbie Zelizer, *Remembering to Forget. Holocaust Memory Through the Camera's Eye*. Chicago, University of Chicago Press, 1998.

89. T. W. Adorno, *Dialéctica negativa*, Madrid, Taurus, 1984, p. 362.

90. David C. Berliner, "*The Abuses of Memory: Reflections on the Memory Boom in Anthropology*," *Anthropological Quarterly*, 78, 1 (Winter 2005): 197–211.

91. See Susan Sontag, *On Photography*, 1977, where she argued that photography had an anesthetic effect that led observers to the point of indifference. For a contrary position, see John Taylor, *Body Horror: Photojournalism, Catastrophe and War*, New York, New York University Press, 1998, especially Chapter 2. Later, Sontag completed her position in *Regarding the Pain of Others*, London, Penguin, 2003, especially pp. 72*ff*, where she speaks of how pain is transformed, through its materialization, into a consumer object.

Index

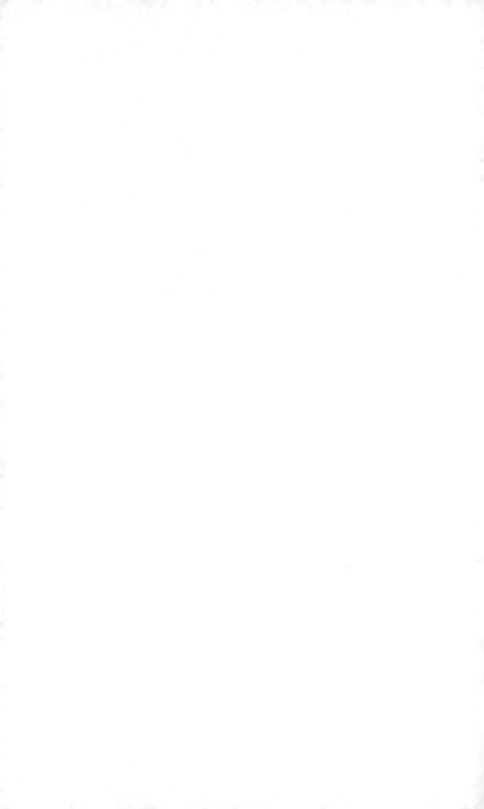

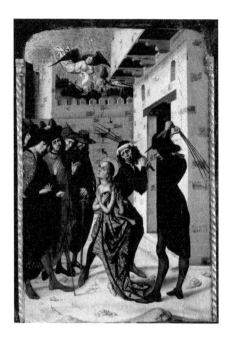

Figure 1 Pedro de Mayorga, Master of Palanquinos, *Altarpiece of Santa Marina*, c. 1500, oil on board, Masaveu Collection, Museo de Bellas Artes de Asturias, Oviedo, Spain.

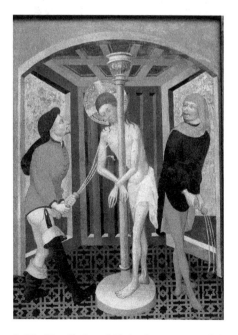

Figure 2 Lluís Borrassà, *The Flagellation of Christ*, first quarter of the 15th century, oil on board, 84 × 61 cm, Goya Museum, Castres, France.

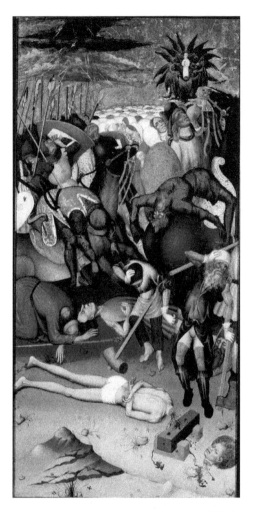

Figure 3 Bernat Martorell, *The Decapitation of St. George*, panel from an altarpiece, 1435, oil on board, 53 × 107 cm, Louvre Museum, Paris © AKG.

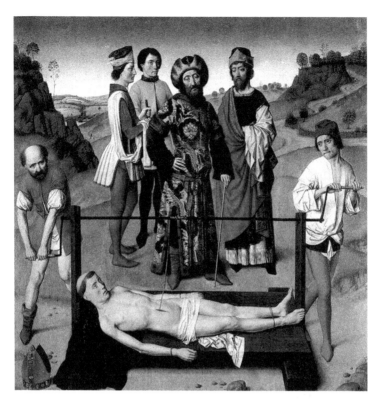

Figure 4   Dieric Bouts, *The Martyrdom of Saint Erasmus*, central panel from the Triptych of Saint Erasmus, 1460, oil on canvas, St. Peter's Cathedral, Louvain, Belgium.

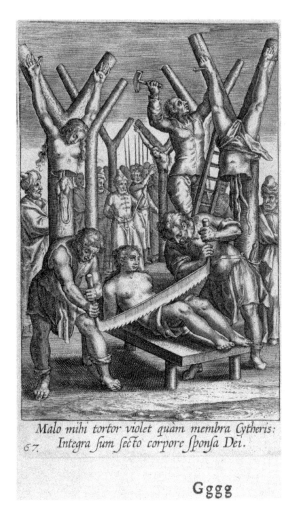

Malo mihi tortor violet quam membra Cytheris:
67. Integra fum fecto corpore fponfa Dei.

Gggg

Figure 5 Petrus Biverus, "Illustration showing women being cut in half and their torsos and legs nailed to posts," in *Sacrum Sanctuarium crucis et patientiae crucifixorum et cruciferorum*, 1634, B. Moretus, Antwerp, opposite page 600, Wellcome Library, London.

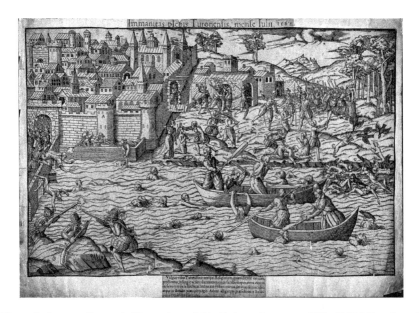

Figure 6 Jacques Tortorel, "Inmanitas plebis Torinensis, mense Ulii, 1562," *Premier volume contenat quarente tableaux ou Histoires diverses qui sont memorable touchant les guerres, massacres et troubles advenus en France en ces dernières années*, 1569–1570, Wellcome Library, London.

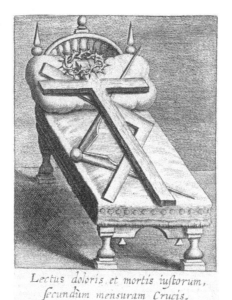

Figure 7 Petrus Biverus, Sacrum Sanctuarium crucis et patientiae crucifixorum et cruciferorum, 1634, B. Moretus, Antwerp, obverse page 600, Wellcome Library, London.

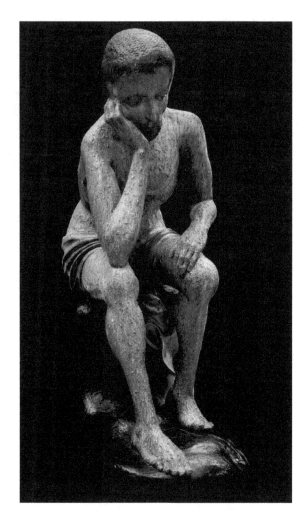

Figure 8 [Anonymous], *Christ in Distress*, c. 1500, polychrome wood, 117 cm, National Museum, Warsaw, Poland © Photograph by Javier Moscoso.

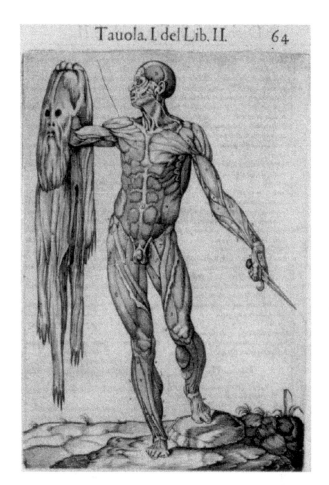

Figure 9   Juan Valverde de Hamusco, "Male figure showing muscles," *History of the Composition of the Human Body*, Rome: A. Salamanca and A. Lafreri, 1556, Wellcome Library, London.

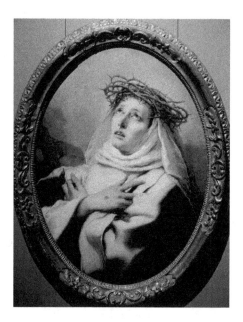

Figure 10 Giovanni Battista Tiepolo, *St. Catherine of Siena*, 1746, 70 × 52 cm, Kunsthistorisches Museum, Vienna © AKG.

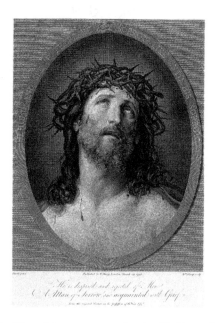

Figure 11 *Christ as the Man of Sorrows*, engraving by W. Sharp, 1798, from a work by Guido Reni, 1575–1642, Wellcome Library, London.

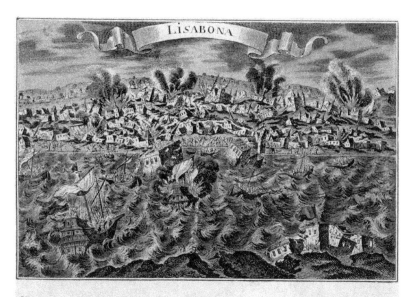

Vorstellung und Beschreibung des ganz erschröcklichen Erdbebens, wodurch die Königl. Portugiesische Residenz-Stadt Lissabon samt dem grösten Theil der Einwohnern zu grunde gegangen.

Figure 12 "Image and Description of the Violent Earthquake that Destroyed Lisbon." 1755, engraving, leaflet by Georg Caspar Pfauntz, Augsburg, Germany © AKG.

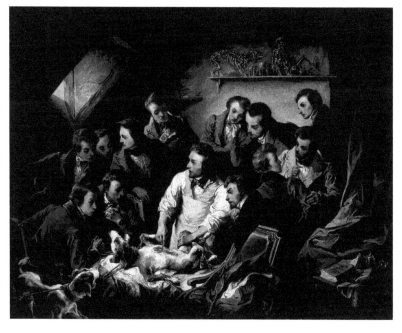

Figure 13 Emile-Edouard Mouchy, *Physiological Demonstration through the Vivisection of a Dog*, oil on canvas, 112 × 143 cm, Wellcome Library, London.

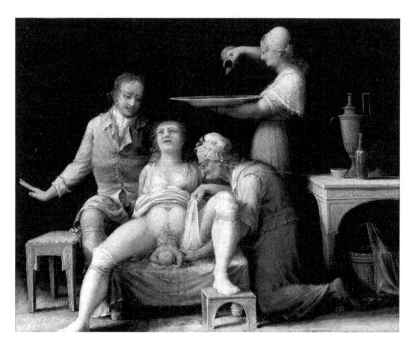

Figure 14 Unknown French painter, A birth scene. 1800, oil on paper stuck to wood, 44. 1 × 56. 6 cm, Wellcome Library, London.

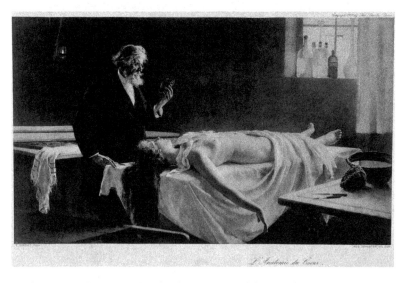

Figure 15 Enrique Simonet y Lombardo, *Anatomy of the Heart*, originally entitled *"And She Had a Heart!"* 1899, engraving by P. Fruhauf, 31 × 54 cm, Wellcome Library, London.

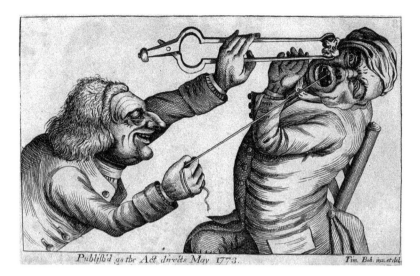

Figure 16 John Collier, A sadistic tooth-drawer terrifies his patient with a piece of burning coal so as to be able to take out a tooth more easily, 1773, engraving, 12.6 × 20.3 cm, Wellcome Library, London.

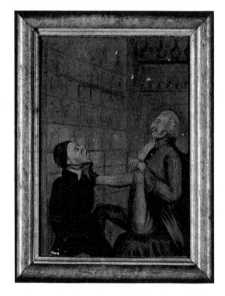

Figure 17 Anonymous, A pharmacist surgeon extracts a man's tooth, oil on panel, 34.0 × 24.5 cm, Wellcome Library, London.

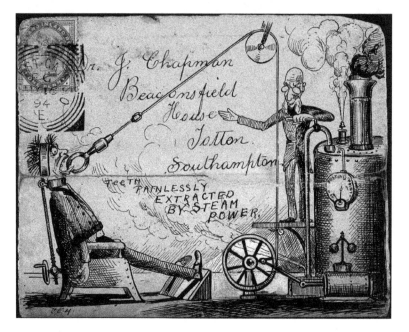

Figure 18   C. E. H., Scientist using a vapor machine with a pulley to extract a tooth from a man, 1894, Wellcome Library, London. The drawing, done on the back of an envelope, says "Teeth painlessly extracted by steam power."

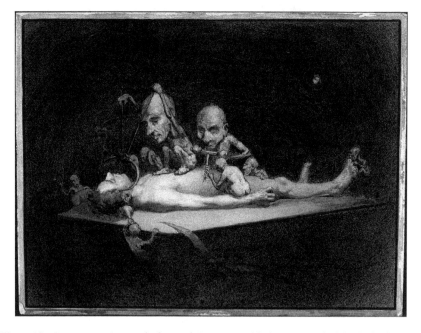

Figure 19   An unconscious naked man lying on a table being attacked by little demons armed with surgical instruments; symbolizing the effects of chloroform on the human body. Watercolor by Richard Tenant Cooper, c. 1912. Wellcome Library, London.

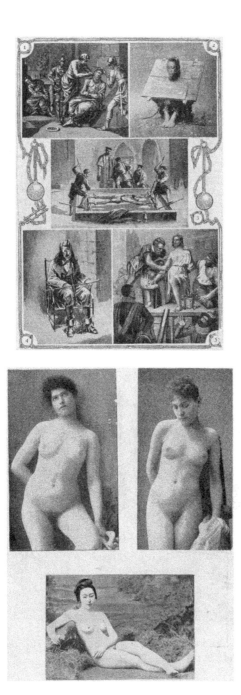

Figure 20 Edwin Nichol Fallaize, pasteboard with halftone ink, 25 × 40 cm, *recto and verso*, Wellcome Library, London.

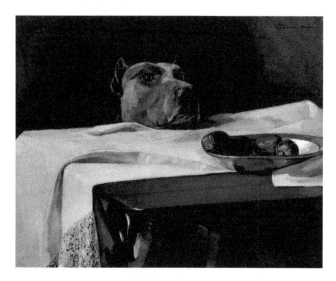

Figure 21 Wilhelm Trübner, *Caesar before the Rubicon*, c. 1878, oil on canvas, 48.5 × 61.0 cm, Österreichische Galerie Belvedere.

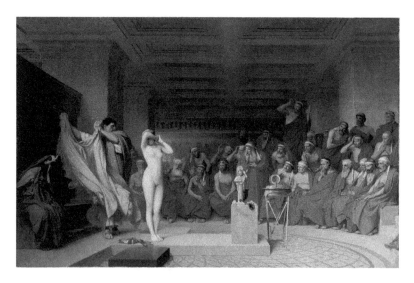

Figure 22 Jean-Léon Gérôme, *Phryne before the Areopagus*, 1861, oil on canvas, 80.5 × 128.0 cm, Hamburguer Kunsthalle, Hamburg © BAG.

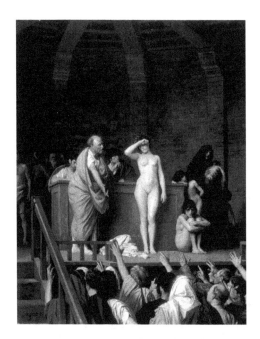

Figure 23 Jean-Léon Gérôme, *Selling Slaves in Rome*, 1884, 92 × 74 cm., Hermitage Museum, Saint Petersburg © AKG.

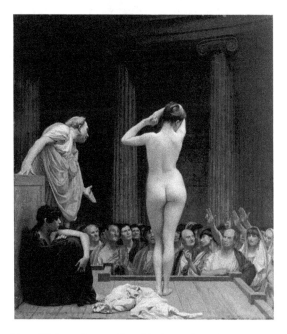

Figure 24 Jean-Léon Gérôme, *Roman Slave Market*, 1884, oil on canvas, 64 × 57 cm, The Walters Art Gallery, Baltimore, USA © BAG.

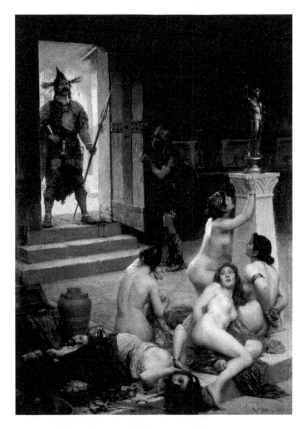

Figure 25 Paul-Joseph Jamin, *Brenin and his Share of the Plunder*, 1893, oil on canvas, 162 × 118 cm, Museum of Fine Arts, La Rochelle, France.

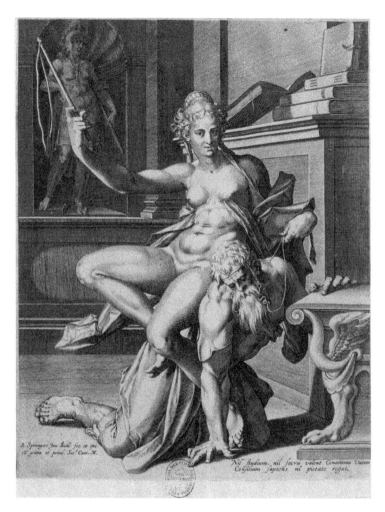

Figure 26 Jan Sadeler, engraving by Bartholomaeus Spranger, *Aristotle and Phyllis*, c. 1587–1593, National Library, Madrid, Spain.

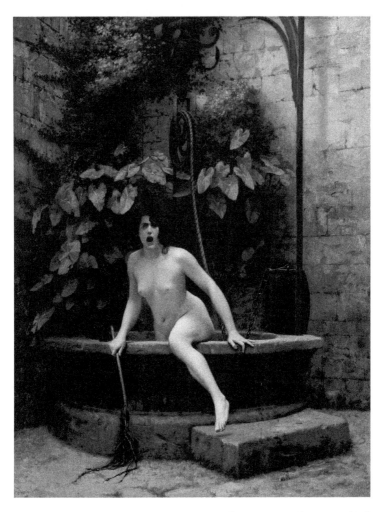

Figure 27 Jean-Léon Gérôme, *Truth Coming Out of Her Well to Shame Mankind*, 1896, Collection du Musée Anne-de-Beaujeu, Moulins, France © Jérôme Modière.

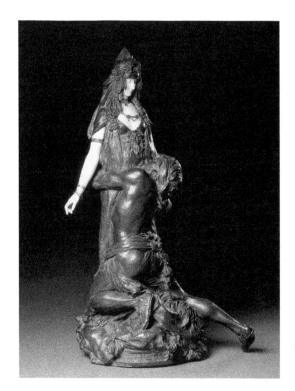

Figure 28 Théodore Rivière, *Salammbô and Matho, I love you, I love you!* 1895, small group in bronze, ivory, gold, and turquoise, 40.0 × 21.4 × 19.0 cm, Musée d'Orsay, Paris. Photograph by Hervé Lewandowski.

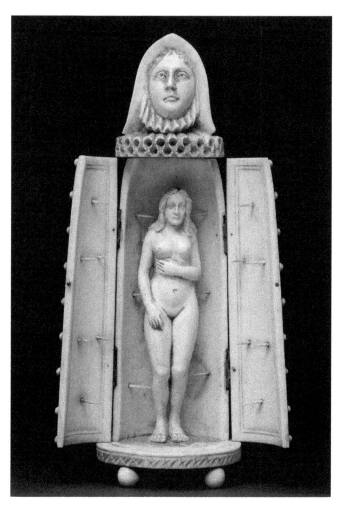

Figure 29 Figure of a woman inside an "Iron Maiden," ivory, Science Museum, Wellcome Collection, London.

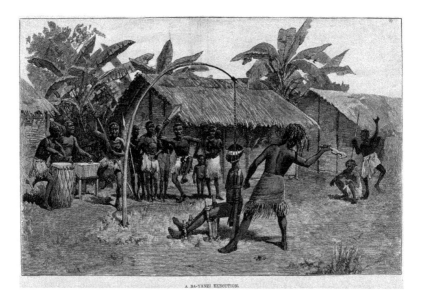

Figure 30 E. J. Glave and H. Ward, Ba-Yanzi execution, in which the head of the victim is held to an artifact that catapults it when the body is decapitated, leaving the rest of the body tied to the floor, color engraving, 15. 4 × 23. 5 cm, Wellcome Library, London.

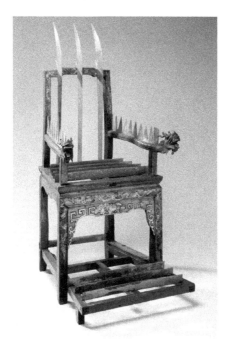

Figure 31 Chinese torture chair in wood and steel. Wellcome Collection, London.

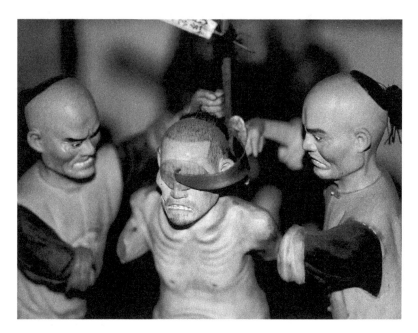

Figure 32   Death by one hundred cuts, Chinese miniature, Science Museum, London.

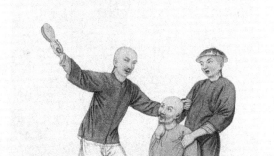

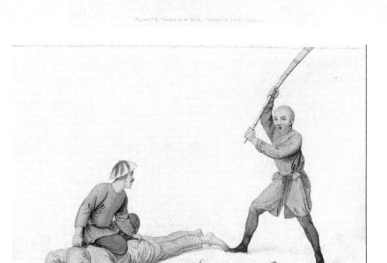

Figure 33   J. Dadley, "Punishment of a boatman. Obliged to kneel, one of the officials prevents him protecting himself while the other pulls his hair and hits him various times on both sides of his face with a kind of double oar made of solid leather," and "Cutting the ankles of a bandit," illustration from the book by George Henry Mason, *Punishment in China*, 1801, Wellcome Library, London.

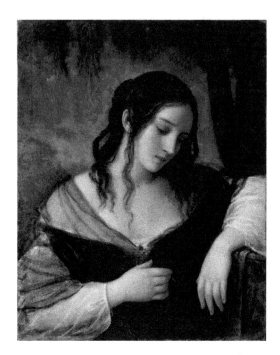

Figure 34 Natale Schiavoni, *Sadness*, 1841, oil on canvas, Österreichische Galerie, Belvedere, Vienna, Austria.

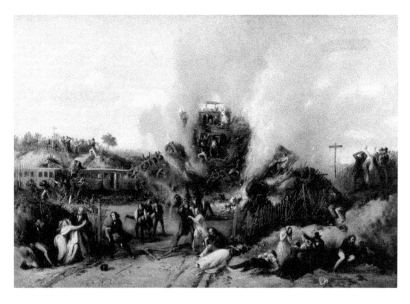

Figure 35 A. P. Provost, *Accident on the Railway between Versailles and Bellevue*, 8 May 1842, Musée de l'île-de-France, Sceaux, France © BAG.

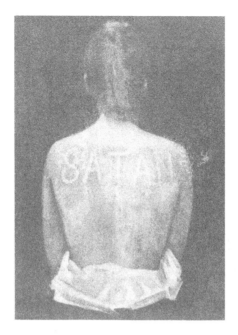

Figure 36 T. Barthélémy, Etude sur le dermographisme (1893), Wellcome Library, London.

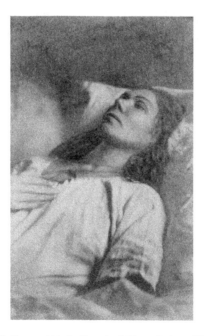

Figure 37 "Hysterical Epilepsy, Attack, Terminal Phase," sheet XVIII of the *Iconographie Photographique de La Salpêtrière*, edited by Désiré-Magloire Bourneville and Paul Regnard, Paris, 1876 © BAG.

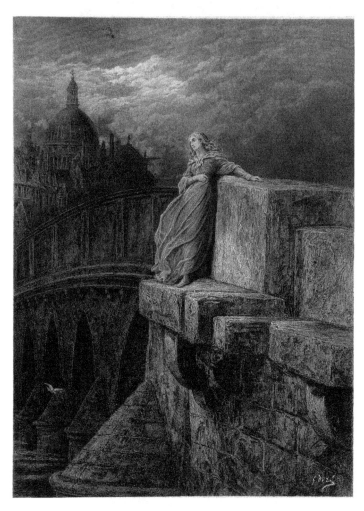

Figure 38   T. Godfrey, according to the work by G. Doré, *An Afflicted Woman Considers Suicide from the Edge of a Bridge* [s.n.][s.l.], mezzotint, Wellcome Library, London.

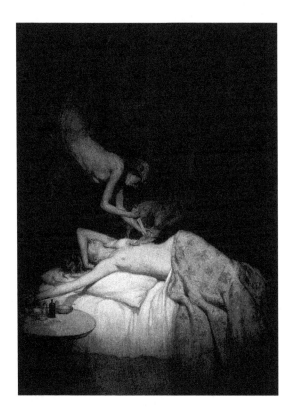

Figure 39 Richard Tennant Cooper, A giant claw pierces the breast of a sleeping naked woman, while another naked woman swoops down stabbing the claw with a knife, symbolizing science's fight against cancer, twentieth century, watercolor, Wellcome Library, London.

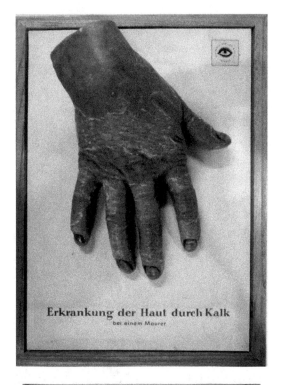

Erkrankung der Haut durch Kalk
bei einem Maurer

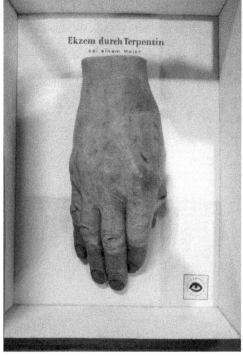

Ekzem durch Terpentin
bei einem Maler

Figure 40 Anatomical models in wax, twentieth century, Museum of Hygiene, Dresden.

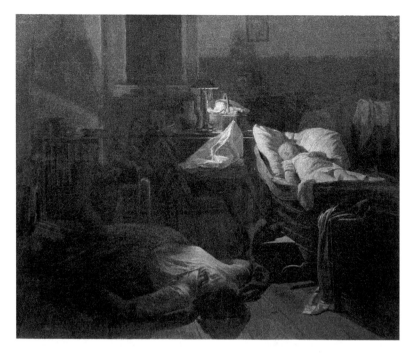

Figure 41 Ferdinand Georg Waldmüller, Exhaustion, 1854, oil on canvas, 63.0 × 75.5 cm, Österreichische Galerie, Vienna.

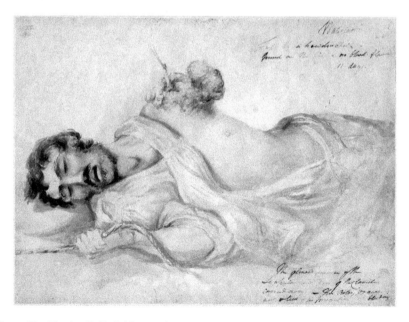

Figure 42 Charles Bell, Soldier with missing arm, lying on his side, grasping a rope. Watercolour. 1815. Wellcome Library, London.

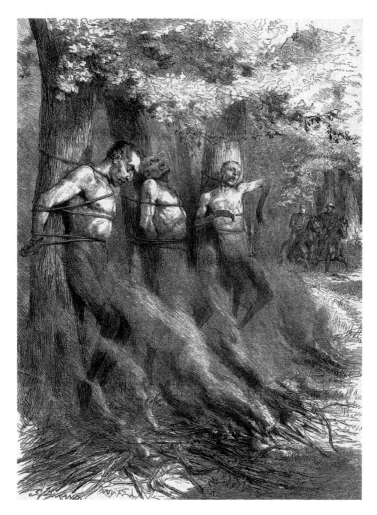

Figure 43 Godefroy Durand, Three naked men tied to trees with a bonfire between them that is threatening to burn or asphyxiate them, engraving on wood, 30.0×22.5 cm, Wellcome Library, London.

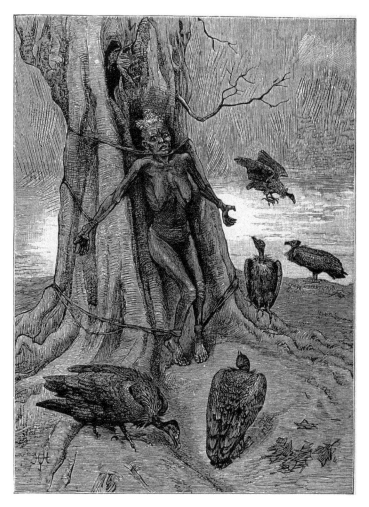

Figure 44 The naked body of a woman tied to a tree and surrounded by vultures awaiting her imminent death, engraving, 15.4 × 11.7 cm, Wellcome Library, London.

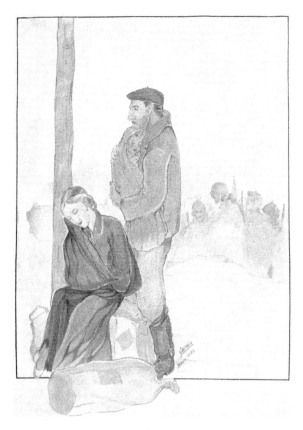

Figure 45 Luis Sarabia, In the Port. Notes by a Deployed member of the Red Navy, 1937–1939. Private Collection, Madrid.

CPSIA information can be obtained
at www.ICGtesting.com
Printed in the USA
LVHW052121190919
631608LV00013B/1066/P